SECOND EDITION

MULTIPLE MYELOMA: A TEXTBOOK FOR NURSES

EDITED BY
JOSEPH D. TARIMAN, PHD, ANP-BC
BETH FAIMAN, PHD, APRN-BC, AOCN®

ONS Publications Department
Publisher and Director of Publications: William A. Tony, BA, CQIA
Managing Editor: Lisa M. George, BA
Assistant Managing Editor: Amy Nicoletti, BA, JD
Acquisitions Editor: John Zaphyr, BA, MEd
Copy Editors: Vanessa Kattouf, BA, Andrew Petyak, BA
Graphic Designer: Dany Sjoen
Editorial Assistant: Judy Holmes

Copyright © 2015 by the Oncology Nursing Society. All rights reserved. No part of the material protected by this copyright may be reproduced or utilized in any form, electronic or mechanical, including photocopying, recording, or by an information storage and retrieval system, without written permission from the copyright owner. For information, visit www.ons.org/sites/default/files/Publication%20Permissions.pdf, or send an email to pubpermissions@ons.org.

Library of Congress Cataloging-in-Publication Data

Multiple myeloma (Tariman)
  Multiple myeloma : a textbook for nurses / edited by Joseph D. Tariman, Beth Faiman. – Second edition.
    p. ; cm.
  Includes bibliographical references and index.
  ISBN 978-1-935864-60-8
  I. Tariman, Joseph D., editor. II. Faiman, Beth, editor. III. Oncology Nursing Society, issuing body. IV. Title.
  [DNLM: 1. Multiple Myeloma–nursing. 2. Oncology Nursing–methods. WY 156]
  RC280.B6
  616.99'418–dc23
                                                                                          2015013670

Publisher's Note

This book is published by the Oncology Nursing Society (ONS). ONS neither represents nor guarantees that the practices described herein will, if followed, ensure safe and effective patient care. The recommendations contained in this book reflect ONS's judgment regarding the state of general knowledge and practice in the field as of the date of publication. The recommendations may not be appropriate for use in all circumstances. Those who use this book should make their own determinations regarding specific safe and appropriate patient care practices, taking into account the personnel, equipment, and practices available at the hospital or other facility at which they are located. The editors and publisher cannot be held responsible for any liability incurred as a consequence from the use or application of any of the contents of this book. Figures and tables are used as examples only. They are not meant to be all-inclusive, nor do they represent endorsement of any particular institution by ONS. Mention of specific products and opinions related to those products do not indicate or imply endorsement by ONS. Websites mentioned are provided for information only; the hosts are responsible for their own content and availability. Unless otherwise indicated, dollar amounts reflect U.S. dollars.

ONS publications are originally published in English. Publishers wishing to translate ONS publications must contact ONS about licensing arrangements. ONS publications cannot be translated without obtaining written permission from ONS. (Individual tables and figures that are reprinted or adapted require additional permission from the original source.) Because translations from English may not always be accurate or precise, ONS disclaims any responsibility for inaccuracies in words or meaning that may occur as a result of the translation. Readers relying on precise information should check the original English version.

Printed in the United States of America

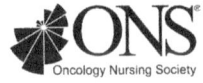

Integrity • Innovation • Stewardship • Advocacy • Excellence • Inclusiveness

This book is dedicated to my partner, Todd Babcock,
who understands and cares so much about what are personally
and professionally important matters to me.
Joseph

Thank you to all my family, friends, colleagues,
and patients. Without their ongoing support, this book
would not have been possible.
Beth

Contributors

Editors

Joseph D. Tariman, PhD, ANP-BC
Assistant Professor
School of Nursing
DePaul University
Chicago, Illinois
Chapter 1. Myeloma Care: Challenges and Opportunities; Chapter 10. On the Horizon: Advances in Genomics and Biomarkers; Chapter 12. Clinical Trials

Beth Faiman, PhD, APRN-BC, AOCN®
Nurse Practitioner, Multiple Myeloma Program
Cleveland Clinic
Cleveland, Ohio
Chapter 1. Myeloma Care: Challenges and Opportunities; Chapter 6. Treatment of Newly Diagnosed, Transplant-Ineligible Patients; Chapter 10. On the Horizon: Advances in Genomics and Biomarkers

Authors

Kevin Brigle, PhD, ANP
Oncology Nurse Practitioner
Massey Cancer Center
Virginia Commonwealth University Health System
Richmond, Virginia
Chapter 7. Treatment of Relapsed and Refractory Multiple Myeloma

Ima N. Garcia, MSN, RN, ACNP-BC, AOCNP®
Nurse Practitioner
Section of Hematology/Oncology
University of Chicago Medical Center
Chicago, Illinois
Chapter 5. High-Dose Therapy and Stem Cell Transplantation

Charise Gleason, MSN, NP-BC, AOCNP®
Nurse Practitioner
The Winship Cancer Institute of Emory University
Atlanta, Georgia
Chapter 4. Epidemiology

Sandra Kurtin, RN, MS, AOCN®, ANP
Nurse Practitioner
University of Arizona Cancer Center
Clinical Assistant Professor of Medicine
University of Arizona
Tucson, Arizona
Chapter 8. Living With Multiple Myeloma

Kimberly Noonan, MS, RN, ANP, AOCN®
Nurse Practitioner
Dana-Farber Cancer Institute
Boston, Massachusetts
Chapter 2. Anatomy and Physiology; Chapter 3. Pathophysiology

Tiffany Richards, MS, ANP-BC, AOCNP®
Nurse Practitioner
Department of Lymphoma/Myeloma
University of Texas MD Anderson Cancer Center
Houston, Texas
Chapter 9. Nursing Research

Sandra Rome, RN, MN, AOCN®, CNS
Hematology/Oncology BMT Clinical Nurse
 Specialist
Cedars-Sinai Medical Center
Los Angeles, California
Chapter 11. Patient Teaching

Disclosure

Editors and authors of books and guidelines provided by the Oncology Nursing Society are expected to disclose to the readers any significant financial interest or other relationships with the manufacturer(s) of any commercial products.

A vested interest may be considered to exist if a contributor is affiliated with or has a financial interest in commercial organizations that may have a direct or indirect interest in the subject matter. A "financial interest" may include, but is not limited to, being a shareholder in the organization; being an employee of the commercial organization; serving on an organization's speakers bureau; or receiving research funding from the organization. An "affiliation" may be holding a position on an advisory board or some other role of benefit to the commercial organization. Vested interest statements appear in the front matter for each publication.

Contributors are expected to disclose any unlabeled or investigational use of products discussed in their content. This information is acknowledged solely for the information of the readers.

The contributors provided the following disclosure and vested interest information:
Kevin Brigle, PhD, ANP: Millennium, Celgene, Incyte, honoraria
Charise Gleason, MSN, NP-BC, AOCNP®: Takeda, Onyx, consultant or advisory role
Sandra Kurtin, RN, MS, AOCN®, ANP: Myelodysplastic Syndromes Foundation, International Myeloma Foundation, Advanced Practitioner Society for Hematology and Oncology, leadership position; Celgene, Takeda, Bristol-Myers Squibb, consultant or advisory role; Celgene, Takeda, Onyx, Incyte, TEVA, honoraria
Tiffany Richards, MS, ANP-BC, AOCNP®: Onyx, Celgene, consultant or advisory role, honoraria

Table of Contents

Foreword xi
Preface xiii
Acknowledgments xvii

Chapter 1. Myeloma Care: Challenges and Opportunities 1
    The Basics: What Is Multiple Myeloma? 1
    Welcoming the Era of Novel Therapeutics 2
    Building Lifelong Partnerships and Collaboration 3
    Finding a New Path to a Cure 4
    Promoting Nursing Research to Support Evidence-Based Myeloma Nursing Care 5
    Overcoming Clinical Challenges 6
    References 6

Chapter 2. Anatomy and Physiology 11
    The Immune System 11
    Innate and Acquired Immunity 11
    Adaptive Immunity: Humoral and Cellular 14
    Organs of the Immune System 15
    Cells Involved in Innate Immunity 16
    Cells Responsible for Adaptive Immunity 17
    Cytokines 27
    Adhesion Molecules 31
    Conclusion 32
    References 32

Chapter 3. Pathophysiology 35
    Introduction 35
    The Role of Genetics 35
    Conclusion 48
    References 49

Chapter 4. Epidemiology 53
    Introduction 53
    Etiology 53
    Incidence 54
    Risk Factors 54
    Conclusion 63
    References 64

viii MULTIPLE MYELOMA: A TEXTBOOK FOR NURSES (SECOND EDITION)

Chapter 5. High-Dose Therapy and Stem Cell Transplantation 71
    Introduction 71
    Evolution of High-Dose Therapy for Multiple Myeloma 72
    Transplantation Process 73
    Types of Autologous Transplantation and Novel Therapies 87
    Transplantation in Patients With Relapsed/Refractory Myeloma 93
    Nonmyeloablative or Reduced-Intensity Allogeneic Stem Cell Transplantation 95
    Transplantation in Older Adults 97
    Late Effects of Stem Cell Transplantation 97
    Post-Transplantation Needs 98
    Conclusion 103
    References 104

Chapter 6. Treatment of Newly Diagnosed, Transplant-Ineligible Patients 113
    Introduction 113
    A New Era 114
    Standard Autologous Stem Cell Transplant 114
    A Philosophical Divide 115
    Reduced-Intensity Autologous Stem Cell Transplant 116
    Conventional Therapies 117
    Maintenance Therapy 138
    Conclusion 141
    References 142

Chapter 7. Treatment of Relapsed and Refractory Multiple Myeloma 149
    Introduction 149
    Clinical and Biochemical Relapse 150
    Imaging Patients With Relapsed Multiple Myeloma 151
    Bisphosphonates in Relapsed Multiple Myeloma 152
    Radiation Therapy in Relapsed Multiple Myeloma 154
    Choice of Therapy for Relapsed Multiple Myeloma 155
    Conclusion 172
    References 173

Chapter 8. Living With Multiple Myeloma 181
    Introduction 181
    Who Are Multiple Myeloma Survivors? 181
    Survivorship: Historical Perspective and Future Directions 183
    The Hybrid Survivorship Model for Myeloma 186
    Phases of Survivorship and Episodes of Care for the Multiple Myeloma Survivor:
        A Chronic Disease Model 188
    Living While Surviving Multiple Myeloma 189
    Managing Comorbid Conditions and Late Effects of Treatment 194
    Cancer Surveillance 194
    Key Supportive Care Issues 200
    Care for the Family Unit: Caregivers and Households 207
    Conclusion 209
    References 210

Chapter 9. Nursing Research 215
    Introduction 215
    Nursing Research Topics in Multiple Myeloma 216
    Gaps in the Literature 227
    Future Scenario of Nursing Research in Myeloma 228
    Conclusion 228
    References 229

Chapter 10. On the Horizon: Advances in Genomics and Biomarkers 231
    Introduction 231
    Overview of Multiple Myeloma Biomarkers and Genomics 232
    Genomic-Based Risk Stratification Techniques 236
    Additional Biologically Based Prognostic Factors 237
    Implications for Treatment Decision Making 238
    Implications for Nursing Practice 239
    Conclusion 241
    References 241

Chapter 11. Patient Teaching 245
    Introduction 245
    Assessment 247
    Setting Goals and Desired Outcomes 250
    Methods and Interventions 252
    What to Teach 258
    Long-Term and Late Side Effects and Survivorship 283
    Palliative Care and Hospice 283
    Evaluation 284
    Conclusion 285
    References 285

Chapter 12. Clinical Trials 293
    Introduction 293
    Ongoing Research Studies 293
    Recently Approved Agent: Panobinostat 294
    Promising Clinical Trials 295
    Conclusion 299
    References 300

Index 305

Foreword

Advancing the science and care of individuals with multiple myeloma has been the unwavering commitment of the two well-recognized nurse experts who are the editors of this second edition of *Multiple Myeloma: A Textbook for Nurses*: Joseph Tariman, PhD, ANP-BC, and Beth Faiman, PhD, APRN-BC, AOCN®. Both Tariman and Faiman have extensive experience in patient care, nursing and clinical trial research, student and staff education, and service on national boards and panels addressing myeloma advances. They have tapped into a broad network of knowledgeable and accomplished nurse experts in multiple myeloma to author the chapters contained in this book.

The book provides a comprehensive review of the challenges and the opportunities encountered throughout the journey of the patient with multiple myeloma from diagnosis through survivorship. The second edition builds upon the foundation established by the previous edition, which was the first-ever textbook about multiple myeloma written by nurses for nurses.

The updated edition of *Multiple Myeloma: A Textbook for Nurses* will serve as an invaluable resource for oncology nurses seeking in-depth knowledge and a specialized resource on multiple myeloma. The book is well referenced and presented in a manner that will benefit both novice and expert nurses.

Throughout the second edition, there is a focused emphasis on nursing research and evidence-based care of patients with multiple myeloma. In addition to extensive updates in every chapter, there are two new chapters in the second edition. New chapters address the advances in genomics and biomarkers and review promising clinical trial discoveries and breakthroughs. With advances in the understanding and treatment of multiple myeloma escalating exponentially in the past 10 years, there is clearly a need for this specialized resource.

On behalf of oncology nurses, I would like to both thank and recognize Joseph Tariman and Beth Faiman for their dedication and significant contribution to the body of knowledge that will benefit patients with multiple myeloma and their care providers. Drs. Tariman and Faiman are nurse leaders who have given of their time and talent in many ways to ensure that multiple myeloma patients receive the highest level of care possible. Likewise, the authors of each chapter contained in this book have shared their expertise with great skill and passion.

To all who read this book, I am sure you will gain knowledge about multiple myeloma and hope that you continue in your commitment to advancing myeloma nursing care.

Margaret Frogge, RN, MSN
Former editor, *Cancer Nursing: Principles and Practice*
Senior Vice President
Riverside Medical Center
Kankakee, Illinois

Preface

When a patient newly diagnosed with cancer is informed by the physician that he or she has multiple myeloma, the physician often gets the question, "What is multiple myeloma?" Most of these patients and their families have never heard of multiple myeloma before, and they have no idea what part of the body is involved in the disease. In contrast, when patients are diagnosed with breast cancer, they immediately recognize the area involved, and most patients have known of someone in their family or circle of friends who has been touched by this disease, or have at least been exposed to stories about it in the media. This lack of familiarity with multiple myeloma poses great challenges to oncology nurses who are responsible for providing disease information to patients and their caregivers.

A recent study on treatment decision making in older adults newly diagnosed with symptomatic multiple myeloma uncovered that patients often are in a state of shock upon hearing the diagnosis of multiple myeloma, and the disease is unknown to most of them. Furthermore, some patients are dealing with treatment decision making immediately after confirmation of a multiple myeloma diagnosis because of end-organ damage, such as bone or kidney damage, requiring urgent initiation of therapy. These newly diagnosed patients with symptomatic illness still likely have very little knowledge about the disease and the different treatment options available to them, so they simply have to put a lot of trust in their physicians (Tariman, Doorenbos, Schepp, Becker, & Berry, 2014).

The clinical scenario and study findings described here are some of the realities that patients with multiple myeloma are experiencing in contemporary clinical practice. They portray a lot of challenges but also many opportunities for oncology nurses and other oncology clinicians to make a difference in the lives of people diagnosed with multiple myeloma. Patients newly diagnosed with multiple myeloma clearly have information needs related to disease, treatment, and possible treatment side effects that must be met to empower them throughout their cancer journey. One other top priority information need for older patients newly diagnosed with symptomatic multiple myeloma is how to maintain self-care while managing the disease (Tariman, Doorenbos, Schepp, Singhal, & Berry, 2015) from the time of diagnosis to the end of life.

The science of multiple myeloma has rapidly evolved over the past decade. Since the publication of the first edition of this book in 2010, three additional new drugs, namely carfilzomib (The Medical Letter, Inc., 2012), pomalidomide (Elkinson & McCormack, 2013), and panobinostat (U.S. Food and Drug Administration [FDA], 2015) have been approved by the FDA. The list of novel agents to treat multiple myeloma currently undergoing phase I, II, and III clinical trials is growing in an unprecedented fashion (International Myeloma Foundation, 2014). Significant advances also are occurring in the understanding of the pathobiology of multiple myeloma at the genetic, epigenetic, and molecular levels (Dhodapkar et al., 2014; Rajkumar et al., 2013). These advances and breakthroughs have driven the updates made by the editors and authors of the second edition of this textbook.

This second edition addresses the need for disease-related information and treatment-focused and evidence-based care of patients with multiple myeloma throughout the care continuum. Providing basic disease- and treatment-related information remains paramount in the care of patients with multiple myeloma in the era of shared decision making. Moreover, maximizing the therapeutic benefits of every novel agent for multiple myeloma presents a major clinical challenge for oncology clinicians. Patients diagnosed with multiple myeloma are dealing with the side effects of the novel chemotherapies (Bertolotti et al., 2008), which could affect compliance and adherence if they are not managed effectively and efficiently (Tufail et al., 2012). This edition provides substantial additions related to the care of patients with multiple myeloma undergoing treatment with novel therapies, and two new chapters discuss the advances in multiple myeloma genomics and biomarkers and promising clinical drug trials, covering major breakthroughs in clinical practice. Many significant discoveries and breakthroughs are being made in multiple myeloma care, which present great opportunities for oncology nurses to improve outcomes, particularly in quality of life and overall survival of patients with multiple myeloma.

We are pleased to present the second edition of this textbook. The authors have worked hard to bring you the most up-to-date information regarding each aspect of multiple myeloma from the most current information on therapies and pathobiology to cutting-edge diagnostic strategies and survivorship care plans. We hope the information contained within each chapter will provide a foundation for improved understanding of multiple myeloma and empower you to take an active role in the care of patients with multiple myeloma and their caregivers throughout the cancer care continuum.

Joseph D. Tariman, PhD, ANP-BC
Beth Faiman, PhD, APRN-BC, AOCN®

References

Bertolotti, P., Bilotti, E., Colson, K., Curran, K., Doss, D., Faiman, B., ... Westphal, J. (2008). Management of side effects of novel therapies for multiple myeloma: Consensus statements developed by the International Myeloma Foundation's Nurse Leadership Board. *Clinical Journal of Oncology Nursing, 12*(Suppl. 3), 9–12. doi:10.1188/08.CJON.S1.9-12

Dhodapkar, M.V., Sexton, R., Waheed, S., Usmani, S., Papanikolaou, X., Nair, B., ... Barlogie, B. (2014). Clinical, genomic, and imaging predictors of myeloma progression from asymptomatic monoclonal gammopathies (SWOG S0120). *Blood, 123,* 78–85. doi:10.1182/blood-2013-07-515239

Elkinson, S., & McCormack, P.L. (2013). Pomalidomide: First global approval. *Drugs, 73,* 595–604. doi:10.1007/s40265-013-0047-x

International Myeloma Foundation. (2014). Myeloma matrix—Drugs in development or recently approved. Retrieved from http://myeloma.org/ResearchMatrix.action?tabId=4&menuId=206&queryPageID=14

The Medical Letter, Inc. (2012). Carfilzomib (Kyprolis) for multiple myeloma. *Medical Letter on Drugs and Therapeutics, 54*(1406), 103–104.

Rajkumar, S.V., Gupta, V., Fonseca, R., Dispenzieri, A., Gonsalves, W.I., Larson, D., ... Kumar, S.K. (2013). Impact of primary molecular cytogenetic abnormalities and risk of progression in smoldering multiple myeloma. *Leukemia, 27,* 1738–1744. doi:10.1038/leu.2013.86

Tariman, J.D., Doorenbos, A., Schepp, K.G., Becker, P., & Berry, D.L. (2014). Patient, physician and contextual factors are influential in the treatment decision making of older adults newly diagnosed with symptomatic myeloma. *Cancer Treatment Communications, 2*(2–3), 34–47. doi:10.1016/j.ctrc.2014.08.003

Tariman, J.D., Doorenbos, A., Schepp, K.G., Singhal, S., & Berry, D.L. (2015). Treatment, prognosis and self-care are top information need priorities of older adults newly diagnosed with active myeloma. *Journal of the Advanced Practitioner in Oncology, 6,* 14–21.

Tufail, M., Siegel, D.S., McBride, L., Bilotti, E., Bello, E., Anand, P., ... Vesole, D.H. (2012). Phase II trial of syncopated thalidomide, lenalidomide, and weekly dexamethasone in patients with newly diagnosed multiple myeloma. *Clinical Lymphoma, Myeloma and Leukemia, 12,* 186–190. doi:10.1016/j.clml.2012.01.004

U.S. Food and Drug Administration. (2015, February 23). FDA approves Farydak [panobinostat] for treatment of multiple myeloma [Press release]. Retrieved from http://www.fda.gov/NewsEvents/Newsroom/PressAnnouncements/ucm435296.htm

Acknowledgments

Special thanks to DePaul University Center for Writing-based Learning staff, especially Hannah Lee, Bridget Wagner, Patrick Krebs, and director Lauri Dietz, PhD, for their editorial assistance.

CHAPTER 1

Myeloma Care: Challenges and Opportunities

Joseph D. Tariman, PhD, ANP-BC, and Beth Faiman, PhD, APRN-BC, AOCN®

The Basics: What Is Multiple Myeloma?

Multiple myeloma is a B-cell cancer of the most mature form of B lymphocytes called *plasma cells*. The diagnosis of multiple myeloma is confirmed when the classic triad of osteolytic lesions, monoclonal plasmacytosis, and serum or urine monoclonal immune globulin protein is observed clinically (Kyle, Nobrega, & Kurland, 1969). The most common presenting signs and symptoms at initial diagnosis include anemia (73%), bone pain (68%), renal insufficiency with a serum creatinine level of 2 mg/dl or more (19%), and hypercalcemia with serum calcium level of 11 mg/dl or more (13%); less common signs and symptoms include a palpable liver (21%), a palpable spleen (5%), and a 7% incidence of amyloidosis among newly diagnosed patients with multiple myeloma (Kyle, 1975; Kyle et al., 2003). The presenting signs and symptoms of multiple myeloma at the time of diagnosis are quite heterogeneous, and in some patients, symptoms such as hyperviscosity, extramedullary disease, recurrent infections, and neurologic symptoms such as confusion, paraplegia, or polyneuropathy also may be present (Dimopoulos & Terpos, 2010).

According to the most recent cancer statistics report, multiple myeloma remains a rare form of cancer accounting only for approximately 1% of all new cancer cases and 15% of all new hematologic cancer cases. Multiple myeloma has an estimated annual incidence of 26,850 new cases and 11,240 myeloma-related deaths (Siegel, Miller, & Jemal, 2015). Multiple myeloma is the second most common hematologic malignancy after non-Hodgkin lymphoma, and it occurs slightly more often in men (14,090 new cases) than in women (12,760 new cases) based on the most recent National Cancer Institute Surveillance, Epidemiology, and End Results Program data and the National Program of Cancer Registries figures (Siegel et al., 2015). In 2013, the number of new cases of myeloma was 5.9 per 100,000 men and women per year while the number of deaths was 3.4 per 100,000 men and women per year, age-adjusted and based on 2006–2010 censuses of cases and deaths (National Cancer Institute, 2013).

Multiple myeloma affects African Americans two to three times more often than their Caucasian counterparts (Landgren et al., 2006). Thus, a genome-wide association study (GWAS) for African American patients diagnosed with multiple myeloma is very well suited for further investigation. Spearheaded by Dr. Cozen and her colleagues at the University of Southern California, the GWAS study for African American patients was successfully launched in 2010 with more than 12 clinical trial participation sites across the United States. To date, no specific genetic abnormality has been found to explain the excess risk of multiple myeloma in the African American patient population. However, preliminary epidemiologic analysis drawn from this GWAS study showed that an increasing body mass index at age 20 is associated with younger age at diagnosis for both men and women (p = 0.0004), and a similar trend was seen in men only at five years prior to diagnosis (Hwang et al., 2013). Final analysis of this GWAS study in African American patients with multiple myeloma is greatly anticipated and is expected to be published in 2015.

Welcoming the Era of Novel Therapeutics

The discovery of the antitumor activity of thalidomide in relapsed, refractory multiple myeloma (Singhal et al., 1999) marked a new era of novel therapeutic options for patients with multiple myeloma. From 2003 to 2013, five drugs, namely bortezomib, lenalidomide, pegylated liposomal doxorubicin, carfilzomib, and pomalidomide, were approved by the U.S. Food and Drug Administration (FDA) for the treatment of patients diagnosed with multiple myeloma (Anderson et al., 2013; National Comprehensive Cancer Network®, 2014). Another drug, panobinostat, was approved by FDA in February 2015 (U.S. FDA, 2015). The advent of these novel agents unequivocally improved the treatment response rate (RR), duration of remissions, event-free survival (EFS), and overall survival (OS) in patients with multiple myeloma. A recent retrospective analysis of treatment outcomes involving 1,038 patients with multiple myeloma diagnosed between 2001 and 2010 showed significant improvement in six-year OS primarily among patients older than 65 years who were diagnosed in 2006–2010, improving from 31% to 56% ($p < 0.001$) (Kumar et al., 2014). The researchers of this study greatly attributed the improved outcomes to patients' access to novel therapies and the successful completion of the prescribed length of therapy.

Patients with multiple myeloma also are reporting good global quality of life (QOL) outcomes with the use of novel agents such as bortezomib therapy during a long-term follow-up study (Delforge et al., 2012). However, more health-related QOL outcomes should be incorporated in randomized clinical drug trials in multiple myeloma to help physicians and patients choose the best possible therapy with consideration of QOL (Kvam, Fayers, Hjermstad, Gulbrandsen, & Wisloff, 2009). Oncology nurses must continue to advocate for the inclusion of QOL study endpoints in randomized clinical trials of novel drugs and should advise patients with multiple myeloma in considering QOL when making treatment decisions.

Building Lifelong Partnerships and Collaboration

The International Myeloma Foundation (IMF), a nonprofit organization dedicated to improving the lives of patients diagnosed with multiple myeloma, has been building lifelong partnerships and collaboration with the medical and nursing scientific communities. Because of the leadership of Susie Novis and Dr. Brian Durie, IMF has been instrumental in establishing and disseminating information related to the standard of care for multiple myeloma based on strong clinical research evidence through its various journal publications, patient and family seminars, and patient educational materials and handouts. When science is lacking or controversies exist in the care and treatment of patients with multiple myeloma, IMF has been proactive in developing best practice guidelines based on consensus among myeloma experts (Chng et al., 2013; Giralt et al., 2009; Kyle et al., 2010).

In 2007, IMF created and supported the Nurse Leadership Board (NLB) with its flagship project that addressed the need for publishing nursing care guidelines related to the management of side effects associated with novel therapies (Durie, 2008). NLB successfully published nursing care guidelines for the management of peripheral neuropathy (Tariman, Love, McCullagh, Sandifer, & the IMF Nurse Leadership Board, 2008), myelosuppression (Miceli, Colson, Gavino, Lilleby, & the IMF Nurse Leadership Board, 2008), deep vein thrombosis (Rome, Doss, Miller, Westphal, & the IMF Nurse Leadership Board, 2008), steroid-related side effects (Faiman, Bilotti, Mangan, Rogers, & the IMF Nurse Leadership Board, 2008), and gastrointestinal side effects (Smith, Bertolotti, Curran, Jenkins, & the IMF Nurse Leadership Board, 2008). Since the publication of the first edition of this book, NLB has added more publications related to routine health maintenance (Bilotti, Gleason, McNeill, & the IMF Nurse Leadership Board, 2011) and overall survivorship care guidelines for patients with multiple myeloma (Bilotti, Faiman, et al., 2011). Most recently, NLB published nursing guidelines for the care of patients following hematopoietic stem cell transplantation in community practice settings

(Faiman, Miceli, Noonan, & Lilleby, 2013; Mangan, Gleason, & Miceli, 2013; Miceli et al., 2013) and relative to the management of new agents in multiple myeloma (Faiman & Richards, 2014; Kurtin & Bilotti, 2013). IMF has consistently sponsored continuing nursing education programs related to multiple myeloma during regional and national meetings, including a myeloma symposium at the Oncology Nursing Society's annual conference (IMF, 2014). The IMF NLB research team is anticipating the completion and publication of its inaugural nursing research effort aimed at describing the current routine health practices of patients with multiple myeloma. The findings from this study will inform oncology nurses and other oncology clinicians on the strengths and weaknesses related to healthcare maintenance and may provide the framework for the development of an intervention study that will address healthcare maintenance issues in patients with multiple myeloma.

Finding a New Path to a Cure

One of the major recent breakthroughs in cancer care includes molecular classifications of various cancer types, and some researchers are now proposing molecular instead of organ-based cancer classifications (Cortés et al., 2014). In the field of multiple myeloma, researchers are now uncovering new molecular subgroups of multiple myeloma with prognostic significance using a micro-RNA–based classifier leading to an improved OS predictive power when compared to International Staging System/fluorescence in situ hybridization–based and gene expression profiling (GEP)-based models of multiple myeloma risk stratification. In the area of multiple myeloma therapeutics, molecular mechanisms such as the cereblon and one of its downstream targets, interferon regulatory factor 4, are now identified as specific cellular targets explaining the antitumor activities of immune modulator drugs (IMiDs) thalidomide, lenalidomide, and pomalidomide (Zhu, Kortuem, & Stewart, 2013). Cereblon is now being considered as a predictive marker for response or resistance to IMiDs (Gandhi et al., 2014). Discoveries like these could lead to improved therapeutic approaches and eventually forge a new pathway to cure myeloma.

IMF recently launched the Black Swan Research Initiative (BSRI), which focuses on eliminating minimal residual disease (MRD). Armed with a new understanding of myeloma at the cellular and molecular levels, IMF and its team of myeloma experts from the United States and Europe are developing ultra-sensitive tests to accurately measure MRD and define its absence as a cure. The tests that are being proposed to achieve MRD-zero include multiparameter flow cytometry, DNA testing of myeloma bone marrow cells, and combined positron-emission tomography–computed tomography to detect focal myeloma lesions. If all three tests are negative after the completion of therapy, this will be considered MRD-zero, which is a new proposed definition of best treatment response beyond the traditional International Myeloma Working Group (IMWG) complete response criteria. These concepts mentioned in BSRI also are echoed in a recent published paper that suggests a new pathway to cure "early stage" myeloma (Roschewski, Korde, Wu, & Landgren, 2013). An international multicenter clinical trial is expected to be launched very soon to validate the prognostic significance of MRD-zero (IMF, 2013).

Promoting Nursing Research to Support Evidence-Based Myeloma Nursing Care

Significant research relative to the diagnosis, monitoring, and treatment of multiple myeloma has been conducted in the past 20 years. The research has led to an advanced understanding of multiple myeloma science and the underlying pathways in which multiple myeloma develops, yet the preponderance of research has been conducted by physicians. Medical research is highly important, but merit exists in advancing nursing science and finding ways to enhance nursing knowledge in support of multiple myeloma patient care. It remains a sad fact that nursing research to support evidence-based practice in the care of patients with multiple myeloma and ways to manage symptoms remains conspicuously absent. A lack of qualified researchers and sufficient funding for nursing research are two common reasons why multiple myeloma nursing science has not progressed as rapidly as the medical and pathobiological science. The lack of progress with nursing management of multiple myeloma symptoms is disturbing, as effective management of multiple myeloma symptoms, which is secondary to treatment or the disease, is one of the keys to successful patient outcomes.

Symptom research in multiple myeloma is particularly challenging for several reasons. First, longitudinal data are needed to understand and intervene with symptoms (Dodd et al., 2001; Dodd, Miaskowski, & Lee, 2004; Thomas et al., 2014). Multiple factors impact the ability to gather longitudinal data in cancer, such as patient withdrawal from clinical studies, inability to adhere to the intervention, lost to long-term follow-up, and death that occurs from the disease or complications of the disease (Barsevick, Whitmer, Nail, Beck, & Dudley, 2006; Brant, Beck, & Miaskowski, 2010; Thomas et al., 2014). Further, symptoms may occur in clusters and be related to the disease, treatment, or other comorbidities. The symptoms are difficult to delineate or address, as patients often are too frail to adhere to scheduled appointments required for symptom monitoring or study procedures if enrolled in a clinical trial (Jones et al., 2013). Symptom research also often lacks objective measures to quantify symptom burden, given the subjective nature of symptoms and heavy emotional connection of cancer.

Yet, symptom research is especially important in multiple myeloma for several reasons. First, the symptom burden of disease and treatments in multiple myeloma can be substantial and primarily includes bone pain, fatigue, muscle weakness, diarrhea, and peripheral neuropathy (Jones et al., 2013). Cumulative physiologic and psychological effects of these symptoms on individuals can lead to poor QOL and limit patient access to new and yet-undiscovered drugs to treat multiple myeloma. Multiple myeloma also is a chronic illness, with many patients living in excess of 10 years (Kumar et al., 2014). Clusters of complex symptoms may develop throughout the disease trajectory, and the symptoms may interact and progress in a fluid nature through various stages over time (Brant et al., 2010; Dodd et al., 2004). These challenges to conduct symptom management and end-of-life research in patients with multiple myeloma are present but are not insurmountable.

Overcoming Clinical Challenges

Nurses are the critical link to successfully identify and intervene for disease- and treatment-related symptoms. The IMF NLB plans to address the gap in scientific multiple myeloma nursing research with current and future studies. Members of the NLB seek to mentor future researchers with an interest in multiple myeloma in the coming years. Better understanding and measurement of symptoms and the underlying pathology of symptoms are not only necessary but also can lead to targeted and personalized treatment interventions. Future development of new instruments to measure symptom burden and psychometric evaluation of the new instruments are an appropriate priority and will provide an opportunity to better understand the burden of symptoms in multiple myeloma. The symptom science of multiple myeloma is an appropriate priority in nursing research. Thus, NLB is charged with the task to build evidence for the safe care of patients with multiple myeloma and improve the state of the knowledge of multiple myeloma nursing care science.

References

Anderson, K.C., Alsina, M., Bensinger, W., Biermann, J.S., Cohen, A.D., Devine, S., ... Kumar, R. (2013). Multiple myeloma, version 1.2013. *Journal of the National Comprehensive Cancer Network, 11,* 11–17.

Barsevick, A.M., Whitmer, K., Nail, L.M., Beck, S.L., & Dudley, W.N. (2006). Symptom cluster research: Conceptual, design, measurement, and analysis issues. *Journal of Pain and Symptom Management, 31,* 85–95. doi:10.1016/j.jpainsymman.2005.05.015

Bilotti, E., Faiman, B.M., Richards, T.A., Tariman, J.D., Miceli, T.S., & Rome, S.I. (2011). Survivorship care guidelines for patients living with multiple myeloma: Consensus statements of the International Myeloma Foundation Nurse Leadership Board. *Clinical Journal of Oncology Nursing, 15*(Suppl.), 5–8. doi:10.1188/11.S1.CJON.5-8

Bilotti, E., Gleason, C.L., McNeill, A., & the IMF Nurse Leadership Board. (2011). Routine health maintenance in patients living with multiple myeloma: Survivorship care plan of the International Myeloma Foundation Nurse Leadership Board. *Clinical Journal of Oncology Nursing, 15*(Suppl.), 25–40. doi:10.1188/11.S1.CJON.25-40

Brant, J.M., Beck, S., & Miaskowski, C. (2010). Building dynamic models and theories to advance the science of symptom management research. *Journal of Advanced Nursing, 66*, 228–240. doi:10.1111/j.1365-2648.2009.05179.x

Chng, W.J., Dispenzieri, A., Chim, C.S., Fonseca, R., Goldschmidt, H., Lentzsch, S., ... Avet-Loiseau, H. (2013). IMWG consensus on risk stratification in multiple myeloma. *Leukemia, 28*, 269–277. doi:10.1038/leu.2013.247

Cortés, J., Calvo, E., Vivancos, A., Perez-Garcia, J., Recio, J.A., & Seoane, J. (2014). New approach to cancer therapy based on a molecularly defined cancer classification. *CA: A Cancer Journal for Clinicians, 64*, 70–74. doi:10.3322/caac.21211

Delforge, M., Dhawan, R., Robinson, D., Jr., Meunier, J., Regnault, A., Esseltine, D.L., ... San Miguel, J.F. (2012). Health-related quality of life in elderly, newly diagnosed multiple myeloma patients treated with VMP vs. MP: Results from the VISTA trial. *European Journal of Haematology, 89*, 16–27. doi:10.1111/j.1600-0609.2012.01788.x

Dimopoulos, M.A., & Terpos, E. (2010). Multiple myeloma. *Annals of Oncology, 21*(Suppl. 7), vii143–vii150. doi:10.1093/annonc/mdq370

Dodd, M., Janson, S., Facione, N., Faucett, J., Froelicher, E.S., Humphreys, J., ... Taylor, D. (2001). Advancing the science of symptom management. *Journal of Advanced Nursing, 33*, 668–676. doi:10.1046/j.1365-2648.2001.01697.x

Dodd, M.J., Miaskowski, C., & Lee, K.A. (2004). Occurrence of symptom clusters. *Journal of the National Cancer Institute Monographs, 2004*(32), 76–78. doi:10.1093/jncimonographs/lgh008

Durie, B.G. (2008). Oncology nurses take the lead in providing novel therapy guidelines for multiple myeloma. *Clinical Journal of Oncology Nursing, 12*(Suppl. 3), 7–8. doi:10.1188/08.CJON.S1.7-8

Faiman, B., Bilotti, E., Mangan, P.A., Rogers, K., & the IMF Nurse Leadership Board. (2008). Steroid-associated side effects in patients with multiple myeloma: Consensus statement of the IMF Nurse Leadership Board. *Clinical Journal of Oncology Nursing, 12*(Suppl. 3), 53–63. doi:10.1188/08.CJON.S1.53-62

Faiman, B., Miceli, T., Noonan, K., & Lilleby, K. (2013). Clinical updates in blood and marrow transplantation in multiple myeloma. *Clinical Journal of Oncology Nursing, 17*(Suppl.) 33–41. doi:10.1188/13.CJON.S2.33-41

Faiman, B., & Richards, T. (2014). Innovative agents in multiple myeloma. *Journal of the Advanced Practitioner in Oncology, 5*, 193–202.

Gandhi, A.K., Mendy, D., Waldman, M., Chen, G., Rychak, E., Miller, K., ... Chopra, R. (2014). Measuring cereblon as a biomarker of response or resistance to lenalidomide and pomalidomide requires use of standardized reagents and understanding of gene complexity. *British Journal of Haematology, 164*, 233–244. doi:10.1111/bjh.12622

Giralt, S., Stadtmauer, E.A., Harousseau, J.L., Palumbo, A., Bensinger, W., Comenzo, R.L., ... Durie, B.G. (2009). International Myeloma Working Group (IMWG) consensus statement and guidelines regarding the current status of stem cell collection and high-dose therapy for multiple myeloma and the role of plerixafor (AMD 3100). *Leukemia, 23*, 1904–1912. doi:10.1038/leu.2009.127

Hwang, A.E., Ailawadhi, S., Bernal-Mizrachi, L., Zimmerman, T.M., Haiman, C., Van Den Berg, D.J., ... Cozen, W. (2013). Obesity in young adulthood is associated with early onset multiple myeloma in African Americans. Retrieved from https://ash.confex.com/ash/2013/webprogram/Paper60589.html

International Myeloma Foundation. (2013). The International Myeloma Foundation's Black Swan Research Initiative. Retrieved from http://www.myeloma.org/PortalPage.action?tabId=8&menuId=366&portalPadeId=18

International Myeloma Foundation. (2014). IMF satellite symposium at ONS—A huge success! Retrieved from http://myeloma.org/ArticlePage.action?tabId=8&menuId=0&articleId=2064&aTab=-4&gParentType=nugget&gParentId=13&parentIndexPageId=207&parentCategoryId=427

Jones, D., Vichaya, E.G., Wang, X.S., Williams, L.A., Shah, N.D., Thomas, S.K., ... Mendoza, T.R. (2013). Validation of the M.D. Anderson Symptom Inventory multiple myeloma module. *Journal of Hematology and Oncology, 6,* 13. doi:10.1186/1756-8722-6-13

Kumar, S.K., Dispenzieri, A., Lacy, M.Q., Gertz, M.A., Buadi, F.K., Pandey, S., ... Rajkumar, S.V. (2014). Continued improvement in survival in multiple myeloma: Changes in early mortality and outcomes in older patients. *Leukemia, 28,* 1122–1128. doi:10.1038/leu.2013.313

Kurtin, S.E., & Bilotti, E. (2013). Novel agents for the treatment of multiple myeloma: Proteasome inhibitors and immunomodulatory agents. *Journal of the Advanced Practitioner in Oncology, 4,* 307–321.

Kvam, A.K., Fayers, P., Hjermstad, M., Gulbrandsen, N., & Wisloff, F. (2009). Health-related quality of life assessment in randomised controlled trials in multiple myeloma: A critical review of methodology and impact on treatment recommendations. *European Journal of Haematology, 83,* 279–289. doi:10.1111/j.1600-0609.2009.01303.x

Kyle, R.A. (1975). Multiple myeloma: Review of 869 cases. *Mayo Clinic Proceedings, 50,* 29–40.

Kyle, R.A., Durie, B.G., Rajkumar, S.V., Landgren, O., Blade, J., Merlini, G., ... Boccadoro, M. (2010). Monoclonal gammopathy of undetermined significance (MGUS) and smoldering (asymptomatic) multiple myeloma: IMWG consensus perspectives risk factors for progression and guidelines for monitoring and management. *Leukemia, 24,* 1121–1127. doi:10.1038/leu.2010.60

Kyle, R.A., Gertz, M.A., Witzig, T.E., Lust, J.A., Lacy, M.Q., Dispenzieri, A., ... Greipp, P.R. (2003). Review of 1027 patients with newly diagnosed multiple myeloma. *Mayo Clinic Proceedings, 78,* 21–33. doi:10.4065/78.1.21

Kyle, R.A., Nobrega, F.T., & Kurland, L.T. (1969). Multiple myeloma in Olmsted County, Minnesota, 1945–1964. *Blood, 33,* 739–745.

Landgren, O., Gridley, G., Turesson, I., Caporaso, N.E., Goldin, L.R., Baris, D., ... Linet, M.S. (2006). Risk of monoclonal gammopathy of undetermined significance (MGUS) and subsequent multiple myeloma among African American and white veterans in the United States. *Blood, 107,* 904–906. doi:10.1182/blood-2005-08-3449

Mangan, P.A., Gleason, C.L., & Miceli, T. (2013). Autologous hematopoietic stem cell transplantation for multiple myeloma: Frequently asked questions. *Clinical Journal of Oncology Nursing, 17*(Suppl.), 43–47. doi:10.1188/13.CJON.43-47

Miceli, T., Colson, K., Gavino, M., Lilleby, K., & the IMF Nurse Leadership Board. (2008). Myelosuppression associated with novel therapies in patients with multiple myeloma: Consensus statement of the IMF Nurse Leadership Board. *Clinical Journal of Oncology Nursing, 12*(Suppl. 3), 13–20. doi:10.1188/08.CJON.S1.13-19

Miceli, T., Lilleby, K., Noonan, K., Kurtin, S., Faiman, B., & Mangan, P.A. (2013). Autologous hematopoietic stem cell transplantation for patients with multiple myeloma: An overview for nurses in community practice. *Clinical Journal of Oncology Nursing, 17*(Suppl.), 13–24. doi:10.1188/13.CJON.S2.13-24

National Cancer Institute. (2013). SEER stat facts sheet: Myeloma. Retrieved from http://seer.cancer.gov/statfacts/html/mulmy.html

National Comprehensive Cancer Network. (2014). *NCCN Guidelines for Patients®: Multiple myeloma* [v.1.2014]. Retrieved from http://www.nccn.org/patients/guidelines/myeloma/#47/z

Rome, S., Doss, D., Miller, K., & Westphal, J. (2008). Thromboembolic events associated with novel therapies in patients with multiple myeloma: Consensus statement of the IMF Nurse Leadership Board. *Clinical Journal of Oncology Nursing, 12*(Suppl. 3), 21–28. doi:10.1188/08.CJON.S1.21-27

Roschewski, M., Korde, N., Wu, S.P., & Landgren, O. (2013). Pursuing the curative blueprint for early myeloma. *Blood, 122,* 486–490. doi:10.1182/blood-2013-01-481291

Siegel, R.L., Miller, K.D., & Jemal, A. (2015). Cancer statistics, 2015. *CA: A Cancer Journal for Clinicians, 65,* 5–29. doi:10.3322/caac.21254

Singhal, S., Mehta, J., Desikan, R., Ayers, D., Roberson, P., Eddlemon, P., ... Barlogie, B. (1999). Antitumor activity of thalidomide in refractory multiple myeloma. *New England Journal of Medicine, 341,* 1565–1571. doi:10.1056/NEJM199911183412102

Smith, L.C., Bertolotti, P., Curran, K., Jenkins, B., & the IMF Nurse Leadership Board. (2008). Gastrointestinal side effects associated with novel therapies in patients with multiple myeloma: Consensus statement of the IMF Nurse Leadership Board. *Clinical Journal of Oncology Nursing, 12*(Suppl. 3), 37–52. doi:10.1188/08.CJON.S1.37-51

Tariman, J.D., Love, G., McCullagh, E., Sandifer, S., & the IMF Nurse Leadership Board. (2008). Peripheral neuropathy associated with novel therapies in patients with multiple myeloma: Consensus statement of the IMF Nurse Leadership Board. *Clinical Journal of Oncology Nursing, 12*(Suppl. 3), 29–36. doi:10.1188/08.CJON.S1.29-35

Thomas, B.C., Waller, A., Malhi, R.L., Fung, T., Carlson, L.E., Groff, S.L., & Bultz, B.D. (2014). A longitudinal analysis of symptom clusters in cancer patients and their sociodemographic predictors. *Journal of Pain and Symptom Management, 47,* 566–578. doi:10.1016/j.jpainsymman.2013.04.007

U.S. Food and Drug Administration. (2015, February 23). FDA approves Farydak [panobinostat] for treatment of multiple myeloma [Press release]. Retrieved from http://www.fda.gov/NewsEvents/Newsroom/PressAnnouncements/ucm435296.htm

Zhu, Y.X., Kortuem, K.M., & Stewart, A.K. (2013). Molecular mechanism of action of immunemodulatory drugs thalidomide, lenalidomide and pomalidomide in multiple myeloma. *Leukemia and Lymphoma, 54,* 683–687. doi:10.3109/10428194.2012.728597

CHAPTER **2**

Anatomy and Physiology

Kimberly Noonan, MS, RN, ANP, AOCN®

The Immune System

The immune system plays an important role in multiple myeloma pathogenesis. A fundamental understanding of immunity is needed to appreciate the cellular interactions involved in the development and progression of multiple myeloma. Knowledge about the cellular interactions of lymphocytes, plasma cells, and cytokines is essential for oncology nurses to better understand the pathophysiologic changes in patients with multiple myeloma.

A functional immune system is essential to maintain good health. Without a healthy immune system, life will be compromised, plagued by infections and disease. The immune system is composed of a complex array of specific cells and proteins that protect the skin, respiratory and gastrointestinal tracts, and other areas from foreign antigens. The immune system is capable of differentiating self from nonself, and therefore the primary role is to protect the host from pathogens such as viruses, microbes, cancer cells, inflammation, and toxins. Figure 2-1 describes the specific types of pathogens that are destroyed by the immune system. Moreover, the immune system is unique in that a response to an initial encounter of a pathogenic antigen occurs successfully with clear evidence that the memory of this antigen is programmed to destroy future encounters of the particular antigen (Chaplin, 2010; Warrington, Watson, Kim, & Antonetti, 2011).

Innate and Acquired Immunity

The immune system is divided into two lines of responses: innate and acquired (adaptive). Although innate and acquired immunity often are

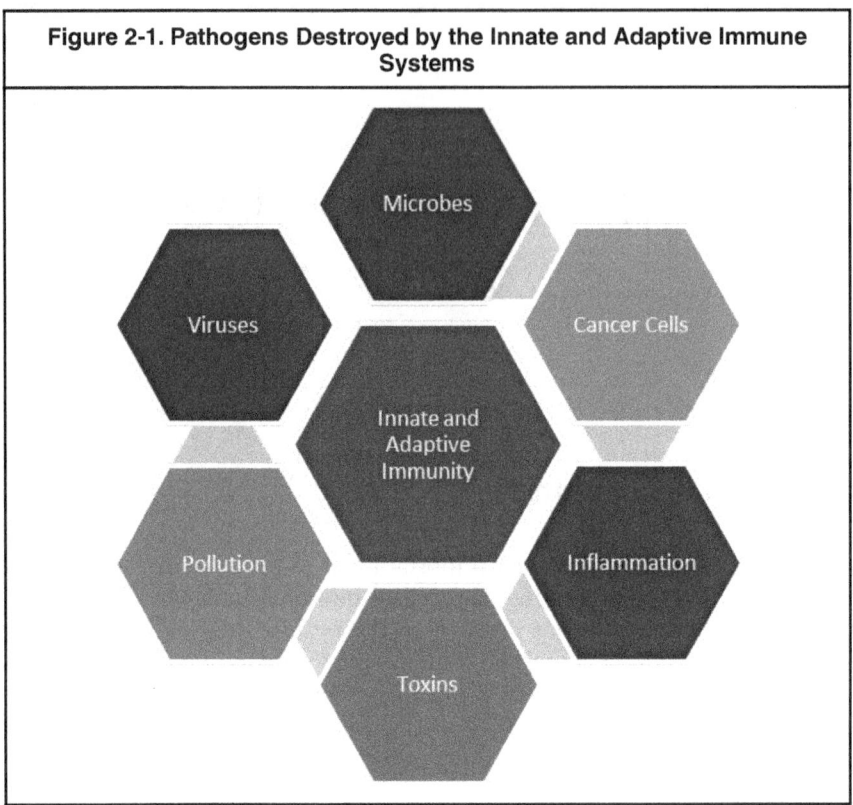

Figure 2-1. Pathogens Destroyed by the Innate and Adaptive Immune Systems

described as separate entities, they frequently interact and can be dependent on each other. Innate immunity represents the first line of defense and involves nonspecific, rapid responses to foreign or nonself substances. Acquired immunity is activated after several days in response to the individual pathogen, toxin, or allergen. The key difference of acquired immunity is the ability to produce long-lived memory cells that persist in a dormant state until the foreign substance is reintroduced to the host, activating acquired immunity (Chaplin, 2010; Post-White & Wu, 2011).

Innate immunity is also called *natural* or *native* immunity. This type of immunity exists in healthy individuals from birth and is the first-line host defense mechanism found in all species (Hoffmann & Akira, 2013). Numerous cells participate during the activation process of innate immunity. These cells are categorized as *hematopoietic* and *nonhematopoietic*. Hematopoietic cells include phagocytic cells (neutrophils, monocytes, and macrophages), cells that release inflammatory mediators (basophils, mast cells, and eosinophils), and natural killer (NK) cells. Nonhematopoietic cells play an important role in innate immunity and include epithelial cells of the skin, respiratory airways, and gastrointestinal tract. Innate immunity also has a humoral component to augment the immune defense. The humoral components include complement proteins, lipopolysaccharide-binding protein (LPS, also known as LBP), C-reactive protein, cytokines, and antimicrobial peptides. The molecular components of innate responses include complement proteins, acute-phase proteins, and cytokines such as interferons (IFNs) (Turvey & Broide, 2010; Warrington et al., 2011).

Epithelial barriers are the first line of defense and consist of the mucous membranes and skin that block the entry of the microbes. Epithelial cells are considered the first line of defense in innate immunity. If microbes do break through these cells, other cells such as phagocytes, NK cells, dendritic cells, and plasma proteins, including the complement system, are activated to destroy the foreign agent (Warrington et al., 2011).

The innate immune system uses several approaches to recognize unwanted microorganisms. The first strategy includes molecular structures that are expressed by a large variety of microbes and referred to as *pathogen-associated molecular patterns* (PAMPs). Examples of these receptors include Toll-like receptors, nucleotide-binding oligomerization domain receptors (or *NOD-like receptors*), and collectin receptors. Another strategy of the innate immune system is the use of damage-associated molecular patterns (DAMPs) to identify microorganisms; these include NOD-like receptors and the receptor for advanced glycation end products (RAGE). The last commonly described approach used by the innate immune system in identifying foreign substances is the detection of "missing self" and involves the major histocompatibility complex (MHC) I–specific inhibitory receptors (Turvey & Broide, 2010).

The second type of immunity is adaptive, or acquired, immunity. Adaptive immunity develops at a slower and more deliberate pace than innate immunity. The primary roles of the adaptive immune response are to accurately recognize a specific nonself antigen and identify effector pathogen pathways that eliminate specific pathogens and develop an immunologic memory that can eliminate a pathogen when an infection occurs (Warrington et al., 2011).

The cells responsible for adaptive immunity include B and T cells (lymphocytes) and antigen-presenting cells (APCs). Lymphocytes and lymphocyte products are involved in adaptive immunity by recognizing substances known as *antigens*, while APCs display the antigen to lymphocytes and collaborate with them in response to antigen. Adaptive immunity involves specificity for its target antigen that has specific receptors, which are expressed on T and B lymphocyte surfaces. Adaptive immune responses are dependent upon the antigen-specific receptors encoded by genes that are assembled by germ-line gene elements to form intact T-cell receptor (TCR) and immunoglobulin (B-cell antigen receptors) genes (Chaplin, 2010; Post-White & Wu, 2011).

Adaptive immune responses are generated in the lymph nodes, spleen, and mucosa-associated lymphoid tissues, which include the tonsils, adenoids, and Peyer patches. T and B cells develop from pluripotent stem cells in the fetal liver and in bone marrow and then circulate throughout the extracellular fluid. B cells reach maturity within the bone marrow, but T cells must travel to the thymus to complete their development (Bonilla & Oettgen, 2010).

Adaptive Immunity: Humoral and Cellular

Humoral Immunity

Adaptive humoral immunity is the main function of the B lymphocytes. It is mediated by antibodies that are produced by plasma cells developed from B cells and under the direction of signals received from T lymphocytes as well as other cells such as dendritic cells. Antibodies or immunoglobulins are molecules including heavy- and light-chain immunoglobulins. Mature B cells (plasma cells) secrete antibodies into the peripheral blood and mucosal fluids. Their functions include recognizing extracellular microbial antigens and neutralizing and eliminating microbes that may be present outside host cells, in the blood, and in the mucosal lumens. Antibodies do not have access to microbes living inside infected cells (Bonilla & Oettgen, 2010).

Cellular Immunity

Cellular immunity, or *cell-mediated immunity*, is primarily a function of the T lymphocytes, which defend the body against microbes such as viruses. Cell-mediated immunity protects an organism by activating antigen-specific cytotoxic T cells. The cytotoxic T cells cause apoptosis of cells displaying epitopes of foreign antigen on their surface. Epitopes are part of an antigen that is recognized by the immune system and elicit an immune response. Cell-mediated immunity also activates macrophages and NK cells. Activated macrophages and NK cells will destroy intracellular pathogens. Lastly, cell-mediated immunity plays a significant role in stimulating cytokine production (Warrington et al., 2011). Some T cells activate phagocytes to destroy microbes that have been ingested by phagocytes into intracellular vesicles. Other T cells kill host cells that harbor infectious microbes in the cytoplasm (Abbas & Lichtman, 2009). Figure 2-2 differentiates the roles of B and T cells in adaptive immunity. Although innate and adaptive immune systems are often perceived as conflicting, they are interdependent, often acting together. The synergy of innate and adaptive immunity is essential for an intact immune system (Chaplin, 2010).

Figure 2-2. Roles of B and T Cells in Adaptive Immunity

Humoral or Antibody-Mediated Immunity
- B lymphocytes, which mature in the bone marrow
- B cells differentiate into plasma cells that secrete immunoglobulins or antibodies.
- Five types of immunoglobulins
- Defends against extracellular microbes such as bacteria and some viruses
- Recognizes many different molecules such as proteins, carbohydrates, and lipids

Cell-Mediated Immunity
- T lymphocytes
- Mature in the thymus
- T cells are activated through the action of antigen-presenting cells.
- Involves cytotoxic T cells (CD8) and helper T cells (CD4)
- Defends against intracellular bacteria, virus-infected cells, and cancer cells
- Cytokine stimulation mediates the immune response.

Note. Based on information from Abbas & Lichtman, 2009; Post-White & Wu, 2011.

Organs of the Immune System

The organs of the immune system comprise the lymph nodes, bone marrow, thymus, spleen, tonsils, and appendix. Bone marrow and the thymus create an environment for immune cell production and maturation. Lymph nodes are nodular aggregates of lymphoid tissue with defined T- and B-cell dependent compartments. Lymph nodes are located throughout the body along lymphatic channels and function to purify lymph, the cellular content of the lymphatic circulatory system (Abbas & Lichtman, 2009; Harvey & Champe, 2008). They are encapsulated organs, presenting distinct cortical and medullary regions. Lymph nodes remove foreign material from the lymph before it enters the bloodstream and provide an environment for immune responses as well as lymphocyte proliferation. In a normally functioning immune system, lymphocytes reside in the lymph (Owen, Punt, & Stranford, 2013). Fluid from the connective tissues, epithelia, and many parenchymal organs is drained by lymphatics. The drained lymph fluid is transported to the lymph nodes. APCs in the lymph node begin to sample the antigens of microbes. In addition, dendritic cells are capable of transporting antigens to the lymph nodes. As a result, the antigens become concentrated in draining lymph nodes.

The spleen is a secondary lymphoid organ and is essential in fighting infections and filtering antigens from the blood. Blood flows through a network of channels or sinusoids in the spleen, and as antigens become trapped, they are engulfed by phagocytes that ingest and destroy microbes (Abbas & Lichtman, 2009). Other secondary lymphoid tissues include the tonsils, Peyer patches in the small intestine, and the appendix. These tissues contain the essential B and T lymphocytes needed to mount an immune response (Post-White & Wu, 2011).

Cells Involved in Innate Immunity

Neutrophils, Monocytes/Macrophages, and Dendritic Cells

The discussion of white blood cells involved in the innate immune response can be confusing and complicated because many of these cells are involved in both innate and adaptive immune responses. Numerous white blood cells are involved in innate immunity. These cells include phagocytes, dendritic cells, mast cells, basophils, eosinophils, NK cells, and lymphocytes (T cells). Phagocytes are categorized into two main cell types, neutrophils and macrophages. Both of these cells engulf or phagocytose microbes.

Neutrophils play a fundamental role in defending the body against infections. Neutrophils are recruited into sites of infection or inflammation because they have the ability to destroy bacterial and fungal pathogens. Neutrophils destroy these pathogens by releasing enzymes and reactive oxygen, causing damage to the surrounding tissue. Neutrophils are powerful phagocytes, capable of being released rapidly into peripheral circulation in response to an immunologic need. They have a short life span, approximately 6–48 hours. Neutrophils express innate pathogen recognition receptors, and these receptors detect PAMPs. When activated, neutrophils undergo proinflammatory changes such as phagocytosis and cytokine secretion. Specific cytokines secreted include tumor necrosis factor (TNF) and interleukin (IL)-1 (Li & Ng, 2012).

Macrophages are derived from the bone marrow as immature monocytes. Upon circulating in the blood, monocytes migrate into tissues, where they differentiate into macrophages. The overall function of macrophages is to promote homeostasis to the host after infection or tissue injury. This is accomplished by engulfing and removing large particulate matter. Unlike neutrophils, monocytes/macrophages live for months to years and have a greater capacity to secrete high levels of cytokines (Verschoor, Puchta, & Bowdish, 2012). Macrophages are identified by the residing tissue. Macrophages found in the liver are called *Kupffer cells*, while macrophages in the connective tissue are named *histiocytes* (Warrington et al., 2011). There are two types of macrophages: M1 and M2. M1 macrophages are induced by IFN, LPS, or proinflammatory cytokines including IL-1, IL-6, IL-12, IL-23, and TNF-α. M1 macrophages express high levels of MHC I and II antigens and secrete complement factors that induce phagocytosis. In contrast, the role of the M2 macrophage reduces the expression of certain cytokines (IL-12, IL-23) while upregulating other cytokines such as IL-10 (Traves, Luque, & Hortelano, 2012).

Dendritic cells are a group of phagocytic cells with both lymphoid and myeloid origin. They also phagocytose and function as APCs, acting as an important communicator between innate and adaptive immunity. Dendritic cells are known for their branch-like cytoplasmic projections and are identified throughout the body (Warrington et al., 2011). Dendritic cells are similar to macrophages because of their ability to promote Toll-like receptor and inhibit IFN-α and IFN-β immune responses (Traves et al., 2012). Dendritic cells are often referred to as *mononuclear phagocytes* and play an integral role in regulating a delicate balance between immunity and tolerance (Chung, Ysebaert, Berneman, & Cool, 2013; Lech, Grobmayr, Weidenbusch, & Anders, 2012).

Eosinophils, Basophils, and Mast Cells

Eosinophils are granulocytes that have the ability to phagocytize toxins and play an important role in parasitic destruction. They are easily recognized by their cytoplasmic granules that contain toxic molecules and enzymes that are active against allergic reactions and asthma. Eosinophils are produced in the bone marrow and live approximately 8–12 days but circulate for only 4–5 hours (Chaplin, 2010; Warrington et al., 2011). Mast cells and basophils are morphologically similar and are instrumental in responding to an acute inflammatory situation such as allergy or asthma. Basophils reside in the bloodstream, whereas mast cells are found in connective tissue. Mast cells and basophils possess high-affinity immunoglobulin E receptors. Both cells play an integral role in immediate hypersensitivity because of histamine release and other lipid mediators that stimulate tissue inflammation, edema, and smooth muscle contraction. Although primarily found in peripheral blood, basophils can make their way to tissue and express integrins and chemokine receptors. These receptors are capable of infiltrating airways, which become compromised by allergies, as well as the skin of patients with atopic dermatitis (Stone, Prussin, & Metcalfe, 2010). Mast cells play a crucial role and provide an explanation of the pathogenesis of the diseases of immediate hypersensitivity and mastocytosis as well as autoimmune diseases, fibrosis, and wound healing. Mast cells and basophils release the cytokine IL-4, which stimulates allergic immune responses (Gilfillan, Austin, & Metcalfe, 2011; Stone et al., 2010).

Cells Responsible for Adaptive Immunity

Adaptive immunity is activated when innate immunity is ineffective in eliminating foreign substances. The primary function of adaptive immunity is to recognize nonself-antigens in the presence of self-antigens. Lymphocytes are the key component in adaptive immunity and are categorized as T or B lymphocytes. Lymphocytes develop in the bone marrow as a pluripotent hematopoietic stem cell that is differentiated as a lymphoid progenitor cell. Lymphoid progenitors are differentiated into one of four mature lymphocyte populations: B cells, T cells, NK cells, and natural killer T (NKT) cells (Chaplin, 2010). Lymphocytes are the primary mediators of adaptive immunity and are also the only cells that produce specific receptors for antigens. T lymphocytes are activated through the action of APCs, and B lymphocytes produce antibodies. The other important immune system cells are the effector cells. B-cell antibody production is involved in antibody-mediated or humoral immunity, whereas cell-mediated immunity response encompasses T cells, APCs, and NK cells.

Antigens

Antigens are substances foreign to the host, and they stimulate a response from the immune system. They can be microbial or nonmicrobial. Microbial antigens include bacteria, fungi, viruses, protozoa, and parasites. Examples of nonmicrobial antigens are resin (such as plant pollen), insect venom, and transplanted organs. The smallest identifiable section of an antigen bound by a receptor is known as an epitope, which is also referred to as an *antigenic determinant* (Harvey & Champe, 2008). Surface proteins located on lymphocytes, called *CD* (or cluster of differentiation), are used to identify a specific cell type or stage of cellular differentiation that is displayed on a cell membrane. For example, B lymphocytes have surface proteins that are CD20+, and T lymphocytes have surface proteins identified as CD4+ or CD8+. The Human Cell Differentiation Molecules has defined more than 350 CD antigens (Chaplin, 2010).

Lymphocytes

B Lymphocytes

Lymphocytes represent 25%–35% of blood leukocytes. B lymphocytes comprise 10%–20% of circulating lymphocytes and have many functions (Warrington et al., 2011). B-cell differentiation is a complicated process that encounters an expression of specific sets of transcription factors, immunoglobulin gene products, and cell surface molecules. If deficiencies of transcription factors occur, B-cell production is inhibited. B-lymphocyte development requires the action of cytokines and transcription factors that positively and negatively organize gene expression (Vale & Schroeder, 2010). B lymphocytes are derived from the bone marrow; 1% of B lymphocytes will develop into plasma cells through programmed steps. One activated B cell may generate up to 4,000 plasma cells and produces approximately 10^{12} antibody molecules per day (Abbas & Lichtman, 2009). This calculation helps to explain why humoral immunity can defend against rapidly dividing microbes. B lymphocytes link innate and acquired adaptive immunity by using specific receptors expressed only on B cells.

The role of B cells, independent of antibody production, is crucial to a normal immune response. B cells are not only responsible to B-lymphocyte activity but also to T-cell responses in the immune system. B cells aid in the activation, anergy (no response to antibody or antigen), differentiation, and expansion of T cells. B-cell receptors (BCRs) are composed of monomeric immunoglobulin with disulfide-linked heterodimers called *immunoglobulin alpha* and *immunoglobulin beta*. When a BCR binds to an epitope, B-cell activation is initiated because of the immunoglobulin α and immunoglobulin β intracellular signaling cascade (Bonilla & Oettgen, 2010; Jang, Machtaler, & Matsuuchi, 2010).

Other B cells require help from T cells that form highly selective antibodies. APCs regulate both the rapid antibody response and T-cell–dependent pathways. The T-cell–dependent pathway cells may differentiate into memory B cells. The function of stored memory cells is to mediate rapid and enhanced responses to second and subsequent exposures to antigens. Memory cells survive in a quiescent state for many years after the antigen is destroyed. The exact mechanism of reactivation of memory cells is unclear. Naïve lymphocytes are responsible for the interaction of the primary immune response (Abbas & Lichtman, 2009; Post-White & Wu, 2011). One of the most important functions of memory B cells is antigen presentation. Memory B cells are known to be long-lived, but they undergo homeostatic self-renewal.

Activated B lymphocytes are also responsible for the production of proinflammatory cytokines such as IL-1 and IL-6 as well as granulocyte macrophage–colony-stimulating factor and TNF. Data also suggest that the role of B cells in inhibiting immune responses is implicated in the development of autoimmune diseases such as rheumatoid arthritis, systemic lupus erythematosus, and multiple sclerosis (Blüml, McKeever, Ettinger, Smolen, & Herbst, 2013; Klinker & Lundy, 2012).

Hematopoietic stem cells begin in the bone marrow where they mature into progenitor B cells, precursor B cells, and immature B cells. Figure 2-3 describes B-cell development. Immature B cells enter into circulation as transitional B cells, migrating to secondary lymphoid organs. B cells are capable of producing cytokines with immunosuppressive, polarizing, inflammatory, and tissue organizing properties (Anolik, Looney, Lund, Randall, & Sanz, 2009).

B lymphocytes are the only cells capable of producing antibodies, and they are responsible for creating humoral immunity. Humoral immunity prevents viral infections, eliminates bacterial invaders, neutralizes bacterial toxins, and responds to certain allergic reactions. Proteins called *antibodies* or *immunoglobulins*, which are secreted by plasma cells into peripheral blood and mucosal fluids, mediate this type of immunity. Immunoglobulins will be discussed later in this chapter. It is important to note that B cells recognize membrane forms of antibodies that become receptors for antigens and ultimately initiate the activation process (Anolik et al., 2009; Warrington et al., 2011). Their function is to neutralize and eliminate microbes that may be present outside host cells, in the blood, and in the mucosal lumens, such as

Figure 2-3. Maturation Process of a Plasma Cell

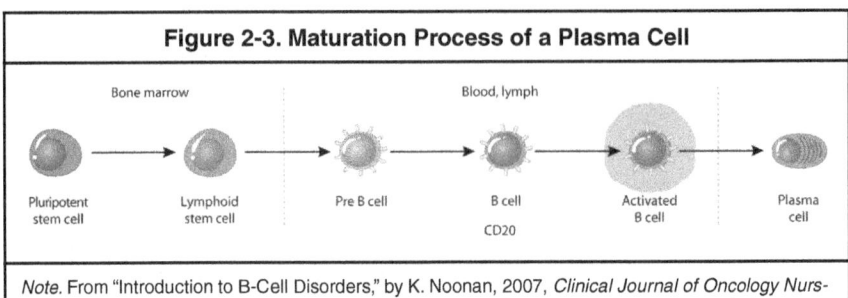

Bone marrow — Pluripotent stem cell → Lymphoid stem cell → Pre B cell | Blood, lymph — B cell (CD20) → Activated B cell → Plasma cell

Note. From "Introduction to B-Cell Disorders," by K. Noonan, 2007, *Clinical Journal of Oncology Nursing, 11*(Suppl. 1), p. 4. Copyright 2007 by Oncology Nursing Society. Reprinted with permission.

the respiratory or gastrointestinal system. Their main function is to recognize extracellular microbial antigens (Anolik et al., 2009).

T Lymphocytes

T cells are derived from hematopoietic stem cells in bone marrow and migrate and mature in the thymus. T lymphocytes have a unique antigen-binding receptor on their membrane that is called the *TCR* and requires the APCs to recognize a specific antigen. The APC cell-surface proteins are known as the *MHCs* and, as previously mentioned, are categorized as class I and class II. Class I MHCs are also known as *human leukocyte antigens* (HLAs) A, B, and C. Class I MHC molecules are found on all nucleated cells in the body and are capable of alerting the immune system of any cell changes such as viruses, intracellular bacteria, or cancer. Class II MHCs are found on certain cells such as macrophages, dendritic cells, and B cells. Class II MHC molecules communicate with the antigen receptor and CD4 molecule on the helper T lymphocytes (Th) (Bonilla & Oettgen, 2010; Chaplin, 2010).

T cells become activated after an encounter with an APC that is detected on an antigen with antigen fragments that are bound to its MHC molecule. This display causes the MHC-antigen complex to activate the TCR, and the T cell secretes cytokines. This response stimulates T cells to differentiate into either cytotoxic T (CD8) or T helper (Th or CD4) cells. Cytotoxic T and Th cells have two distinct roles. Cytotoxic T cells are primarily involved in cellular destruction of foreign agents. Clonal expansion of cytotoxic T cells produces effector cells that are responsible for lysis of target cells (Chaplin, 2010; Post-White & Wu, 2011).

Th or CD4+ cells are responsible for establishing and maximizing the immune response. There are four subsets of CD4+ T cells: Th1, Th2, Th17, and Treg (Veldhoen, 2009). They mediate the immune response by directing other cells to perform specific tasks. Th cells are activated via the class II MHC molecules through antigen recognition. Activated Th cells release cytokines that influence cellular activities. APCs induce two types of Th cell responses. The Th1 response activates bactericidal activities of macrophages and other cytokines that induce B cells to coat and neutralize antibodies. Th2 responses release cytokines involved in the activation of immunoglobulin E antibody–producing B cells, mast cells, and eosinophils that are crucial in initiating the acute inflammatory responses (Abbas & Lichtman, 2009; Warrington et al., 2011).

NK cells, another type of lymphocyte, are functionally and phenotypically different from T and B lymphocytes. NK cells are also known as *large granular lymphocytes* (LGLs). The function of the NK cell is to destroy tumor cells, virus-infected cells, and intracellular microbes. The NK cell is thought to be programmed to kill foreign cells automatically, in contrast to the CD8+ T cells, which require activation to become cytotoxic (Warrington et al., 2011).

NKT cells represent a subset of T cells that recognize nonpeptide antigens presented by nonclassical MHC molecules of the CD1 family. Activated NKT cells are responsible for the production of cytokines, including IL-4, which is involved in allergic reactions (Bonilla & Oettgen, 2010).

Antigen-Presenting Cells

APCs are located in the epithelium and capture antigens so that they are presented to the lymphocytes. Dendritic cells, macrophages, and B cells are examples of APCs. APCs are often located in the skin (fibroblasts), gastrointestinal tract (pancreatic beta cells), and respiratory tract (certain activated epithelial cells). APCs are essential in recognizing specific antigens. The surfaces of APCs express class I and class II MHCs. T cells become activated when they encounter an APC that is bound to its MHC molecule (Chaplin, 2010; Xu & Banchereau, 2014).

Effector Cells

Effector cells consist of lymphocytes and other leukocytes that are primarily responsible for eliminating microbes. In humoral immunity, activated B cells produce effector cells called *plasma cells*, which secrete protein molecules called *antibodies* or *immunoglobulins* (Abbas & Lichtman, 2009; Owen et al., 2013).

There are two types of T-lymphocyte effector cells. The first type is CD4+, or helper T cells, which produce cytokines. These specific cytokines activate B cells and macrophages. The second type is CD8+ T lymphocytes, which have the ability to kill infected host cells. Both B and T effector cells generally are short-lived, with the exception of a few (Bonilla & Oettgen, 2010). Figure 2-2 describes the roles of B and T cells in adaptive immunity. Table 2-1 outlines the cells of immunity.

Plasma Cells

Plasma cells are the effector cells that originate and develop from the B lymphocytes. Plasma cells are recognized as the basis of humoral immu-

Table 2-1. Cells of Immunity

Cells	Function
Lymphocytes: B cells, T cells, and natural killer (NK) cells	**Lymphocytes recognize antigens.**
• B cells mature in bone marrow.	B cells become plasma cells, which create antibodies or immunoglobulins in humoral immunity.
• T cells mature in the thymus.	T cells are the mediators for cell-mediated immunity. Two types of T lymphocytes exist: helper and cytotoxic T cells. NK cells are involved in innate immunity.
Antigen-presenting cells (APCs): macrophages, B cells, and dendritic cells, specifically follicular dendritic cells	APCs capture antigens for lymphocytic display. Dendritic cells initiate T-cell responses.
Effector cells: T lymphocytes, macrophages, and granulocytes	**Effector cells eliminate antigens.** T lymphocytes: CD4, or helper, T cells and CD8, or cytotoxic, T lymphocytes Macrophages and monocytes: Part of the mononuclear-phagocyte system Granulocytes: Eosinophils, basophils

Note. Based on information from Abbas & Lichtman, 2009; Owen et al., 2013; Warrington et al., 2012.

nity (Oracki, Walker, Hibbs, Corcoran, & Tarlinton, 2010). They are antibody-producing cells and have the same specificity as the naïve B-cell membrane receptors that are responsible for antigen recognition that initiates response (Abbas & Lichtman, 2009; Oracki et al., 2010). Plasma cells appear larger on a peripheral smear with abundant cytoplasm, which also distinguishes them from T and B lymphocytes. The nuclei of normal, mature plasma cells have no nucleoli, but the nuclei of neoplastic plasma cells such as those seen in multiple myeloma have conspicuous nucleoli (Cruse & Lewis, 2009).

Plasma cells synthesize immunoglobulin in response to stimulation by an antigen. An immunoglobulin is a characteristic four-polypeptide structure consisting of at least two identical antigen-binding sites. Antibodies are applied to an immunoglobulin molecule with specificity for an epitope of molecules that make up antigens. Antibodies bind to antigens to immobilize them, render them harmless, or tag the antigen for destruction. The antigen is removed by the complement cascade (Abbas & Lichtman, 2009; Warrington et al., 2011). Immunoglobulins are divided into five classes and often function as B-cell receptors.

Antibody responses can be short- or long-lived and are differentiated into T-cell dependent (TD) and T-cell independent (TI) and are determined by where the B cells are located in the lymphoid. B cells become activated following contact of the BCR with a specific antigen in either TD or TI response. Most plasma cells are derived from TD responses involving germinal center reactions. Short-lived plasma cells are generated by TI responses in the extrafollicular foci of the peripheral lymphoid organs such as the lymph nodes, spleen, Peyer patches, and tonsils. APCs also play a role in B cell–differentiating plasma cells. APCs including dendritic cells and macrophages initiate adaptive immunity by signaling TD and TI responses (Xu & Banchereau, 2014). Plasma cells differ in life span and localization of cell surface markers. Conditions that may influence plasma cell differentiation include the nature of the antigen, the subset from which the B cell is drawn, the location where the antigen interaction occurred, and the accessory cells involved. Marginal-zone B cells located in the marginal zone of the splenic white pulp respond to blood-borne polysaccharide antigens and to nonprotein antigens in the mucosal tissues and peritoneum. Marginal-zone antigens do not require T-cell help to create an antibody (Abbas & Lichtman, 2009; Oracki et al., 2010).

Independent B-cell development is unique as the process is directed by several transcription factors, such as PU.1, IKAROS, E2A, EBD, PAX5, and IRF8. In the bone marrow, B cells pass through several distinct developmental stages and will acquire their antigen specificity. After exiting the marrow, development to a mature or naïve stage is completed, as noted by the appearance of immunoglobulin D and immunoglobulin M on the cell surface (Bonilla & Oettgen, 2010).

Immunoglobulins

Understanding the concept of immunoglobulins, including what they are and how they work, is essential in relating to the pathophysiology of multiple myeloma. *Antibody* and *immunoglobulin* definitions are used interchangeably because antibody molecules are immunoglobulins of defined specificity produced by plasma cells. Immunoglobulins are protein molecules with multifunctional tools used by cells to mediate interactions of antigen molecules with a variety of cellular and humoral effector mechanisms. They are complex and individualized structures that are specific to particular antigens. An individual immunoglobulin not only binds to a defined set of ligands but also can bind to an unlimited array of antigens sharing little or no similarity. This property of adjustable binding may alter the DNA of the individual B cells. Immunoglobulins provide two important functions, namely the recognition of cell-surface receptors for antigen, permitting cell signaling and cell activation, and serving as effector molecules that individually bind and neutralize antigens at a distance (Schroeder & Cavacini, 2010).

Immunoglobulins belong to the eponymous immunoglobulin super-family (IgSF). They are composed of four polypeptide chains, which include two identical heavy chains (H) and two identical light chains (L). Light-chain regions are identified as either variable (V) kappa or V lambda. The four chains are assembled to form a Y-shaped molecule and are linked by disulfide bonds to form a monomeric unit. Both heavy and light chains are divided into variable and constant (C) regions. The V portions are designated as heavy (V_H), kappa, or lambda. The juxtaposition of the one V_H and one of the V lambda chains creates the antigen-binding portion of the intact immunoglobulin (Ig) molecule. The variable regions of the heavy and light chains contain three subregions that are extremely variable between different antibody molecules. The hypervariable sequences form the antigen-binding domain of the molecules. Therefore, the immunoglobulin has two identical antigen-binding sites. The two heavy chains are attached to each other, and each individual heavy and light chain can be subdivided into regions known as *immunoglobulin domains* (Chaplin, 2010). There are five types of heavy chains: mu (IgM), delta (IgD), gamma (IgG), epsilon (IgE), and alpha (IgA). They are all encoded on chromosome 14. Light chains contain one constant and one variable domain. This differs from a heavy-chain structure, which consists of one variable and four constant domains (Abbas & Lichtman, 2009; Chaplin, 2010). Table 2-2 lists the types and subtypes of immunoglobulins and their functions.

Immunoglobulins are divided into fragments, with each fragment determining the biologic properties that are characteristic of a particular class of immunoglobulin. Figure 2-4 provides an explanation of light and heavy chains, as well as fragments of immunoglobulin. The components of a full immunoglobulin structure are as follows (Abbas & Lichtman, 2009; Schroeder & Cavacini, 2010).

- **Fab**, or antigen-binding fragment; each fragment has an epitope-binding site.
- **Fc**, or constant fragment, is responsible for many biologic activities that occur following engagement of an epitope.
- **Fd** is the heavy-chain section of Fab.
- **Fd¢** is a heavy-chain portion of Fab with an extra amino acid.
- **F(ab¢)2** is a dimeric molecule containing two segments with epitope-binding sites.
- **Hinge region** is the area where the disulfide bonds join the heavy chain.

Heavy-Chain Immunoglobulins

Immunoglobulins are categorized in domains. Light chains have two domains, whereas heavy chains have four or five domains. The molecular weight of heavy chains is approximately 55 kilodaltons (kd) (Abbas & Lichtman, 2009; Owen et al., 2013). See Figure 2-4 to identify the heavy-chain region on the immunoglobulin. Heavy-chain isotypes determine the class,

Table 2-2. Types and Subtypes of Immunoglobulins and Their Functions

Immunoglobulin (Ig)	Subtypes	Function
IgM	None	First immunoglobulin expressed during B cell development Complement activation, opsonizing antigen for destruction
IgA	IgA 1, 2	Mucosal immunity and complement activation
IgD	None	Function unclear but appears to be involved in homeostasis Naïve B-cell antigen receptor
IgG	IgG 1–4	Complement activation, opsonization, and neutralization of microorganisms and viruses; antibody-dependent cell-mediated cytotoxicity, neonatal immunity, feedback inhibition of B cells
IgE	None	Mast cell and basophil activation trigger histamine and other inflammatory mediators needed for hypersensitivity protection, helminthic parasites.

Note. Based on information from Abbas & Lichtman, 2009; Post-White & Wu, 2011; Warrington et al., 2011.

or isotype. The five types of immunoglobulin are IgG, IgA, IgM, IgD, and IgE. The presence of a specific type of proteins, known as a *monoclonal protein* (M protein), is indicative of a clonal plasma cell proliferative disorder that is often detected in myeloma, monoclonal gammopathy of undetermined significance, Waldenström macroglobulinemia, or other lymphomas. Further clinical investigation is warranted to distinguish among the various plasma cell disorders. The most abundant immunoglobulin is IgG. IgG is present in body fluids and can easily enter body tissue. IgG is the only immunoglobulin that crosses the placenta and transfers immunity from mother to fetus. These immunoglobulins protect against bacteria, toxins, and viruses, play a significant role in hypersensitivity, and are responsible for initiating antibody-dependent cell-mediated cytotoxicity. IgG has four subclasses, IgG1 through IgG4. IgA is a secretory immunoglobulin with two isoforms, alpha 1 and alpha 2. IgA can be found in saliva, tears, colostrum, and secretions found in the bronchus, gastrointestinal tract, prostate, and vagina. IgA prevents the attachment of viruses and bacteria to epithelial cells. IgM is the first immunoglobulin to be formed following antigenic stimulation. The function of IgM is to immobilize the antigen and activate the pathway of complement. IgM is the first antibody type produced by a newborn and does not cross the placenta. Most B cells

Figure 2-4. The Immunoglobulin Structure

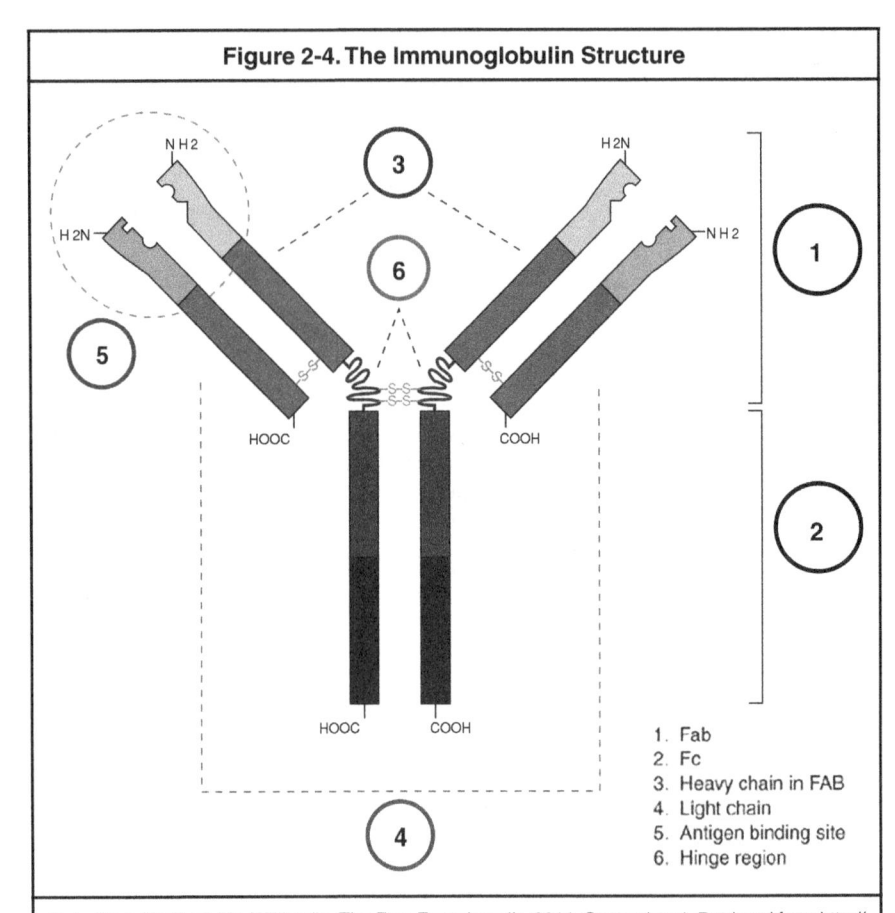

1. Fab
2. Fc
3. Heavy chain in FAB
4. Light chain
5. Antigen binding site
6. Hinge region

Note. From "Antibody," in *Wikipedia, The Free Encyclopedia*, 2014, September 4. Retrieved from http://en.wikipedia.org/w/index.php?title=Antibody&oldid=335724201. Open access artwork used under the terms of the GNU Free Documentation License (http://commons.wikimedia.org/wiki/Commons:GNU_Free_Documentation_License) and the Creative Commons Attribution ShareAlike 3.0 (http://creativecommons.org/licenses/by-sa/3.0).

display IgM on their cell surfaces. IgD is found on the cell membranes of B lymphocytes and serves as an antigen receptor for initiating the differentiation of B cells. Little is known about the function of IgD. IgE has the lowest concentration of the five immunoglobulins subtypes and has the shortest half-life of approximately five days. IgE is involved in inflammation, allergic responses, and attack on parasitic infections. IgE binds to mast cells and basophils. The binding of antigen triggers cells to release histamine and other mediators that are important in the process of inflammation and allergic responses. IgE levels are thought to be influenced by genetic makeup, race, and immune status as well as environmental factors

(Stone, Prussin, & Metcalfe, 2010). Table 2-2 describes each immunoglobulin and the pertinent characteristics of each isotype.

Light-Chain Immunoglobulins

Light chains are polypeptides that are synthesized by plasma cells. Light chains unite with heavy chains to create classes of immunoglobulins. They are found on the outer portion of the immunoglobulin (see Figure 2-4). Light chains are categorized as κ or λ and are found on chromosomes 2 and 22, respectively. They are further divided into 10 subtypes consisting of four κ and six λ. An individual immunoglobulin molecule possesses two light chains that are either κ or λ, but not a mixture of the two. This κ or λ restriction is helpful in determining the M protein of the plasma cells in multiple myeloma.

In a healthy state, the majority of light chains in serum are bound to heavy chains, making the serum level of the unbound light chains, or free light chains (FLCs), low in concentration. Low levels of FLCs can also be measured in urine, cerebrospinal fluid, and synovial fluid. In certain diseases, an overproduction of FLC can occur. When an M protein or monoclonal gammopathy is detected in diseases such as multiple myeloma, primary systemic amyloidosis (AL amyloidosis), and nonamyloid light-chain deposition disease (NALCDD), the levels of monoclonal FLCs are significantly increased. FLCs may be increased in certain inflammatory or autoimmune diseases such as multiple sclerosis, systemic lupus erythematosus, AIDS, POEMS syndrome (polyneuropathy, organomegaly, endocrinopathy, monoclonal plasma-proliferative disorder, and skin changes), and Sjögren disease (Kaplan, Livneh, & Sela, 2011). Approximately 20% of patients with plasma cell disease only have an overproduction of light chains without an increase in heavy-chain production (Kaplan et al., 2011).

Immunoglobulins can bind to a wide variety of antigens. They are capable of binding to macromolecules as well as to small molecules. The antigen-binding region on the antibody molecule forms a flat surface capable of accommodating many different shapes. Epitopes or determinants located on antigens are recognized by antibodies. These determinants may be recognized by chemical sequences or shapes. The strength by which an antigen-binding surface of an antibody binds to one epitope of an antigen is known as the *affinity of the interaction* (Abbas & Lichtman, 2009).

Cytokines

Cytokines are low-molecular-weight regulatory proteins that are mostly soluble and produced during all phases of an immune response. Cytokines are secreted proteins that possess multifunctional capabilities involved in the growth, differentiation, and activation to regulate and determine the nature of immune responses. There are six cytokine families: the IL-1 family, the Hematopoietin (class I) family, the IFN (class II) cytokine family, the TNF family, the IL-17 family, and the Chemokine family (Commins, Borish, & Steinke, 2010; Owen et al., 2013).

The main responsibility of cytokines is to communicate among cells of the immune system. Cytokines are integral in the process of inflammation and immune responses, particularly during the initiation, perpetuation, and downregulation of both innate and adaptive immune responses. The immune system is dependent upon consistent and accurate intracellular communication by cytokines. Because cytokine interactions are a key component of myeloma cell survival, many novel multiple myeloma therapies are directed at interrupting cytokine pathways (Liu, Suksanpaisan, Chen, Russell, & Peng, 2013).

Cytokines are derived from mononuclear phagocytic cells, dendritic cells, and other APCs. Cytokines released from these cell types have the ability to activate an entire network of interacting cells. Cytokines can be grouped by those that are predominantly APCs or T lymphocytes that are associated with cell-mediated, humoral, cytotoxic, or allergic immunity responses (Commins et al., 2010; Owen et al., 2013). The antigens are taken up by APCs and are processed and presented to Th lymphocytes. This provides one of the many pathways for this class of cytokine production. Another pathway involves monocytes, triggering the production of cytokines through the innate immune system. APCs trigger and produce cytokines through pattern recognition receptors, yet another common pathway of cytokine production (Commins et al., 2010).

Cytokines are potent mediators of immune cells. The interaction of a cytokine with its receptor on a target cell can cause changes in the expression of adhesion molecules and promote mobility of the cell. Cytokines can signal an immune cell to increase or decrease the activity of specific enzymes, potentially causing a change in the effector function. Cytokines also have the ability to instruct cellular survival and death. They often are considered the hormones of the immune system. Cytokines bind to high-affinity surface receptors and are produced by non–immune cells such as fibroblast or endothelial cells (Owen et al., 2013).

Cytokines are often described by their specific cellular interactions. Most cytokines act on cells that produce them, known as *autocrines*. *Paracrines*, on the other hand, are cytokines that act on adjacent cells. *Endocrines* are cytokines that are found distant from their sites of secretion. In innate immune reactions, enough dendritic cells and macrophages may be activated to create large amounts of cytokine production that is dispersed in many body regions, thus making endocrine actions possible (Abbas & Lichtman, 2009; Owen et al., 2013).

It is interesting to note that cytokines typically affect more than one cell type and have more than one physiologic cellular effect. Certain cytokines have biologic roles that overlap and develop into a cascade where one cytokine interaction is dependent upon another. In addition to positive feedback cytokine loops, many negative feedback signals regulate the immune system. Such mechanisms are essential in preventing a response from overwhelming the host. Excessive cytokine production is associated with illnesses and conditions such as septic shock, cancer, and asthma (Commins et al., 2010).

Cytokines have different functions in innate and adaptive immunity. IL-1, -6, and -12, TNF, and IFNs α and β are involved in innate immunity. They play important roles in inflammation, as well as in controlling viral infections and intracellular parasites. IL-12 is a key inducer of adaptive cell-mediated immunity and indirectly of inflammation; it also has the ability to influence the cytolytic potential of cytotoxic T cells and NK cells (Commins et al., 2010).

Cytokines activate the immune cells in adaptive immunity by aiding in the proliferation and differentiation of the appropriate development of effector and memory cells. Cytokines such as IFN-γ and IL-2, -4, and -10 are essential for these interactions. IL-2 is necessary for the proliferation and function of helper T and cytotoxic T cells, B lymphocytes, and NK cells. IL-2 also interacts with T lymphocytes by binding to specific membrane receptors present on activated T cells. Additionally, IL-2 receptors can trigger class II MHC interactions. Sustained T-cell proliferation relies on both IL-2 and IL-2 receptors. If either is missing, cell proliferation is not possible. IL-4 is a cytokine that regulates molecules that direct B cells needed to produce immunoglobulin E antibodies. IL-5 is an activator of eosinophils and works with IgE antibodies to control parasitic infections. IFN-γ is the key macrophage-activating cytokine that aids both adaptive cell-mediated immunity and innate immune responses. Macrophages and NK cells are activated by IFN-γ to kill microbes more efficiently (Abbas & Lichtman, 2009; Owen et al., 2013).

Many cytokines stimulate bone marrow pluripotent stem cells and progenitor or precursor cells to produce white blood cells, red blood cells, dendritic cells, and platelets. The colony-stimulating factors, such as granulocyte progenitor cells and granulocyte-monocyte progenitor cells, were named according to the type of cell that they target. IL-11 stimulates thrombocyte production, and erythropoietin stimulates red blood cell production (Post-White & Wu, 2011). Table 2-3 lists and describes cytokines and their biologic activities.

Chemokines are cytokines that are chemoattractants. Chemoattractants are molecules that attract cells that influence the assembly, disassembly, and cytoskeletal protein contractility and the expression of cell surface adhesion molecules. *Chemokine* specifically refers to a subpopulation of cytokines that share a specific purpose of mobilizing immune cells from one organ or from one part of an organ to another. IL-1 and TNF are examples of chemokines. An example of chemokine response can be seen as leukocytes accumulate at an infected area and vascular dilation and fluid accumulation occur, along

Table 2-3. Types of Cytokines, Cell Sources, and Biologic Effects

Cytokine	Cell Sources	Target and Biologic Effects
Interleukin (IL)-2	Activated T cells	Growth factor for T cells; activates cytotoxic T and natural killer (NK) cells
IL-3	Helper T cells	Growth factor for progenitor hematopoietic cells
IL-4	Helper T cells	Promotes growth and survival of T, B, and mast cells; activates B cells and eosinophils; induces IgE-type responses
IL-5	Helper T cells	Induces eosinophil growth; induces IgA production in B cells
IL-6	Mononuclear phagocytes, endothelial cells, and fibroblasts	Stimulates liver to produce acute-phase response; induces proliferation of antigen-presenting cells and especially antibody-producing B cells
IL-7	Bone marrow stromal cells	Stimulates survival and expansion of immature precursor B and T cells
IL-10	Mononuclear macrophages, dendritic cells, and some helper T cells	Decreases inflammation and inhibits activated macrophages
IL-12	Mononuclear phagocytes and dendritic cells	Mediator of the innate immune response to intracellular microbes; key inducer of cell-mediated immune responses to microbes; activates NK cells; promotes interferon-γ production by NK and T cells
IL-15	Macrophages	NK and T-cell proliferation
IL-18	Macrophages	Interferon production in NK and T cells
Tumor necrosis factor	Macrophages and T cells	Inflammation; neutrophil activation; fever; synthesis of acute-phase proteins, fat catabolism, and apoptosis
Interferon-α and -β	Dendritic cells, macrophages, and fibroblasts	Antiviral; increase class I major histocompatibility complex and NK activation
Interferon-γ	NK and T cells	Activates macrophages and stimulates antibody responses

(Continued on next page)

Table 2-3. Types of Cytokines, Cell Sources, and Biologic Effects *(Continued)*

Cytokine	Cell Sources	Target and Biologic Effects
Chemokines	Macrophages, dendritic cells, endothelial cells, T cells, fibroblasts, and platelets	Increase leukocyte integrin affinity, chemotaxis, and activation
Colony-stimulating factors (CSFs) (granulocyte-CSF [G-CSF], granulocyte macrophage–CSF [GM-CSF], macrophage-CSF [M-CSF])	Activated T cells, macrophages, and endothelial cells; bone marrow stromal fibroblasts (GM-CSF and M-CSF)	G-CSF promotes growth and maturation of granulocytes. GM-CSF promotes growth and maturation of granulocytes and monocytes. M-CSF promotes growth and maturation of monocytes.

Note. Based on information from Abbas & Lichtman, 2009; Owen et al., 2013; Schroeder & Cavacini, 2010.

with protein buildup causing inflammation. Chemokines are instrumental in attracting the innate immune system to the infection site and inducing T-cell movement toward APCs found in the lymphoid tissues (Commins et al., 2010; Owen et al., 2013).

Cytokines are used in oncologic as well as nononcologic practices. IFN is used for the treatment of many types of cancers, including melanoma, Kaposi sarcoma, renal cell cancer, and hematologic malignancies. IFN also is used for multiple sclerosis, hepatitis C, atopic dermatitis, and chronic granulomatous disease. Antitumor necrosis factor is used to treat rheumatoid arthritis. Cytokines continue to be studied in many clinical settings, and the use of cytokines to treat various diseases is likely to increase (Abbas & Lichtman, 2009; List & Neri, 2013).

Adhesion Molecules

Adhesion molecules are cell surface molecules involved in the binding of cells to extracellular matrix or to neighboring cells, where the principal function is adhesion, rather than cell activation. Examples of adhesion molecules are integrins and selectins. One of the most important functions of adhesion molecules is to ensure that cells are mobilized to a specific location. Adhesion molecules on T cells recognize ligands located on an APC and stabilize the process of binding the T cell and APC (Abbas & Lichtman, 2009).

Conclusion

The immune system is an interconnected and complex system that is vital to our survival. Immunity develops in two specific pathways: innate and acquired. Innate immunity is native immunity, whereas acquired immunity develops slowly. Acquired immunity is categorized into humoral and cell-mediated. B lymphocytes are responsible for humoral immunity, and T lymphocytes are responsible for cell-mediated immunity. B and T lymphocytes are essential to the immune system. B lymphocytes are the only cells capable of producing antibody-secreting plasma cells. Antibodies produced by plasma cells secrete immunoglobulin (sometimes expressed as Ig). The role of antibodies is to bind with the antigen, immobilize the antigen, and ultimately cause antigenic destruction.

Immunoglobulins are composed of four polypeptide chains. These chains include two identical heavy chains and two identical light chains. Light chains are categorized as κ or λ and are found on chromosomes 2 and 22, respectively. Heavy chains are more complicated, as there are five types: IgM, IgD, IgG, IgE, and IgA. Immunoglobulins are divided into fragments, and each fragment determines the biologic properties that are characteristic of a particular class of immunoglobulin. Figure 2-4 explains the immunoglobulin fragments.

Cytokines are low-molecular-weight regulatory proteins that are produced during all phases of an immune response. They play an essential role in initiation, perpetuation, and downregulation of immune responses, innate and adaptive immunity, and inflammation. Cytokines often are categorized and described by their specific cellular interactions. They are crucial to the immune system interactions.

Patients with multiple myeloma will experience a dysfunctional immune system. Understanding the immune system is critical when caring for people with multiple myeloma. Although the impact of a compromised immune system can be devastating to patients, knowledge of immunity will help nurses in identifying strategies that will aid in the care provided to these patients.

References

Abbas, A.K., & Lichtman, A.H. (2009). Introduction to the immune system. In A.K. Abbas & A.H. Lichtman (Eds.), *Basic immunology: Functions and disorders of the immune system* (3rd ed., pp. 1–23). Philadelphia, PA: Elsevier Saunders.

Anolik, J.H., Looney, R.J., Lund, F.E., Randall, T.D., & Sanz, I. (2009). Insights into the heterogeneity of human B cells: Diverse functions, roles in autoimmunity, and use as therapeutic targets. *Immunologic Research, 45,* 144–158. doi:10.1007/s12026-009-8096-7

Blüml, S., McKeever, K., Ettinger, R., Smolen, J., & Herbst, R. (2013). B-cell targeted therapeutics in clinical development. *Arthritis Research and Therapy, 15*(Suppl. 1), S4. doi:10.1186/ar3906

Bonilla, F.A., & Oettgen, H.C. (2010). Adaptive immunity. *Journal of Allergy and Clinical Immunology, 125*(Suppl. 2), S33–S40. doi:10.1016/j.jaci.2009.09.017

Chaplin, D.D. (2010). Overview of the immune response. *Journal of Allergy and Clinical Immunology, 125*(Suppl. 2), S3–S23. doi:10.1016/j.jaci.2009.12.980

Chung, C.Y., Ysebaert, D., Berneman, Z.N., & Cool, N. (2013). Dendritic cells: Cellular mediators for immunological tolerance. *Clinical and Developmental Immunology,* Article ID 972865. doi:10.1155/2013/972865

Commins, S.P., Borish, L., & Steinke, J.W. (2010). Immunologic messenger molecules: Cytokines, interferons, and chemokines. *Journal of Allergy and Clinical Immunology, 125*(Suppl. 2), S53–S72. doi:10.1016/j.jaci.2009.07.008

Cruse, J.M., & Lewis, R.E. (2009). *Illustrated dictionary of immunology* (3rd ed.). Boca Raton, FL: CRC Press. doi:10.1201/9780849379888

Gilfillan, A.M., Austin, S.J., & Metcalfe, D.D. (2011). Mast cell biology: Introduction and overview. *Advances in Experimental Medicine and Biology, 716,* 2–12. doi:10.1007/978-1-4419-9533-9_1

Harvey, R.A., & Champe, P.C. (2008). Cells and organs. In R.A. Harvey & P.C. Champe (Eds.), *Lippincott's illustrated reviews: Immunology* (pp. 77–88). Philadelphia, PA: Lippincott Williams & Wilkins.

Hoffmann, J., & Akira, S. (2013). Innate immunity. *Current Opinion in Immunology, 25,* 1–3. doi:10.1016/j.coi.2013.01.008

Jang, C., Machtaler, S., & Matsuuchi, L. (2010). The role of Ig-α/β in B cell antigen receptor internalization. *Immunology Letters, 134,* 75–82. doi:10.1016/j.imlet.2010.09.001

Kaplan, B., Livneh, A., & Sela, B.A. (2011). Immunoglobulin free light chain dimers in human diseases. *Scientific World Journal, 22,* 726–735. doi:10.1100/tsw.2011.65

Klinker, M.W., & Lundy, S.K. (2012). Multiple mechanisms of immune suppression by B lymphocytes. *Molecular Medicine, 18,* 123–137. doi:10.2119/molmed.2011.00333

Lech, M., Grobmayr, R., Weidenbusch, M., & Anders, H.J. (2012). Tissues use resident dendritic cells and macrophages to maintain homeostasis and to regain homeostasis upon tissue injury: The immunoregulatory role of changing tissue environments. *Mediators of Inflammation,* Article ID 951390. doi:10.1155/2012/951390

Li, J.L., & Ng, L.G. (2012). Peeking into the secret life of neutrophils. *Immunologic Research, 53,* 168–181. doi:10.1007/s12026-012-8292-8

List, T., & Neri, D. (2013). Immunocytokines: A review of molecules in clinical development for cancer therapy. *Clinical Pharmacology: Advances and Applications, 5*(Suppl. 1), 29–45. doi:10.2147/CPAA.S49231

Liu, C., Suksanpaisan, L., Chen, Y.W., Russell, S.J., & Peng, K.W. (2013). Enhancing cytokine-induced killer cell therapy of multiple myeloma. *Experimental Hematology, 41,* 508–517. doi:10.1016/j.exphem.2013.01.010

Oracki, S.A., Walker, J.A., Hibbs, M.L., Corcoran, L.M., & Tarlinton, D.M. (2010). Plasma cell development and survival. *Immunological Reviews, 237,* 140–159. doi:10.1111/j.1600-065X.2010.00940.x

Owen, J.A., Punt, J., & Stranford, S.A. (2013). *Kuby immunology* (7th ed.). New York, NY: W.H. Freeman.

Post-White, J., & Wu, S.B. (2011). Immunology. In C.H. Yarbro, D. Wujcik, & B.H. Gobel (Eds.), *Cancer nursing: Principles and practice* (7th ed., pp. 23–36). Burlington, MA: Jones & Bartlett Learning.

Schroeder, H.W., Jr., & Cavacini, L. (2010). Structure and function of immunoglobulins. *Journal of Allergy and Clinical Immunology, 125*(Suppl. 2), S41–S52. doi:10.1016/j.jaci.2009.09.046

Stone, K.D., Prussin, C., & Metcalfe, D.D. (2010). IgE, mast cells, basophils, and eosinophils. *Journal of Allergy and Clinical Immunology, 125*(Suppl. 2), S73–S80. doi:10.1016/j.jaci.2009.11.017

Traves, P.G., Luque, A., & Hortelano, S. (2012). Macrophages, inflammation, and tumor suppressors: ARF, a new player in the game. *Mediators of Inflammation,* Article ID 568783. doi:10.1155/2012/568783

Turvey, S.E., & Broide, D.H. (2010). Innate immunity. *Journal of Clinical Immunology, 125*(Suppl. 2), S24–S32. doi:10.1016/j.jaci.2009.07.016

Vale, A.M., & Schroeder, H.W., Jr. (2010). Clinical consequences of defects in B-cell development. *Journal of Allergy and Clinical Immunology, 25,* 778–787. doi:10.1016/j.jaci.2010.02.018

Veldhoen, M. (2009). The role of T helper subsets in autoimmunity and allergy. *Current Opinion in Immunology, 21,* 606–611. doi:10.1016/j.coi.2009.07.009

Verschoor, C.P., Puchta, A., & Bowdish, D.M. (2012). The macrophage. *Methods in Molecular Biology, 844,* 139–156. doi:10.1007/978-1-61779-527-5_10

Warrington, R., Watson, W., Kim, H.L., & Antonetti, F.R. (2011). An introduction to immunology and immunopathology. *Allergy, Asthma and Clinical Immunology, 7*(Suppl. 1), S1. doi:10.1186/1710-1492-7-S1-S1

Xu, W., & Banchereau, J. (2014). The antigen presenting cells instruct plasma cell differentiation. *Frontiers in Immunology, 4,* 504. doi:10.3389/fimmu.2013.00504

CHAPTER 3

Pathophysiology

Kimberly Noonan, MS, RN, ANP, AOCN®

Introduction

Multiple myeloma is a clonal malignancy of plasma cells that is characterized by plasmacytosis in bone marrow, production of monoclonal proteins, osteolytic bone lesions, renal disease, anemia, hypercalcemia, and immunodeficiency. The development of multiple myeloma is a complex multistep process involving both early and late genetic changes in the tumor cell, as well as unique supportive conditions within the bone marrow microenvironment (Rajkumar et al., 2013). Multiple myeloma is the second most common hematologic neoplasm after lymphoma. To date, multiple myeloma is incurable; however, as treatments have improved, patients are living longer and dying with their disease and not of their disease (Kumar et al., 2014; Mikhael et al., 2013).

The development of myeloma is an interdependent multistep process beginning with the emergence of a limited number of monoclonal plasma cells. During the early phase of development, less than 10% of these monoclonal plasma cells can be present without end-organ damage or specifically without CRAB symptoms (i.e., hyperCalcemia, Renal impairment, Anemia, and Bone lytic lesions) and less than 3 g/dl of a monoclonal (M) spike (Berenson et al., 2010). This condition is categorized as monoclonal gammopathy of undetermined significance (MGUS). MGUS is a well-described premalignant condition of multiple myeloma and has a conversion rate of 1% per year into malignant myeloma (Sawyer, 2011).

The Role of Genetics

Research over the past decade has revealed numerous overlapping and nonoverlapping genetic abnormalities in patients with multiple myeloma.

These genetic findings have had a significant impact on patient survival (Avet-Loiseau et al., 2007; Kumar et al., 2012). In the past, detection of conventional cytogenetic abnormalities was limited by the low proliferation of multiple myeloma tumor cells because only dividing tumor cells could be analyzed. Today, this is less of a problem with the advent of fluorescence in situ hybridization (FISH), multicolor spectral karyotyping, comparative genomic hybridization, and gene expression profiling (Lawasut et al., 2013; Sawyer, 2011; Walker et al., 2010).

Currently, cytogenetic abnormalities are categorized in groups. The first group is described as a *nonhyperdiploid group* where the majority has a translocation involving the immunoglobulin heavy locus on chromosome 14 and 1 of the 5 recurrent translocation partners (chromosomes 4, 6, 11, 16, or 20). Another group is identified as the *hyperdiploid group*, which is characterized by trisomies of one or more odd-numbered chromosomes such as 3, 7, 9, 11, or 17. Another group of cytogenetic abnormalities consists of a deletion in chromosomes such as deletion (also called *monosomy*) of chromosome 17, leading to the loss of p53, monosomy of chromosome 13, or interstitial deletion, involving 13q. The final cytogenetic abnormalities involve the *MYC* deletion and are considered to be secondary abnormalities that increase as the disease evolves (Kumar et al., 2012).

In a study by Avet-Loiseau et al. (2007), chromosomal abnormalities were examined in newly diagnosed patients with multiple myeloma using FISH on bone marrow plasma cells and screened for genomic abnormalities. Chromosomal abnormalities were detected in 90% of 1,064 patients enrolled in the study. These abnormalities included del(13) (48% of patients), t(11;14) (21%), t(4;14) (14%), hyperdiploidy (39%), *MYC* translocation (13%), and del(17p) (11%). After 41 months of follow-up, statistical analyses showed that del(13), t(4;14), nonhyperdiploidy, *MYC* translocation, and del(17p) were associated with a negative event-free survival and overall survival, while t(11;14) and *MYC* translocation did not influence the prognosis. Similar cytogenetic findings were reported in patients newly diagnosed with smoldering multiple myeloma comparing t(4;14) cytogenetic abnormalities to t(11;14). Median survival was 105 versus 147 months, respectively (Rajkumar et al., 2013).

It is believed that primary translocations occur early in the development of multiple myeloma, whereas secondary translocations occur later as the disease progresses (Kuehl & Bergsagel, 2002). Hyperdiploid cytogenetic findings are associated with an improved survival compared to nonhyperdiploid abnormalities (Fonseca et al., 2009; Kumar et al., 2012). The incidence of immunoglobulin heavy-chain translocations increases as multiple myeloma progresses from approximately 50% in MGUS to 90% in multiple myeloma. Nearly all MGUS and multiple myeloma tumors have cyclin D dysregulation, which is suggestive of an early pathogenetic event. The transformation of MGUS to multiple myeloma may result from secondary cytogenetic changes (Lopez-Corral et al., 2011).

The identification of genetic abnormalities in patients with multiple myeloma plays a crucial role in the treatment of this disease (Rajkumar, 2012). The Mayo Stratification of Myeloma and Risk-Adapted Therapy (mSMART) guidelines suggest that high- and intermediate-risk FISH abnormalities include del(17p), t(4;14), t(14;16), t(14;20), cytogenetic deletion 13, cytogenetic hypodiploidy, and plasma cell labeling index of greater than 3%. Standard genetic risk includes hyperdiploidy, t(11;14), and t(6;14) (Kumar et al., 2014). The ability to identify high- and standard-risk genetic features will have an impact on treatment options and potentially on the outcome of patients with multiple myeloma.

Plasma Cell Development

The differentiation of stem cells to immature B lymphocytes and then to plasma cells originates in the bone marrow. This is where the plasma cells undergo immunoglobulin (Ig) heavy-chain gene rearrangement, which ultimately causes an expression of surface IgM. The B cells then migrate as naïve B lymphocytes to the secondary lymphoid tissue, and antigen stimulation occurs and causes proliferation. It is at this stage that the cells' immunoglobulin heavy-chain and light-chain genes contribute to the selection of B-cell clones that express immunoglobulin. The cells may leave the secondary lymphoid organs and circulate as memory B cells or differentiate into plasmablasts following a switch of immunoglobulin class from IgM to IgG, IgA, IgD, or IgE. Plasmablasts migrate back to the bone marrow and undergo terminal differentiation into plasma cells. During this stage, cell surface markers are identified. These markers, along with the heavy-chain immunoglobulin, define the nature of the malignant cells. Normal and malignant plasma cells express CD138, which is the universal marker. They also express CD38; however, the levels of CD38 vary between normal and abnormal plasma cells (Owen, Punt, & Stranford, 2013; Tariman & Faiman, 2011; Zhao et al., 2012).

Myeloma Cells and Bone Marrow Microenvironment Interplay

The concept of tumor microenvironment interaction is closely linked to multiple myeloma, but it is also shared by a wide spectrum of other hematologic malignancies. A better understanding of the interplay between myeloma cells and the bone marrow microenvironment has been the source of new molecular targets and therapeutic strategies, leading to several clinical trials (Andrews, Kabrah, May, Donaldson, & Morse, 2013). Figure 3-1 illustrates the interaction of myeloma cells and their bone marrow microenvironment, validating the current therapeutic targets for the disease.

The main pathophysiologic changes in multiple myeloma relate to the abnormalities within the bone marrow microenvironment, bone marrow

Figure 3-1. Signaling Cascades in Myeloma Cells in the Bone Marrow Microenvironment

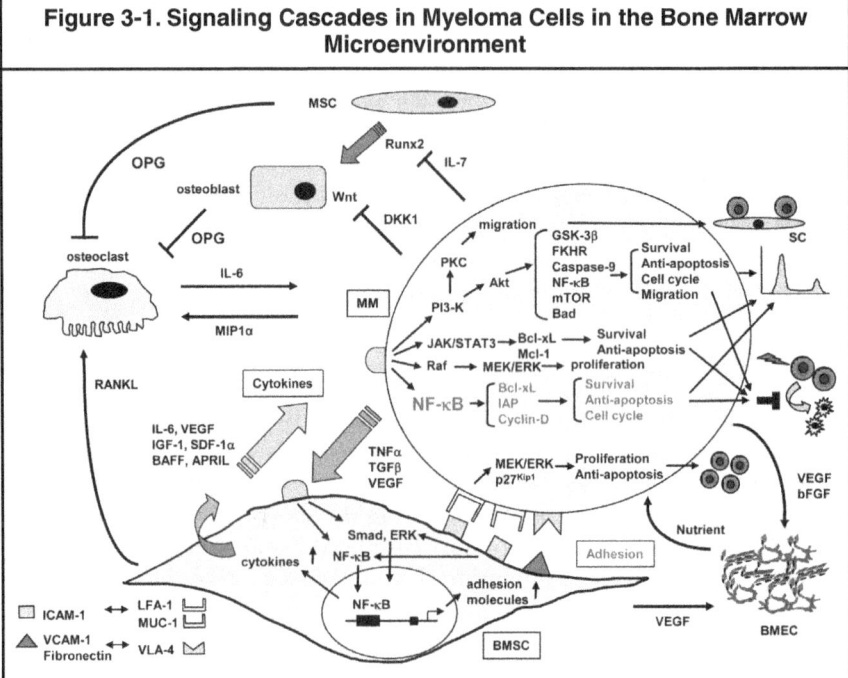

APRIL—a proliferation-inducing ligand; BAFF—B-cell activating factor; bFGF—basic fibroblast growth factor; BMEC—bone marrow endothelial cell; BMSC—bone marrow stromal cell; ERK—extracellular signal-regulated kinase; GSK—glycogen synthetase kinase; ICAM—intracellular adhesion molecule; IGF—insulin-like growth factor; IL—interleukin; LFA—lymphocyte function-associated antigen; MIP—macrophage inflammatory protein; MM—multiple myeloma; MSC—mesenchymal stromal cell; mTOR—mechanistic target of rapamycin; NF-κB—nuclear factor–kappa-B; OPG—osteoprotegerin; PI3-K—phosphatidylinositol-3 kinase; PKC—protein kinase C; RANKL—receptor activator of nuclear factor–kappa-B ligand; Runx2—runt-related transcription factor 2; SDF—stromal-derived factor; TGF—transforming growth factor; TNF—tumor necrosis factor; VCAM—vascular cell adhesion molecule; VEGF—vascular endothelial growth factor; VLA—very late antigen; Wnt—Wingless-type signaling pathway

Note. Figure courtesy of T. Hideshima. From "Understanding Multiple Myeloma Pathogenesis in the Bone Marrow to Identify New Therapeutic Targets," by T. Hideshima, C. Mitsiades, G. Tonon, P.G. Richardson, and K.C. Anderson, 2007, *Nature Reviews Cancer, 7,* p. 588. Copyright 2007 by Macmillan Publishers Ltd; and "Advances in Biology of Multiple Myeloma: Clinical Applications," by T. Hideshima, P.L. Bergsagel, W.M. Kuehl, and K.C. Anderson, 2004, *Blood, 104,* p. 611. Copyright 2003 by American Society of Hematology. Adapted with permission.

stromal cells (BMSCs), and cytokine interactions that cause disease progression and resistance to chemotherapy. BMSCs, such as fibroblastic stromal cells, osteoblasts, osteoclasts, vascular endothelial cells, and lymphocytes, play a significant role in myeloma pathogenesis by contributing to the growth and proliferation of myeloma cells. The interaction of BMSCs with malignant plasma cells is required for the homing and growth of malignant plasma cells and osteoblasts, the bone-forming cells. In a collaborative fashion, cytokines also contribute to the growth, progression, and dissemination of the myeloma cells in conjunction with BMSCs (Borrello, 2012; Oranger, Carbone, Izzo, & Grano, 2013). It is important to consider that pathophysiologic abnormalities are interdependent, and therefore information in this text may be repeated to enhance the explanation of other complicated concepts.

The interaction of myeloma cells with the bone marrow microenvironment involves the activation by cytokines, growth factors, and/or adhesion molecules of a cascade series that add to the proliferation and antiapoptosis of myeloma cells (Hengeveld & Kersten, 2015). Signaling cascades are activated by cytokines, growth factors, and/or adhesion molecules in multiple myeloma cells. Some of these signaling pathways are listed and explained in Table 3-1, including phosphatidylinositol-3 kinase (PI3K)/Akt, inhibitor kappa-B (IκB) kinase, nuclear factor–kappa-B (NF-κB), Ras/Raf/mitogen-activated protein kinase (MAPK), mitogen-activated kinase (MEKK)/extracellular signal-regulated kinase (ERK), Janus kinase (JAK)-2/signal transducer and activator of transcription (STAT)-3, and Wingless-type (Wnt) pathway. Other pathways include protein kinase C (PKC) and heat-shock proteins (HSPs) (Andrews et al., 2013; Bi & Chng, 2014; Hengeveld & Kersten, 2015). Figure 3-2 lists additional factors associated with the growth and proliferation of myeloma cells.

Bone Marrow Microenvironment

The bone marrow appears to play a vital role in the differentiation, migration, proliferation, survival, and drug resistance of malignant plasma cells. Understanding the interaction between multiple myeloma cells and the bone marrow microenvironment is the basis for myeloma treatment advances. The bone marrow microenvironment is composed of a variety of extracellular matrix (ECM) proteins, such as fibronectin, collagen, laminin, osteopontin, proteoglycans, and glycosaminoglycans, as well as cell components, including hematopoietic stem cells, progenitor and precursor cells, immune cells, erythrocytes, bone marrow endothelial cells, and BMSCs (Fowler, Edwards, & Croucher, 2011; Oranger et al., 2013). Bone marrow comprises three types of cells: self-renewing stem cells, differentiated progenitor cells, and functional mature blood cells. Erythrocytes, myelocytes, lymphocytes, and megakaryocytes are derived from a small population of primitive cells called the *pluripotent stem cells*. Cytokines produced by BMSCs control the regulation of blood cells. ECM proteins provide a protective foundation for the microenvironment cellular components to perform the function they are assigned (Bianchi, Kumar, Ghobrial, & Roccaro, 2012). ECM cells also secrete growth and antiapoptotic cytokine factors known as interleukin-6 (IL-6), insulin-like growth factor-1 (IGF-1), vascular endothelial growth factor (VEGF), and tumor necrosis factor-alpha (TNF-α).

Table 3-1. Survival Pathways in Multiple Myeloma

Pathway	Functions
Phosphatidylinositol-3 kinase (PI3K/Akt) Threonine protein kinase	Activate downstream targets Prevent the degradation of nuclear factor–kappa-B Regulate cell proliferation by targeting the activity of glycogen synthase kinase B Prevent cyclin D1 degradation
Mitogen-activated protein kinases (MAPKs) Types: • Extracellular signal-regulated kinase (ERK) family • P38 MAPK family • Jun amino-terminal kinases (JNK) family—c-Jun NH2 terminal kinase	Regulate the production and secretion of cytokines Regulate key cellular processes, such as cell cycle progression, growth, differentiation, motility, and apoptosis
Notch pathway	Induces apoptosis of multiple myeloma cells by upregulating Noxa, a proapoptotic protein Receptor/transcriptional regulator that is important for tumor survival
Janus kinase-2/signal transducer and activator of transcription-3 (JAK2/STAT3)	JAK2 is a no-receptor tyrosine kinase highly expressed on multiple myeloma cells. IL-6 activates JAK2, which induces phosphorylation of tyrosine followed by the activation of STAT3. Activation associated with multiple myeloma cell survival
Wingless-type (Wnt) pathway	Regulates plasma and B-cell motility Plays a key role in bone disease by prompting proliferation and survival of osteoblastic cells DKK1 elevated in patients with multiple myeloma, inhibits Wnt pathway, and blocks transcription factor Runx2/Cbfa1 necessary for osteoblast cell differentiation

Note. Based on information from Leleu & Anderson, 2008; Li et al., 2010.

Nonhematopoietic and hematopoietic cells, as well as an extracellular and a liquid compartment of the bone marrow microenvironment, are organized in a complex structure of subhelminthic parasitic microenvironments or niches within protective mineralized bone. Within this well-orchestrated system, niches remain quiescent and preserved until there is an insult, such as the development of myeloma cells, creating a significant imbalance. In multiple myeloma, homeostasis between the cellular, extracellular, and liquid compartments within the bone marrow is disrupted. Multiple myeloma

> **Figure 3-2. Contributing Factors of Multiple Myeloma Growth and Proliferation**
>
> - Homing and adhesion of myeloma cells to the bone marrow via bone marrow stromal cells or extracellular matrix proteins
> - Spread of tumor via the bloodstream from one site to another site within the bone marrow
> - Paracrine factors involved in survival, differentiation, and proliferation of myeloma cells
> - Angiogenesis
> - Osteoclastogenesis and osteolysis
> - Suppression of osteoblastogenesis
> - Humoral and cellular immunodeficiency
>
> *Note.* Based on information from Ghobrial, 2012; Manier et al., 2012; Yaccoby, 2010.

cells home to the bone marrow and adhere to the ECM proteins and to the BMSCs. The homing of malignant multiple myeloma cells allows the progression or metastasis of the disease to new bone marrow sites (Bianchi et al., 2012; Ghobrial, 2012).

The interactive binding of the multiple myeloma cells to bone marrow cells is reported to increase autocrine and paracrine production and increase the secretion of IL-6, stromal-derived factor-1 (SDF), VEGF, fibroblast growth factor (FGF), IGF-1, TNF-α, and transforming growth factor-beta (TGF-β) (Hengeveld & Kersten, 2015). Figure 3-3 categorizes the cellular and noncellular elements found in the bone marrow microenvironment of patients with multiple myeloma.

Bone Marrow Stromal Cells

BMSCs include fibroblastic stromal cells, osteoblasts, osteoclasts, vascular endothelial cells, and lymphocytes. They play a critical role of linking the myeloma cells to the bone marrow microenvironment. The interaction of malignant plasma cells with BMSCs is essential for the homing and growth of plasma cells. This interaction is also involved in the impairment of osteoclasts, the bone-resorbing cells, and osteoblasts, the bone-forming cells. The interaction of plasma cells and BMSCs can alter the host's immune cells and prevent immune-mediated tumor rejection, contributing to multiple myeloma disease progression (Oranger et al., 2013).

BMSCs have shown to provide efficient support for the survival and proliferation of myeloma cells by producing high levels of cytokines, specifically NF-κB signaling pathways and IL-6, further promoting myeloma cell growth, survival, drug resistance, and migration. IL-6 enhances the production and secretion of VEGF by multiple myeloma cells (Manier et al., 2012). The BMSC-multiple myeloma interaction is also mediated through a pathway known as

> **Figure 3-3. Cellular and Noncellular Elements of the Bone Marrow**
>
> **Cellular**
> - Hematopoietic cells
> - Hematopoietic stem cells
> - Progenitor/precursor cells
> - Natural killer cells
> - Macrophages
> - Platelets
> - Megakaryocytes
> - Erythrocytes
> - Lymphocytes
> - Dendritic cells
> - Nonhematopoietic cells (bone marrow stromal cells)
>   – Fibroblasts
>   – Chondrocytes
>   – Osteoclasts
>   – Osteoblasts
>   – Endothelial cell precursors
>
> **Noncellular**
> - Noncellular or extracellular matrix
>   – Collagen
>   – Fibronectin
>   – Laminin
>   – Proteoglycans
>   – Glycosaminoglycans
> - Liquid (cytokines)
>   – IL-6, VEGF, IGF-1, TNF-α
>   – IGF-2, IL-21, HGF, bFGF
>   – IL-1, IL-10, IL-11, SDF-1α
>   – CD40, TNF, Wnt, MIP-1α
>   – TGF-β, IL-15
>
> CD—cluster of differentiation; bFGF—basic fibroblast growth factor; HGF—hepatocyte growth factor; IGF—insulin-like growth factor; IL—interleukin; MIP—macrophage inflammatory protein; SDF—stromal-derived factor; TGF—transforming growth factor; TNF—tumor necrosis factor; VEGF—vascular endothelial growth factor; Wnt—Wingless-type signaling pathway
>
> *Note.* Based on information from Bi & Chng, 2014; Garcia-Gomez et al., 2014; Oranger et al., 2013.

Notch. The interaction of Notch with Notch ligand will activate pathways that will cause the secretion of IL-6, VEGF, and IGF-1, promoting cellular proliferation and improving the survival of multiple myeloma cells (Li et al., 2010). All of these molecular interactions are triggered either directly via cell adhesion molecule–mediated interactions of myeloma cells with BMSCs and ECM or indirectly by growth factors released by BMSCs or myeloma cells.

It is conceivable that BMSCs use similar molecular mediators such as cytokines, growth factors, and adhesion molecules to interact with normal hematopoietic cells, as well as myeloma cells. Growth factors can also modulate adhesion molecule profiles on myeloma cells and BMSCs. The relationship of growth factors, myeloma cells, and BMSCs in the bone marrow milieu promotes the growth, survival, and migration of myeloma cells. The combined interaction contributes to the progression and resistance to conventional therapies. In fact, BMSCs attenuate the response to conventional chemotherapy, such as corticosteroids and cytotoxic chemotherapy (Bianchi & Anderson, 2014; Bianchi et al., 2012).

Myeloma Cells' Interaction With Osteoclasts and Osteoblasts

A distinct characteristic of multiple myeloma is the induction of bone disease. Osteolytic bone resorption is caused by the stimulation of osteoclastogenesis and the suppression of osteoblastogenesis adjacent to the area of the tumor location. Growth factors such as IL-6, IL-1, VEGF, stromal-derived factor-1-alpha (SDF-1α), and macrophage inflammatory protein-1-alpha (MIP-1α) also stimulate osteoclastogenesis. It is common for myeloma cells to migrate to bone structures in the body. Osteoclastic cells remove bone tissue as bone remodeling occurs, whereas osteoblastic cells build bone. Many stimuli, such as cytokines, hormones, calcium, phosphate, and mechanical stress, activate osteoclastic bone resorption and osteoblastic bone formation (Roodman, 2010; Terpos, Berenson, Raje, & Roodman, 2014). A key question remains unanswered as to whether skeletal lesions are caused by the fertile "soil" provided by myeloma cells or if the bone marrow microenvironment attracts myeloma cells more than other tissues do. No matter what the reason is, BMSCs play a critical role in bone destruction in patients with multiple myeloma. Skeletal involvement in this patient population is obviously related to the increased activity of osteoclasts but, arguably, is equally related to the lack of appropriate compensatory osteoblastic responses. Osteoclast activation and formation are involved in the development of osteolytic lesions that are characteristic in patients with multiple myeloma (Buckle et al., 2012).

Osteoblastic cells regulate bone resorption by two processes. The first process is through osteoprotegerin (OPG, also called *osteoclastogenesis inhibitory factor*), a member of the TNF receptor family (Roodman, 2010; Weitzmann, Roggia, Toraldo, Weitzmann, & Pacifici, 2002). The second process is the receptor activator of the NF-κB ligand (RANKL). RANKL is a transmembrane signaling receptor, also a member of the TNF superfamily, and is found on the surface of osteoclasts. The RANK/RANKL signaling pathway is an important pathway of normal and malignant bone remodeling (Roodman, 2011; Yaccoby, 2010). OPG binds to RANKL and inhibits bone resorption. RANKL stimulates osteoclast differentiation and activity, whereas OPG inhibits these processes. These two processes are a crucial development found in myeloma bone pathobiology. In multiple myeloma, the balance of RANKL and OPG is disrupted, leading to the activation of osteoclasts and bone destruction (Schmiedel et al., 2013).

BMSCs secrete OPG, which prevents excessive activation of osteoclasts by serving as a decoy receptor and competing with RANK for binding RANKL. The blockade of RANKL binding to RANK or the binding of OPG to RANKL inhibits osteoclast maturation and bone destruction. Elevated levels of soluble RANKL (sRANKL) in patients with multiple myeloma were associated with disease activity and prognosis (Terpos et al., 2003). The important point is that myeloma cells affect the OPG:RANKL ratio in the bone marrow microenvironment, which causes bone disease in patients with myeloma (Yaccoby, 2010). Figure 3-4 explains the OPG and RANKL abnormality that occurs in patients with multiple myeloma.

The interaction of adhesion molecules and cytokines with BMSCs is another important interaction found during the multiple myeloma bone destruction process. As the multiple myeloma cells home to the marrow, they adhere to BMSCs by the binding of vascular cell adhesion molecule-1

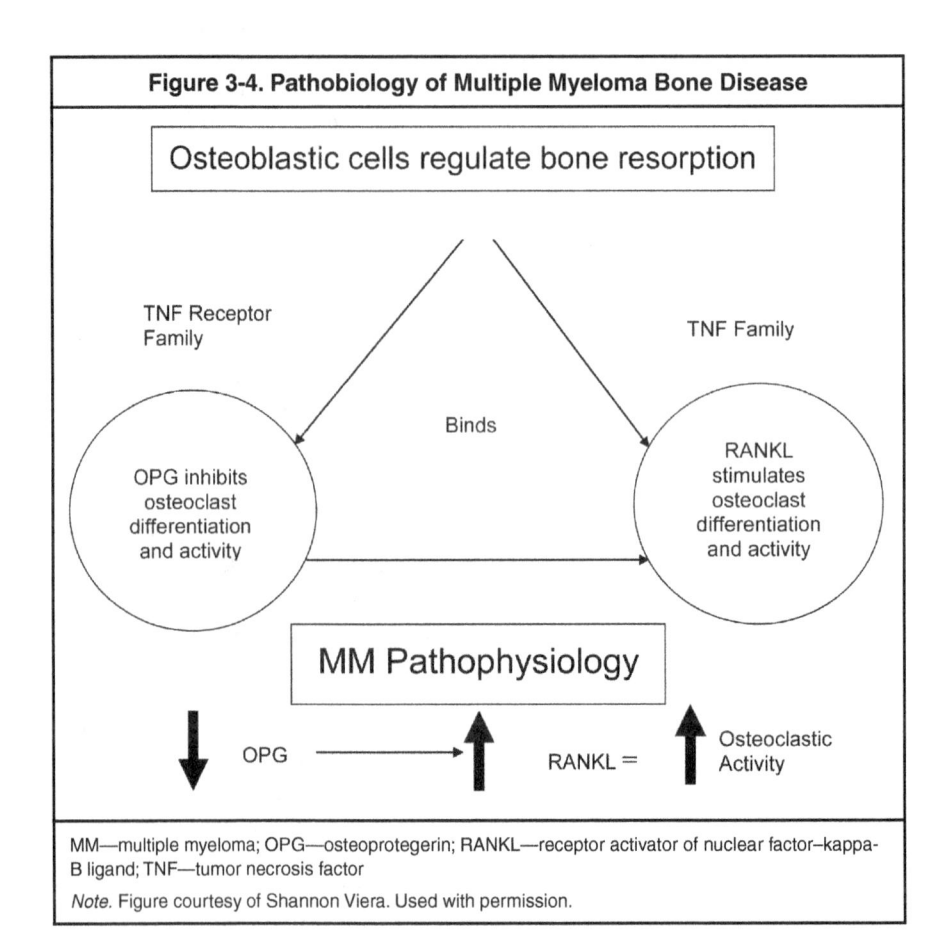

Figure 3-4. Pathobiology of Multiple Myeloma Bone Disease

MM—multiple myeloma; OPG—osteoprotegerin; RANKL—receptor activator of nuclear factor–kappa-B ligand; TNF—tumor necrosis factor

Note. Figure courtesy of Shannon Viera. Used with permission.

(VCAM-1). Macrophage inflammatory protein-1-beta (MIP-1β) is a chemokine that is produced by multiple myeloma cells in 70% of patients and induces the development of osteolytic bone lesions by stimulating IL-6 and potentiating RANKL (Manier et al., 2012).

Malignant plasma cells secrete molecules responsible for the inhibition of osteoblastic activity. Some of these cytokines include frizzled-related proteins 2 and 3, Dickkopf-1 (DKK1), and sclerostin, which are all implicated in the Wingless-type (Wnt) signaling pathway (Oranger et al., 2013). The formation and differentiation of osteoblasts from mesenchymal cells requires the interaction from the transcription factor with runt-related transcription factor 2/core binding factor alpha 1 (RUNX2/Cbfa1). Osteoblastic differentiation is associated with an increased RUNX2/Cbfa1. Myeloma cells secrete soluble factors such as DKK1 and IL-7, which also inhibit RUNX2/Cbfa1 and ultimately cause the activation of the Wnt signaling pathway (Giuliani, Rizzoli, & Roodman, 2006; Nierste, Glackin, & Kirschner, 2014).

T lymphocytes could impact osteoclast and osteoblast development by contributing to bone remodeling in both healthy people as well as those with myeloma. A subclass of CD4+ cells, T regulatory cells (Tregs), has been identified in multiple myeloma. The presence of Tregs is associated with a poor prognosis (Bryant et al., 2013). Tregs are instrumental in the maintenance of tolerance to self-antigens. They suppress self-reactive T cells and also may impair tumor-specific immune responses and therefore contribute to tumor tolerance (Zhou & Levitsky, 2007).

Cytokines

The bone marrow microenvironment consists of cytokines and growth factors. Myeloma cells and BMSCs trigger the paracrine and autocrine production and secretion of cytokines and growth factors into the bone marrow microenvironment. Some of these cytokines include IL-6, SDF-1, VEGF, FGF, IGF-1, TNF-α, and TGF-β (Bianchi et al., 2012). Cytokines contribute to myeloma pathogenesis directly and indirectly. Cytokines directly affect multiple myeloma growth by triggering key tumor cell responses and adding to the growth, survival, migration, and drug resistance of myeloma cells. Indirectly, cytokines modify the tumor microenvironment by increasing tumor angiogenesis and bone resorption. Figure 3-5 lists cytokines that play a significant role in multiple myeloma development (Andrews et al., 2014; Roodman, 2010).

Interleukin-6

IL-6 is an important cytokine in normal hematopoiesis as well as in the development of multiple myeloma. IL-6 promotes differentiation of

Figure 3-5. Cytokines With a Role in Multiple Myeloma Development
• Interleukin (IL)-6 • Insulin-like growth factor-1 (IGF-1) • Vascular endothelial growth factor (VEGF) • Tumor necrosis factor-alpha (TNF-α) • Stromal-derived factor-1-alpha (SDF-1α) • Transforming growth factor-beta (TGF-β) • Basic fibroblast growth factor (bFGF) • Macrophage inflammatory protein-1-alpha (MIP-1α) • Stem cell factor (SCF) • Hepatocyte growth factor (HGF) • IL-1b • IL-3 • IL-10 • IL-15 • IL-21 • Ang-1 • B-cell activating factor (BAFF) • Matrix metalloproteinases-2 (MMP2) • Matrix metalloproteinases-9 (MMP9) • A proliferation-inducing ligand (APRIL)
Note. Based on information from Andrews et al., 2014; Roodman, 2010; Tariman & Faiman, 2011.

normal B-cell lineage cells, which ultimately leads to an increased production of immunoglobulin by plasma cells. IL-6 stimulates the proliferation and drug resistance of malignant plasma cells in myeloma. If not the most essential cytokine involved in myeloma production, it is a key growth and survival factor in the disease. IL-6 is produced and secreted by BMSCs and osteoblasts. IL-6 production increases in myeloma and is secreted by multiple myeloma tumor cells in an autocrine manner (Hideshima, Nakamura, Chauhan, & Anderson, 2001). As IL-6 production increases, tumor cell mass increases. IL-6 induces the expression of a transcription factor, Xbp-1, which is involved in plasma cell/myeloma differentiation. IL-6 triggers the activation of many myeloma pathways, including MEK/MAPK, JAK/STAT3 and PI3K/Akt (Burger, 2013; Garcia-Gomez, Sanchez-Guijo, Del Cañizo, San Miguel, & Garayoa, 2014).

Most IL-6 in the bone marrow milieu is secreted by BMSCs. The transcription and secretion of IL-6 are augmented by the binding capacity of myeloma tumor cells and the secretion of other cytokines such as TNF-α, VEGF, and TGF-β. It is interesting to note that TNF-α-induced IL-6 in BMSCs is mediated via NF-κB activation. This is an important sequencing of events, as it displays and exemplifies the interconnection of several cytokines on one specific pathway (Manier et al., 2012). Figure 3-6 depicts the interaction of IL-6 with other cytokines.

Figure 3-6. Interaction of IL-6 With Other Cytokines

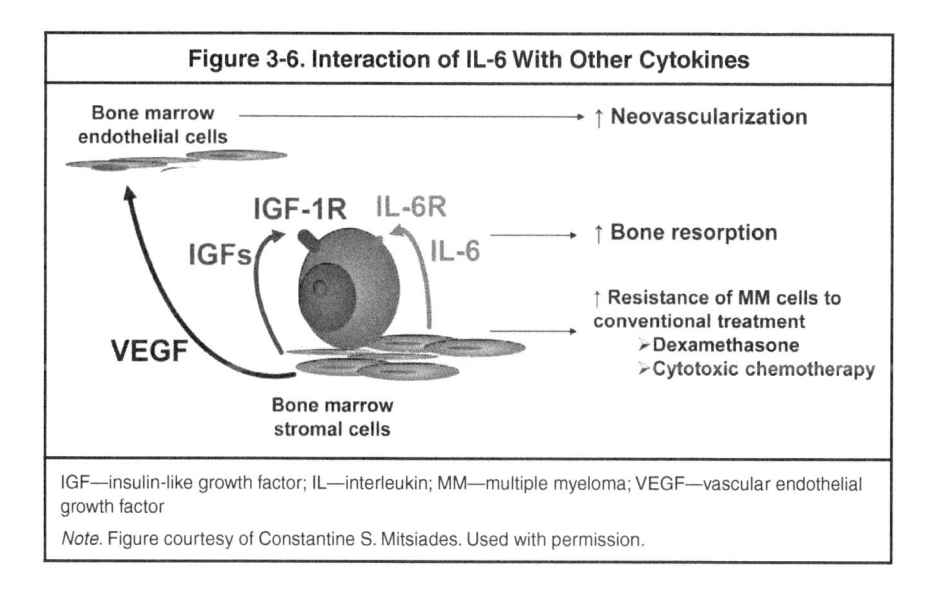

[Figure: Bone marrow endothelial cells → ↑ Neovascularization; IGFs, IGF-1R, IL-6R, IL-6, VEGF, Bone marrow stromal cells → ↑ Bone resorption; ↑ Resistance of MM cells to conventional treatment ➤ Dexamethasone ➤ Cytotoxic chemotherapy]

IGF—insulin-like growth factor; IL—interleukin; MM—multiple myeloma; VEGF—vascular endothelial growth factor

Note. Figure courtesy of Constantine S. Mitsiades. Used with permission.

Vascular Endothelial Growth Factor

The proangiogenic activity of myeloma cells is supported by VEGF production, and myeloma cells directly produce VEGF. VEGF produced by myeloma cells stimulates IL-6, and VEGF secretion by BMSCs induces VEGF production by myeloma cells in a paracrine fashion (Giuliani, Storti, Bolzoni, Palma, & Bonomini, 2011). VEGF-1 is expressed by myeloma cells in autocrine signaling pathways such as PI3K/protein kinase Ca-dependent cascade, MEK/ERK, and Mcl-1, leading to myeloma cell proliferation and survival. VEGF also affects osteoblasts, NK cells, monocytes, and endothelial progenitors (Giuliani et al., 2011).

Tumor Necrosis Factor-Alpha

TNF-α is a combination cytokine known as the *TNF-α superfamily*. A superfamily is a large group of related proteins or molecules. TNF-α is elevated in patients with myeloma. The level of TNF-α in the marrow microenvironment also is increased (Galson, Silbermann, & Roodman, 2012). TNF-α has multiple functions in myeloma bone disease. TNF-α increases marrow stromal cell production of RANKL, IL-6, and other osteoclastogenic cytokines.

TNF-α also is a potent inducer of osteoclast formation itself and can either directly increase osteoclast formation or enhance the effects of RANKL. TNF-α can block osteoblast differentiation from BMSCs by decreasing the expression of critical osteoblast transcription factors (Roodman, 2010).

Cluster of Differentiation-40

CD40, a member of the TNF-α superfamily, is expressed by antigen-presenting cells (APCs) and T cells, as well as B-cell malignancies. This superfamily member mediates PI3K/Akt and NF-κB pathways, as well as increases the cellular growth in p53-dependent multiple myeloma and triggers VEGF secretions. B-cell activating factor (BAFF) and a proliferation-inducing ligand (APRIL) protect myeloma cells from apoptosis induced by IL-6 deprivation and dexamethasone. They promote cellular growth and adhesion to BMSCs. These processes are mediated through NF-κB, PI3K/Akt, and MAPK pathways. CD40-activated multiple myeloma cells adhere to fibronectin and target CD40-signaling multiple myeloma cells. CD40 and fibronectin inhibit immunoglobulin secretion (Garcia-Gomez et al., 2014; Tai & Anderson, 2011).

Insulin-Like Growth Factor-1

IGF-1 is a multifunctional peptide that regulates cell proliferation, differentiation, and apoptosis. It is an important paracrine growth factor that induces proliferation, survival, migration, and drug resistance in myeloma cells (Sprynski et al., 2009; Tagoug et al., 2013). In addition to an autocrine effect based on production of IGF by myeloma cells, activation of the IGF-1 receptor results from the interaction between myeloma cells and BMSCs.

IGF-1 promotes proliferation and drug resistance in myeloma cells through the activation of MAPK and PI3K/Akt signaling cascades. IGF-1 induces cell migration and invasion via a PI3K-dependent pathway, through the Akt1-independent pathway, and through protein kinase D, RhoA, and b1-integrin. IGF-1 appears to be a more potent inducer of Akt signaling than IL-6. IGF-1 has also been shown to activate NF-κB signaling (Mitsiades et al., 2002). IGF-1 increases the content of antiapoptotic proteins such as Bcl-2, Bcl-xL, and FLIP (Birmann et al., 2009; Tagoug et al., 2013).

Conclusion

The pathophysiology of multiple myeloma is a complicated but well-orchestrated and organized sequence of interactions. Many of these interactions are linked together and are interdependent. Understanding the interconnections involved in the development of myeloma, as well as the complicated pathways, is a critical step in treating and managing patients with this disease. Better understanding of the pathobiologic changes in multiple myeloma has led to improved therapies using combination regimens that target multiple pathways of myeloma cell survival. As the knowledge of multiple myeloma grows and research progresses, the goal of finding a cure may be a not-so-distant reality.

References

Andrews, S.W., Kabrah, S., May, J.E., Donaldson, C., & Morse, H.R. (2013). Multiple myeloma: The bone marrow microenvironment and its relation to treatment. *British Journal of Biomedical Science, 70*, 110–120.

Avet-Loiseau, H., Attal, M., Moreau, P., Charbonnel, C., Garban, F., Hulin, C., ... Mathiot, C. (2007). Genetic abnormalities and survival in multiple myeloma: The experience of the Intergroupe Francophone du Myélome. *Blood, 109*, 3489–3495. doi:10.1182/blood-2006-08-040410

Berenson, J.R., Anderson, K.C., Audell, R.A., Boccia, R.V., Coleman, M., Dimopoulos, M.A., ... Kyle, R.A. (2010). Monoclonal gammopathy of undetermined significance: A consensus statement. *British Journal of Haematology, 150*, 28–38. doi:10.1111/j.1365-2141.2010.08207.x

Bi, C., & Chng, W.J. (2014). MicroRNA: Important player in the pathobiology of multiple myeloma. *Biomedical Research International, 2014*, Article ID 521586. doi:10.1155/2014/521586

Bianchi, G., & Anderson, K.C. (2014). Understanding biology to tackle the disease: Multiple myeloma from bench to bedside and back. *CA: A Cancer Journal for Clinicians, 64*, 422–444. doi:10.3322/caac.21252

Bianchi, G., Kumar, S., Ghobrial, I.M., & Roccaro, A.M. (2012). Cell trafficking in multiple myeloma. *Open Journal of Hematology, 3*(Suppl. 1). doi:10.13055/ojhmt_3_S1_04.120221

Birmann, B.M., Tamimi, R.M., Giovannucci, E., Rosner, B., Hunter, D.J., Kraft, P., ... Colditz, G.A. (2009). Insulin-like growth factor-1- and interleukin-6-related gene variation and risk of multiple myeloma. *Cancer Epidemiology, Biomarkers and Prevention, 18*, 282–288. doi:10.1158/1055-9965.EPI-08-0778

Borrello, I. (2012). Can we change the disease biology of multiple myeloma? *Leukemia Research, 36*(Suppl. 1), S3–S12. doi:10.1016/S0145-2126(12)70003-6

Bryant, C., Suen, H., Brown, R., Yang, S., Favaloro, J., Aklilu, E., ... Joshua, D.E. (2013). Longterm survival in multiple myeloma is associated with a distinct immunological profile, which includes proliferative cytotoxic T-cell clones and a favourable Treg/Th17 balance. *Blood Cancer Journal, 3*, e148. doi:10.1038/bcj.2013.34

Buckle, C.H., De Leenheer, E., Lawson, M.A., Yong, K., Rabin, N., Perry, M., ... Croucher, P.I. (2012). Soluble rank ligand produced by myeloma cells causes generalised bone loss in multiple myeloma. *PLOS ONE, 7*, e41127. doi:10.1371/journal.pone.0041127

Burger, R. (2013). Impact of interleukin-6 in hematological malignancies. *Transfusion Medicine and Hemotherapy, 40*, 336–343. doi:10.1159/000354194

Fonseca, R., Bergsagel, P.L., Drach, J., Shaughnessy, J., Gutierrez, N., Stewart, A.K., ... Avet-Loiseau, H. (2009). International Myeloma Working Group molecular classification of multiple myeloma: Spotlight review. *Leukemia, 23*, 2210–2221. doi:10.1038/leu.2009.174

Fowler, J.A., Edwards, C.M., & Croucher, P.I. (2011). Tumor–host cell interactions in the bone disease of myeloma. *Bone, 48*, 121–128. doi:10.1016/j.bone.2010.06.029

Galson, D.L., Silbermann, R., & Roodman, G.D. (2012). Mechanisms of multiple myeloma bone disease. *Bonekey Reports, 1*, 135. doi:10.1038/bonekey.2012.135

Garcia-Gomez, A., Sanchez-Guijo, F., Del Cañizo, M.C., San Miguel, J.F., & Garayoa, M. (2014). Multiple myeloma mesenchymal stromal cells: Contribution to myeloma bone disease and therapeutics. *World Journal of Stem Cells, 6*, 322–343. doi:10.4252/wjsc.v6.i3.322

Ghobrial, I.M. (2012). Myeloma as a model for the process of metastasis: Implications for therapy. *Blood, 120,* 20–30. doi:10.1182/blood-2012-01-379024

Giuliani, N., Rizzoli, V., & Roodman, G.D. (2006). Multiple myeloma bone disease: Pathophysiology of osteoblast inhibition. *Blood, 108,* 3992–3996. doi:10.1182/blood-2006-05-026112

Giuliani, N., Storti, P., Bolzoni, M., Palma, B.D., & Bonomini, S. (2011). Angiogenesis and multiple myeloma. *Cancer Microenvironment, 4,* 325–337. doi:10.1007/s12307-011-0072-9

Hengeveld, B.J., & Kersten, M.J. (2015). B-cell activating factor in the pathophysiology of multiple myeloma: A target for therapy? *Blood Cancer Journal, 5,* e282. doi:10.1038/bcj.2015.3

Hideshima, T., Bergsagel, P.L., Kuehl, W.M., & Anderson, K.C. (2004). Advances in biology of multiple myeloma: Clinical applications. *Blood, 104,* 607–618. doi:10.1182/blood-2004-01-0037

Hideshima, T., Mitsiades, C., Tonon, G., Richardson, P.G., & Anderson, K.C. (2007). Understanding multiple myeloma pathogenesis in the bone marrow to identify new therapeutic targets. *Nature Reviews Cancer, 7,* 585–598. doi:10.1038/nrc2189

Hideshima, T., Nakamura, N., Chauhan, D., & Anderson, K.C. (2001). Biologic sequelae of interleukin-6 induced PI3-K/Akt signaling in multiple myeloma. *Oncogene, 20,* 5991–6000. doi:10.1038/sj.onc.1204833

Kuehl, W.M., & Bergsagel, P.L. (2002). Multiple myeloma: Evolving genetic events and host interactions. *Nature Reviews Cancer, 2,* 175–187. doi:10.1038/nrc746

Kumar, S.K., Dispenzieri, A., Lacy, M.Q., Gertz, M.A., Buadi, F.K., Pandey, S., ... Rajkumar, S.V. (2014). Continued improvement in survival in multiple myeloma: Changes in early mortality and outcomes in older patients. *Leukemia, 28,* 1122–1128. doi:10.1038/leu.2013.313

Kumar, S., Fonseca, R., Ketterling, R.P., Dispenzieri, A., Lacy, M.Q., Gertz, M.A., ... Rajkumar, S.V. (2012). Trisomies in multiple myeloma: Impact on survival in patients with high-risk cytogenetics. *Blood, 119,* 2100–2105. doi:10.1182/blood-2011-11-390658

Lawasut, P., Groen, R.W., Dhimolea, E., Richardson, P.G., Anderson, K.C., & Mitsiades, C.S. (2013). Decoding the pathophysiology and the genetics of multiple myeloma to identify new therapeutic targets. *Seminars in Oncology, 40,* 537–548. doi:10.1053/j.seminoncol.2013.07.010

Leleu, X., & Anderson, K.C. (2008). Promising new agents in phase I and II clinical trials in multiple myeloma. In K.C. Anderson & I.M. Ghobrial (Eds.), *Multiple myeloma: Translational and emerging therapies* (pp. 211–242). New York, NY: Informa Healthcare.

Li, M., Chen, F., Clifton, N., Sullivan, D.M., Dalton, W.S., Gabrilovich, D.I., ... Nefedova, Y. (2010). Combined inhibition of Notch signaling and Bcl-2/Bcl-xL results in synergistic antimyeloma effect. *Molecular Cancer Therapeutics, 9,* 3200–3209. doi:10.1158/1535-7163.MCT-10-0372

Lopez-Corral, L., Gutierrez, N.C., Vidriales, M.B., Mateos, M.V., Rasillo, A., Garcia-Sanz, R., ... San Miguel, J.F. (2011). The progression from MGUS to smoldering myeloma and eventually to multiple myeloma involves a clonal expansion of genetically abnormal plasma cells. *Clinical Cancer Research, 17,* 1692–1700. doi:10.1158/1078-0432.CCR-10-1066

Manier, S., Sacco, A., Leleu, X., Ghobrial, I.M., & Roccaro, A.M. (2012). Bone marrow microenvironment in multiple myeloma progression. *Journal of Biomedicine and Biotechnology, 2012,* Article ID 157496. doi:10.1155/2012/157496

Mikhael, J.R., Dingli, D., Roy, V., Reeder, C.B., Buadi, F.K., Hayman, S.R., ... Lacy, M.Q. (2013). Management of newly diagnosed symptomatic multiple myeloma: Updated Mayo stratification of myeloma and risk-adapted therapy (mSMART) consensus guidelines 2013. *Mayo Clinic Proceedings, 88,* 360–376. doi:10.1016/j.mayocp.2013.01.019

Mitsiades, C.S., Mitsiades, N., Poulaki, V., Schlossman, R., Akiyama, M., Chauhan, D., ... Hideshima, T. (2002). Activation of NF-kappa B and upregulation of intracellular anti-apoptotic proteins via the IGF-1/Akt signaling in human multiple myeloma cells: Therapeutic implications. *Oncogene, 21,* 5673–5683. doi:10.1038/sj.onc.1205664

Nierste, B.A., Glackin, C.A, & Kirshner, J. (2014). Dkk-1 and IL-7 in plasma of patients with multiple myeloma prevent differentiation of mesenchymal stem cells into osteoblasts. *American Journal of Blood Research, 4*(2), 73–85.

Oranger, A., Carbone, C., Izzo, M., & Grano, M. (2013). Cellular mechanisms of multiple myeloma bone disease. *Clinical and Developmental Immunology, 2013,* Article ID 289458. doi:10.1155/2013/289458

Owen, J.A., Punt, J., & Stranford, S.A. (2013). *Kuby immunology* (7th ed.). New York, NY: W.H. Freeman.

Rajkumar, S.V. (2012). Multiple myeloma: 2012 update on diagnosis, risk-stratification, and management. *American Journal of Hematology, 87,* 78–88. doi:10.1002/ajh.22237

Rajkumar, S.V., Gupta, V., Fonseca, R., Dispenzieri, A., Gonsalves, W.I., Larson, D., ... Kumar, S.K. (2013). Impact of primary molecular cytogenetic abnormalities and risk of progression in smoldering multiple myeloma. *Leukemia, 27,* 1738–1744. doi:10.1038/leu.2013.86

Roodman, G.D. (2010). Pathogenesis of myeloma bone disease. *Journal of Cellular Biochemistry, 109,* 283–291. doi:10.1002/jcb.22403

Roodman, G.D. (2011). Osteoblast function in myeloma. *Bone, 48,* 135–140. doi:10.1016/j.bone.2010.06.016

Rosean, T.R., Tompkins, V.S., Tricot, G., Holman, C.J., Olivier, A.K., Zhan, F., & Janz, S. (2014). Preclinical validation of interleukin 6 as a therapeutic target in multiple myeloma. *Immunologic Research, 59,* 188–202. doi:10.1007/s12026-014-8528-x

Sawyer, J.R. (2011). The prognostic significance of cytogenetics and molecular profiling in multiple myeloma. *Cancer Genetics, 204,* 3–12. doi:10.1016/j.cancergencyto.2010.11.002

Schmiedel, B.J., Scheible, C.A., Nuebling, T., Kopp, H.G., Wirths, S., Azuma, M., ... Salih, H.R. (2013). RANKL expression, function, and therapeutic targeting in multiple myeloma and chronic lymphocytic leukemia. *Cancer Research, 73,* 683–694. doi:10.1158/0008-5472.CAN-12-2280

Sprynski, A.C., Hose, D., Caillot, L., Reme, T., Shaughnessy, J.D., Jr., Barlogie, B., ... Klein, B. (2009). The role of IGF-1 as a major growth factor for myeloma cell lines and the prognostic relevance of the expression of its receptor. *Blood, 113,* 4614–4626. doi:10.1182/blood-2008-07-170464

Tagoug, I., Jordheim, L.P., Herveau, S., Matera, E.L., Huber, A.L., Chettab, K., ... Dumontet, C. (2013). Therapeutic enhancement of ER stress by insulin-like growth factor I sensitizes myeloma cells to proteasomal inhibitors. *Clinical Cancer Research, 19,* 3556–3566. doi:10.1158/1078-0432.CCR-12-3134

Tai, Y.T., & Anderson, K.C. (2011). Antibody-based therapies in multiple myeloma. *Bone Marrow Research, 2011,* Article ID 924058. doi:10.1155/2011/924058

Tariman, J.D., & Faiman, B. (2011). Multiple myeloma. In C.H. Yarbro, D. Wujcik, & B.H. Gobel (Eds.), *Cancer nursing: Principles and practice* (7th ed., pp. 1513–1545). Burlington, MA: Jones & Bartlett Learning.

Terpos, E., Berenson, J., Raje, N., & Roodman, G.D. (2014). Management of bone disease in multiple myeloma. *Expert Review of Hematology, 7,* 113–125. doi:10.1586/17474086.2013.874943

Terpos, E., Szydlo, R., Apperley, J.F., Hatjiharissi, E., Politou, M., Meletis, J., ... Rahemtulla, A. (2003). Soluble receptor activator of nuclear factor kappaB ligand-osteoprotegerin ratio predicts survival in multiple myeloma: Proposal for a novel prognostic index. *Blood, 102,* 1064–1069. doi:10.1182/blood-2003-02-0380

Walker, B.A., Leone, P.E., Chiecchio, L., Dickens, N.J., Jenner, M.W., Boyd, K.D., ... Morgan, G.J. (2010). A compendium of myeloma-associated chromosomal copy number abnormalities and their prognostic value. *Blood, 116,* e56–e65. doi:10.1182/blood-2010-04-279596

Weitzmann, M.N., Roggia, C., Toraldo, G., Weitzmann, L., & Pacifici, R. (2002). Increased production of IL-7 uncouples bone formation from bone resorption during estrogen deficiency. *Journal of Clinical Investigation, 110,* 1643–1650. doi:10.1172/JCI15687

Yaccoby, S. (2010). Advances in the understanding of myeloma bone disease and tumour growth. *British Journal of Haematology, 149*, 311–321. doi:10.1111/j.1365-2141.2010.08141.x

Zhao, E., Xu, H., Wang, L., Kryczek, I., Wu, K., Hu, Y., ... Zou, W. (2012). Bone marrow and the control of immunity. *Cellular and Molecular Immunology, 9*, 11–19. doi:10.1038/cmi.2011.47

Zhou, G., & Levitsky, H.I. (2007). Natural regulatory T cells and de novo-induced regulatory T cells contribute independently to tumor-specific tolerance. *Journal of Immunology, 178*, 2155–2162. doi:10.4049/jimmunol.178.4.2155

CHAPTER 4

Epidemiology

Charise Gleason, MSN, NP-BC, AOCNP®

Introduction

Multiple myeloma is the second most common hematologic disorder in the United States, constituting approximately 1.4% of new cancer cases (National Cancer Institute, 2014). Great strides have been made in knowledge about the biology and therapeutics for myeloma. These advances are being applied to diagnosis and treatments and have resulted in improved overall survival for patients, yet little is known about the underlying causes. Multiple myeloma represents about 0.8% of all cancers worldwide, with about 114,000 new cases occurring annually (World Cancer Research Fund International, 2014). The number of newly diagnosed cases is highest in North America, Australia, New Zealand, Northern Europe, and Western Europe when compared to Asian countries. A modest increase in incidence and mortality from the disease has occurred in most regions of the world over the past two decades without an obvious explanation (National Cancer Institute, 2014; Parkin, Bray, Ferlay, & Pisani, 2005).

Etiology

The exact etiology of multiple myeloma is unknown, and unlike other types of cancer that have documented risk factors, myeloma has few known predisposing factors for its development. Known risk factors include increasing age, family history, personal history of monoclonal gammopathy of undetermined significance (MGUS), and African American race (National Cancer Institute, 2014). The factors that contribute to the evolution and prevalence of MGUS to multiple myeloma remain unclear (Gerkes, de Jong, Sijmons, & Vellenga, 2007; Lynch et al., 2008), but there is great interest in the role of genetic factors, race, environmental exposures, diet, immunologic function, and infection. Because MGUS is a well-known precursor, this chapter will provide a comprehensive review of the epidemiology of both MGUS and myeloma and the role of genetics, race, environmental factors, diet, immunology, and infection in the development of multiple myeloma.

Incidence

Cancer is the number-two cause of death in the United States with 589,430 deaths estimated for 2015 (approximately 1,600 deaths per day), and 11,240 of those attributable to myeloma (6,240 in men and 5,000 in women) (American Cancer Society, 2015a). Since 1975, myeloma incidence has increased by about 1% annually while mortality rates have declined. The estimated prevalence rate of myeloma in the United States was 89,658 in 2012 (Howlader et al., 2015). An estimated 26,850 new cases occurred in the United States in 2015, with 14,090 in men and 12,760 in women. The disease most commonly affects older adults, with the median age of diagnosis being 69 years; incidence rises exponentially with age (Howlader et al., 2015). In the United States, the lifetime risk of developing myeloma is 1 in 143 (0.7%), and less than 1% of cases are diagnosed before the age of 35 years (American Cancer Society, 2015b).

Incidence rates of myeloma in North America, Australia, New Zealand, and Europe are similar, with an increased incidence in men compared to women and a higher incidence in Blacks (Parkin, Whelan, Ferlay, Teppo, & Thomas, 2002). Within the United States, the incidence is greater in men than in women (7.7 per 100,000 versus 4.9 per 100,000). Among African American men, the myeloma incidence rate is double that of Caucasians (14.8 per 100,000 versus 7.2 per 100,000), whereas people of Asian origin living in the United States have lower rates (National Cancer Institute, 2014). Higher incidence is also observed in the Caribbean and South and Central African countries, which is consistent with the increased risk for myeloma seen in those of African descent (Parkin et al., 2005). Table 4-1 shows incidence by race per the National Cancer Institute's Surveillance, Epidemiology, and End Results (SEER) Program data. In large myeloma centers, half of the patients with monoclonal gammopathy have MGUS, whereas 15%–20% have multiple myeloma (Kyle et al., 2006).

Risk Factors

Risk factors for MGUS are similar to those for multiple myeloma, with age as a predominant factor. MGUS is present in more than 3% of the population older than age 50, with approximately 1% of patients with MGUS

Table 4-1. Incidence of Multiple Myeloma, 2014*

Race/Ethnicity	Male	Female
All races	7.7	4.9
White	7.2	4.3
Black	14.8	10.5
Asian/Pacific Islander	4.5	3.0
American Indian/Alaska Native	4.3	3.5
Hispanic	6.9	4.7
Non-Hispanic	7.8	4.9

*Number of new cases per 100,000 by race/ethnicity and sex, based on data from SEER 18 2007–2011, age-adjusted

Note. From *SEER Stat Fact Sheets: Multiple Myeloma*, by National Cancer Institute Surveillance, Epidemiology, and End Results Program, 2014. Retrieved from http://seer.cancer.gov/statfacts/html/mulmy.html.

progressing to myeloma each year. Because the rate of conversion from MGUS to myeloma does not increase with time, patients with MGUS will need to follow up with their healthcare provider indefinitely or refer to a myeloma center as needed (Kyle & Rajkumar, 2008; Kyle et al., 2002, 2006). In a large population-based study with 21,463 patients in Olmsted County, Minnesota, the prevalence of MGUS was 3.2% in people age 50 or older and 5.3% in residents age 70 or older (Kyle et al., 2002, 2006). It is not clear how many cases of myeloma are preceded by MGUS, as MGUS is not typically found on routine laboratory analysis and patients usually are asymptomatic. The diagnosis of MGUS frequently is a coincidental finding and for the most part is underdiagnosed in the typical clinical setting (Kyle et al., 2006). A study by Weiss, Abadie, Verma, Howard, and Kuehl (2009) looked at the proportion of patients with newly diagnosed myeloma who had preexisting plasma cell disorders (PPCDs). The authors found that myeloma had evolved from PPCD in 27 out of 30 patients (90%), and the researchers suspected that PPCD incidence is even higher. They concluded that nearly all multiple myeloma is preceded by MGUS (Weiss et al., 2009). The main risk factors for progression to a malignant condition are the presence of an abnormal serum free light-chain ratio, a serum monoclonal protein of at least 1.5 g/dl, and a monoclonal immunoglobulin (Ig) other than IgG (Kyle et al., 2006; Rajkumar et al., 2005). These risk factors help to classify which patients with MGUS are at greatest risk for progressing to myeloma. Again, while MGUS is a precursor to developing myeloma, the frequency remains low at around 1% per year (Greenberg, Vachon, & Rajkumar, 2012).

Family History and Genetics

Over the years, reports of myeloma occurring in the same family suggest a possible involvement of genetic factors in its development. Several studies have reported that first-degree relatives of patients with MGUS or myeloma are two to three times more likely to develop MGUS or myeloma than those without the family connection (Greenberg, Rajkumar, & Vachon, 2011; Greenberg et al., 2012; Landgren & Weiss, 2009). Landgren et al. (2006) conducted a large population-based study comparing familial characteristics of autoimmune and hematologic disorders in patients with myeloma. The results showed a threefold increased risk among patients with a history of pernicious anemia and an increased risk in participants who had a history of systemic lupus erythematosus. The researchers reported no significant increased risk among individuals with a first-degree relative with MGUS and an elevated risk among those with first-degree family history of myeloma. Ogmundsdottir et al. (2005) evaluated the occurrence of multiple myeloma in 218 Icelandic patients, noting that the risk for relatives of patients with myeloma developing MGUS was not increased, but there was a significant risk of developing myeloma for females separately and for males and females combined when looking at first-degree relatives of patients with myeloma.

Lynch et al. (2005) conducted a large observational study looking at 39 families with multiple cases of myeloma or related disorders. The authors concluded that a diagnosis of myeloma *does* carry a risk of myeloma to other family members: the odds ratio for myeloma and first-degree relative was 3.7. Their results reflected a lower age at diagnosis in successive generations. Interestingly, they reported on one family in which three siblings had the disease. A diagnosis of myeloma carries a familial risk for other types of cancers, particularly lymphoma and leukemia, as well as certain types of solid tumors (Bourguet, Grufferman, Delzell, Delong, & Cohen, 1985; Eriksson & Hallberg, 1992; Grosbois et al., 1999; Lynch et al., 2005, 2008).

A possible association exists between the human leukocyte antigens (HLAs) and incidence of myeloma. In an early study by Leech et al. (1983), researchers found an increased frequency of HLA-Cw2 allele and the incidence of myeloma in both Black and White men. The associated risk was 5.7 for Blacks and 2.6 for Whites. These studies suggest a possible genetic component, but other factors also play a role, and further studies are needed. To date, about 100 families are noted to have affected members with plasma cell dyscrasias, supporting evidence that there is an inherited link to development of myeloma (Koura & Langston, 2013).

Evidence has demonstrated an increased risk of myeloma in families with cases of breast cancer. *BRCA1* and *BRCA2* mutations among Ashkenazi Jewish patients and an increased risk of myeloma have been reported (Struewing et al., 1997). Sobol et al. (2002) noted that the *BRCA2* nonsense mutation, A10204T, might play a role in the development of a myeloma phenotype. In one family that has been prone to melanoma, a germ-line mutation of the *CDKN2A (p16)* gene was found in a family member who had myeloma. Additionally, researchers found that the wild-type *CDKN2A* allele was lost in malignant plasma cells, suggesting an increased susceptibility to multiple myeloma as well as a few other types of cancer (Dilworth et al., 2000).

Rand et al. (2013) reported the results of a recent meta-analysis of a genome-wide association study in individuals of European ancestry and confirmed the association between multiple myeloma risk and two previously published single-nucleotide polymorphisms (SNPs) (rs4487645, $p = 0.0007$ and rs105251, $p = 0.0044$) reported by Broderick et al. in 2012 and also identified a possible association with a new SNP in chromosome 12q23.1 (rs1345359). According to the investigators of this meta-analysis, this new SNP in chromosome 12q23.1 that is associated with multiple myeloma risk is not located in a gene nor associated with biofeatures in ENCODE. The investigators suggested that additional correlation studies are necessary to identify a functional SNP linked to this locus. Furthermore, a second SNP in chromosome 20q13.2 also requires further validation by conducting larger studies that would improve the discovery of a variant allele with statistically significant association with multiple myeloma disease.

Tewari et al. (2011) reported the results of the 8q24 locus and the risk of acquiring multiple myeloma as demonstrated in the Epilymph study and the Irish myeloma study. Genotyping was done on cancer-specific regions at the 8q24 locus and included rs13254738, rs16901979, rs13281615, rs6983267, rs7000448, and rs1447295. Data from each center were pooled, and their results suggested an association between variants of the 8q24 locus and myeloma, in particular in SNP rs16901979 and rs6983267. Greenberg et al. (2013) have made an association between rs1052501 and multiple myeloma as well as MGUS, but the association of progression from MGUS to multiple myeloma requires further study.

Ongoing studies on genetic variation continue and are very important in understanding the pathogenesis of the disease. Vangsted et al. (2012) investigated variations in the cytokine interleukin-1 beta (IL-1β) and nuclear factor–kappa-B (NF-κB) due to the change in inflammatory response. Their results noted that a genetically low IL-1β was associated with a lower risk of multiple myeloma. These results supported data from Haabeth et al. (2011) indicating an association between high IL-1β and a higher risk of multiple myeloma. Morgan et al. (2014) performed a meta-analysis of two genome-wide association studies that have identified a number of SNPs associated with multiple myeloma. The regions that are mostly associated with myeloma include SNPs at chromosomes 2p23.3, 3p22.1, 3q26.2, 6p21.33, 7p15.3, 17p11.2, and 22q13.1. These studies were performed in Europe but do provide evidence that common genetic variations have an impact on the risk of myeloma.

Race

Although hematopoietic neoplasms are more common in Caucasians, both MGUS and myeloma occur more frequently in African Americans, with the incidence of myeloma being twice as high in African American patients when compared to their Caucasian counterparts (Howlader et al., 2014; Jain, Ascensao, & Schechter, 2009). Most recently, Landgren et al. (2014) looked at the risk of MGUS among African Americans and Caucasians in a large population-based study of 12,482 individuals from the National Health and Nutritional Examination Survey, noting MGUS to be more prevalent in African Americans (3.7%) compared to Caucasians (2.3%) (p = 0.001), and MGUS in African Americans has more features associated with higher risk of progression to multiple myeloma. Moreover, there was a strong geographic disparity in MGUS prevalence between North and Midwest and Southeast and West regions of the United States, which has etiologic implications in terms of the role of environmental factors (Landgren et al., 2014). The authors of the study have long been advocating that the focus of future studies be shifted to examining risk factors for MGUS to better understand the etiology of myeloma (Landgren et al., 2006). Although many accounts exist of familial history of myeloma, most studies have been done with Caucasian families.

Lynch et al. (2008) reported on an African American family that had five cases of multiple myeloma, three cases of MGUS, and five cases of prostate cancer in two generations. In Ghana, the prevalence of MGUS in Black men was twice as high as in White men, supporting the hypothesis that race-related genetic susceptibility might explain the higher rate of MGUS among Blacks (Landgren et al., 2007). In a large population-based study that examined disparities in myeloma incidence by race, researchers noted that Blacks had a four-year earlier onset of disease than their White counterparts, and that over the study period, disease-specific survival was greater for Blacks than Whites (Waxman et al., 2010). The study also noted that survival improvement was less pronounced in the Black population. The authors noted that molecular studies are needed by race, but their findings were consistent with a genetic basis for the development of myeloma (Waxman et al., 2010).

Jain et al. (2009) reported on eight African American families with familial myeloma and MGUS over a 30-year period, which is one of the largest studies to date focusing on the African American population. The eight families were identified over three decades in a medical center whose clinic population was greater than 75% African American. They reported that out of eight families, 20 of 58 (35%) first-degree relatives had plasma cell dyscrasias, including 12 cases of myeloma, 8 cases of MGUS, and 1 case of amyloidosis. In this particular study, the median age at diagnosis for patients with myeloma was 61 years. Some other factors thought to explain the increased risk of MGUS and myeloma in African American patients include environmental factors, diet, tobacco and alcohol use, and socioeconomic factors (Benjamin, Reddy, & Brawley, 2003), although Landgren et al. (2010) noted that the increased risk of MGUS in this population is not explained by differences in socioeconomic factors.

Environmental Factors

It is not unusual for patients to ask what caused their myeloma and whether their occupation or lifestyle choices could be factors. Known suspected risk factors include ionizing radiation and farming and agricultural exposures along with other occupational exposures, including organic solvents and pesticides. Alexander et al. (2007) performed an extensive epidemiologic literature review and noted the small numbers of cases in occupational cohort studies and a lack of statistical power and appearance of bias due to differential recall of exposures between the cases and controls. Although exposures to organic solvents, pesticides, and other chemicals have been studied, results continue to be varied and inconsistent (Alexander et al., 2007; Bergsagel et al., 1999).

Ionizing Radiation

Ichimaru, Ishimaru, Mikami, and Matsunaga (1982) evaluated the relationship between ionizing radiation associated with exposure to an atomic bomb and the incidence of myeloma in a fixed cohort of survivors of the bombings at Hiroshima and Nagasaki and found an increased risk of myeloma. The analysis showed that the standardized relative risk adjusted for city, sex, and age at the time of the bombings increased with marrow-absorbed radiation dose. Furthermore, the researchers noted that the effect of radiation did not become apparent in individuals receiving 50 rad or more until 20 years or more after exposure. In a more recent study looking at the incidence of MGUS and myeloma in atomic bomb survivors, transformation from MGUS to myeloma occurred in 16% of unexposed patients, 17% in dose-unknown patients, and 26% in exposed patients, suggesting that exposure to the radiation accelerated the transformation of MGUS to myeloma (Alexander et al., 2007; Neriishi, Nakashima, & Suzuki, 2003). However, Preston et al. (1994) analyzed the incidence of myeloma after exposure to the atomic bomb through 1987 and found no increased risk.

Occupational Risk Factors

Farmers and agricultural workers have been exposed, for years, to potentially hazardous substances, including pesticides and other chemicals, but they typically have a lower cancer mortality rate when compared to the general population. In a meta-analysis from various epidemiologic studies of agricultural workers published between 1992 and 1998 (Acquavella et al., 1998; Blair, Zahm, Pearce, Heineman, & Fraumeni, 1992; Khuder & Mutgi, 1997), results suggested that the risk of myeloma among farmers is similar to that of the general population. Kachuri et al. (2013) studied pesticide exposure in Canadian men linking the use of carbamate pesticides to a twofold risk of myeloma. A more recent multicenter collaborative study of lifetime occupation and risk of myeloma suggested an increased risk in farmers, cleaning workers, and those with prolonged exposures to pesticides, but additional studies need to be explored (Perrotta et al., 2013).

Pesticides have also been widely examined to evaluate the risk of myeloma based on exposures by agricultural workers and licensed pesticide applicators. An extensive review of the literature by Alexander et al. (2007) revealed inconsistent results, with some studies suggesting a positive correlation and other studies finding no relationship (Blair, Sandler, et al., 2005; Freeman et al., 2005; Rusiecki et al., 2004; Semenciw et al., 1993). In one study, the risk of cancer was low overall, and researchers hypothesized that the cancer rates seemed to be a result of low rates of smoking and other positive lifestyle factors (Lee et al., 2004). Exposure to organic solvents does not appear to be a risk factor for myeloma. Although exposure to high levels of benzene places a person at higher risk for developing acute myeloid leukemia, no evidence exists to support increased risk for developing myeloma (Bertazzi et al., 2001). Gold et al. (2011) looked at evidence from a large case-control study regarding the relationship between six chlorinated solvents and myeloma and found an association between certain chlorinated solvents and increased myeloma risk. The study was limited by relatively low participation.

Approximately three million Americans in the U.S. military who were deployed to Vietnam in the 1960s and early 1970s were exposed to large amounts of defoliant mixtures known as Agent Orange (named as such because of the orange stripe on the container). About 19 million gallons of a 50:50 mixture of two phenoxy herbicides were used on approximately 3.6 million acres in Vietnam and Laos (Frumkin, 2003). Many studies have been done on the relationship between Agent Orange and the development of hematologic malignancies, and the U.S. Department of Veterans Affairs (2014) has presumptively recognized the association of Agent Orange and myeloma as a service connection but also notes that evidence of an association is limited. The study results have yielded limited information on the link of Agent Orange to cancer. Moreover, results have been sparse and inconclusive, but myeloma has been labeled as a cancer with limited evidence of association to Agent Orange (American Cancer Society, 2014; Frumkin, 2003).

Researchers have also studied the relationship between myeloma and personal or occupational exposure to hair coloring and dyes. An increase in the incidence of disease in a small fraction of hair dye users, particularly those using black dye, has been reported, but researchers found no significant exposure to response based on the duration for all hair colors combined (Herrinton et al., 1994; Takkouche, Etminan, & Montes-Martinez, 2005; Thun et al., 1994). Using hair colors that do not contain carcinogens and that have appropriate product warnings helps consumers to reduce their risk. In other environmental studies among rubber workers and people in wood-related occupations (Alder et al., 2006; Demers et al., 1995; Greenberg et al., 2001), results have been inconsistent. Occupational exposure to certain chemicals, solvents, or pesticides may contribute to the development of myeloma, but the evidence remains inconclusive.

Socioeconomic Status and Lifestyle Factors

Baris et al. (2000) evaluated the impact of socioeconomic status (SES) and the incidence of multiple myeloma and observed an inverse correlation between occupation-based SES and the risk for myeloma in both Black and White individuals. Their study found that low occupation-based SES accounted for 37% of myeloma cases in Blacks but only 17% in Whites because of the higher percentage of Black (62.9%) compared to White (34.7%) controls. It remains unclear whether low SES-related factors, such as poor housing, jobs with exposure to occupational carcinogens, unemployment, poor nutrition, and lack of health care, contribute to a higher incidence (Gorey & Vena, 1994). The authors also noted no relationship to lifestyle factors such as tobacco or alcohol use. In a more recent meta-analysis, Rota et al. (2014) concluded that no association exists between alcohol use and myeloma, although interestingly, the dose-risk meta-regression analysis reported a modest decrease in myeloma risk with moderate to heavy alcohol consumption. Further studies are warranted.

Epidemiologists have investigated the correlation between diet and multiple myeloma. Tavani et al. (2000) examined the relationship between red meat consumption and cancer development. Although red meat intake has been associated with digestive tract cancers, it seems to have no relationship to myeloma. In a very large case-control study by Fritschi, Ambrosini, Kliewer, and Johnson (2004), the authors reported that an increase in proportions of total energy and fat from fresh fish seems to protect against the development of hematologic malignancies, including myeloma. Other foods such as grains, meats, vegetables, and dairy products have shown mixed results with no significant increased risk of developing myeloma (Brown et al., 2001; Chatenoud et al., 1998; Negri, La Vecchia, Franceschi, D'Avanzo, & Parazzini, 1991; Tavani et al., 1997, 2000).

Several studies have identified a relationship between obesity and myeloma or MGUS (Landgren et al., 2010; Lichtman, 2010; Samanic, Gridley, Chow, Lubin, & Hoover, 2004). Brown et al. (2001) reported an association between increased obesity trends that may contribute to the incidence of myeloma in both Blacks and Whites. A large Canadian study conducted over eight provinces found an increased risk in both men and women who were obese, but smoking and alcohol use did not modify this association (Pan, Johnson, Ugnat, Wen, & Mao, 2004). The authors noted that the mechanism for the link was unclear and hypothesized that it could be related to a decreased immune response. In an earlier study by Friedman and Herrinton (1994), researchers found the same association between myeloma and obesity, but only in White males.

At the time of this writing, Hwang et al. (2013) are enrolling African American patients with active multiple myeloma to a multicenter collaborative study investigating possible explanations as to why the incidence of myeloma is higher in African American populations. They are looking at active cases of myeloma and whether body mass index (BMI) is associated with risk factors at presentation. Obesity is a well-known risk factor for many cancers, and prior studies have focused on individuals of European descent. To date, 1,044 patients have been enrolled in the study, with 1,014 samples of DNA collected. Patients are asked to fill out a questionnaire that includes information on height and weight at 20 years of age and at five years prior to diagnosis. The results to date suggest an association between increased BMI at age 20 and younger age at multiple myeloma diagnosis. Obesity at a younger age may influence multiple myeloma risk through pathways like IL-6 and insulin-like growth factor, which may contribute to B-cell activation. The study is still recruiting patients, and more data are needed.

Immunologic Factors

Interest exists in exploring the relationship between chronic or recurrent infections and the development of myeloma. Case studies to identify the associations of infections and autoimmune disorders have failed to demonstrate consistent findings, and relationships have been nonspecific (Brown, Gridley, Check, & Landgren, 2008; Goldin & Landgren, 2009; Gramenzi et al., 1991). Research has not shown links between chronic or acute immune stimulation and myeloma, nor between myeloma and certain immunizations, such as those for influenza, polio, smallpox, and tetanus (Alexander et al., 2007; Gramenzi et al., 1991; Lewis et al., 1994).

Several studies have linked AIDS with an increased incidence of MGUS and myeloma, especially in the older adult population. Several studies have shown an increased risk in those living with AIDS (Biggar, Kirby, Atkinson, McNeel, & Engels, 2004; Dezube, Aboulafia, & Pantanowitz, 2004; Frisch, Biggar, Engels, & Goedert, 2001; Grulich et al., 2002). An Australian study found a significantly elevated risk of cancers including myeloma in an Australian cohort of people with AIDS (Grulich, Wan, Law, Coates, & Kaldor, 1999), and a U.S. and Puerto Rican AIDS registry study reported an increased incidence of MGUS, multiple myeloma, and other malignancies following the diagnosis of AIDS (Goedert et al., 1998). It is hypothesized that both the HIV infection and immune dysregulation may lead to a higher prevalence of MGUS in patients with HIV, but the role of HIV infection in the progression of MGUS to myeloma is not clearly understood (Konstantinopoulos, Pantanowitz, & Dezube, 2006).

Conclusion

More than 26,000 new cases of myeloma are expected to be diagnosed in the United States in 2015, and the main identified risk factors include age, sex, race, family history, and personal history of MGUS. The incidence is higher in men and twice as high in African Americans. Unlike other cancers, few predisposing risk factors are known. The etiology remains unknown; hence, no type of screening tool is available, as is the case with other cancers. A positive link has been made to ionizing radiation exposure at higher doses, and some questionable links have been made to environmental factors such as pesticide exposure and occupational hazards. Vietnam veterans who were exposed to Agent Orange have a suggestive association, and per the Department of Veterans Affairs, a presumptive service connection has been made.

The role of genetics is still undefined in myeloma, but several studies have reported an increased risk of developing myeloma when there is a positive family history, such as a first-degree relative. There are known cases of myeloma occurring in the same family over several generations. Race plays a factor in the incidence of MGUS and multiple myeloma, with higher rates occurring in African Americans. MGUS is linked to the subsequent development of myeloma, with higher risk factors including the association of an abnormal free light-chain ratio and a higher level of monoclonal protein at the time of MGUS diagnosis.

Obesity, diet, and exercise may be contributing factors, as well as poor SES, but studies are inconclusive, and these are more likely related to a factor that has yet to be discovered. The final analysis of the association of early-onset multiple myeloma in African Americans who were obese before the age of 20 is an important finding to explore further and currently is the most consistently reported. An increased risk among people with AIDS has been noted, especially as this population ages. As the general population ages, the risk of developing myeloma will continue to rise. Although a wealth of progress has taken place regarding both the biology and treatment of multiple myeloma, continued studies are needed to further understand the disease and associated risk factors. More research efforts are now being devoted to the study of MGUS in African Americans, which could potentially provide more scientific underpinnings on the biologic causes of multiple myeloma.

References

Acquavella, J., Olsen, G., Cole, P., Ireland, B., Kaneene, J., Schuman, S., & Holden, L. (1998). Cancer among farmers: A meta-analysis. *Annals of Epidemiology, 8,* 64–74. doi:10.1016/S1047-2797(97)00120-8

Alder, N., Fenty, J., Warren, F., Sutton, A.J., Rushton, L., Jones, D.R., & Abrams, K.R. (2006). Meta-analysis of mortality and cancer incidence among workers in the synthetic rubber-producing industry. *American Journal of Epidemiology, 164,* 405–420. doi:10.1093/aje/kwj252

Alexander, D.D., Mink, P.J., Adami, H.O., Cole, P., Mandel, J.S., Oken, M.M., & Trichopoulos, D. (2007). Multiple myeloma: A review of the epidemiologic literature. *International Journal of Cancer, 120*(Suppl. 12), 40–61. doi:10.1002/ijc.22718

American Cancer Society. (2014). Agent orange and cancer. Retrieved from http://www.cancer.org/cancer/cancercauses/othercarcinogens/intheworkplace/agent-orange-and-cancer

American Cancer Society. (2015a). *Cancer facts and figures 2015.* Retrieved from http://www.cancer.org/research/cancerfactsstatistics/index

American Cancer Society. (2015b). Multiple myeloma [Detailed guide]. Retrieved from Retrieved from http://www.cancer.org/cancer/multiplemyeloma/detailedguide/index

Baris, D., Brown, L.M., Silverman, D.T., Hayes, R., Hoover, R.N., Swanson, G.M., ... Fraumeni, J.F., Jr. (2000). Socioeconomic status and multiple myeloma among US blacks and whites. *American Journal of Public Health, 90,* 1277–1281. doi:10.2105/AJPH.90.8.1277

Benjamin, M., Reddy, S., & Brawley, O.W. (2003). Myeloma and race: A review of the literature. *Cancer and Metastasis Reviews, 22,* 87–93. doi:10.1023/A:1022268103136

Bergsagel, D.E., Wong, O., Bergsagel, P.L., Alexanian, R., Anderson, K., Kyle, R.A., & Raabe, G.K. (1999). Benzene and multiple myeloma: Appraisal of the scientific evidence. *Blood, 94,* 1174–1182.

Bertazzi, P.A., Consonni, D., Bachetti, S., Rubagotti, M., Baccarelli, A., Zocchetti, C., & Pesatori, A.C. (2001). Health effects of dioxin exposure: A 20-year mortality study. *American Journal of Epidemiology, 153,* 1031–1044. doi:10.1093/aje/153.11.1031

Biggar, R.J., Kirby, K.A., Atkinson, J., McNeel, T.S., & Engels, E. (2004). Cancer risk in elderly persons with HIV/AIDS. *Journal of Acquired Immune Deficiency Syndromes, 36,* 861–868. doi:10.1097/00126334-200407010-00014

Blair, A., Sandler, D.P., Tarone, R., Lubin, J., Thomas, K., Hoppin, J.A., ... Alavanja, M.C.R. (2005). Mortality among participants in the Agricultural Health Study. *Annals of Epidemiology, 15,* 279–285. doi:10.1016/j.annepidem.2004.08.008

Blair, A., Zahm, S.H., Pearce, N.E., Heineman, E.F., & Fraumeni, J.F., Jr. (1992). Clues to cancer etiology from studies of farmers. *Scandinavian Journal of Work, Environment and Health, 18,* 209–215. doi:10.5271/sjweh.1578

Bourguet, C.C., Grufferman, S., Delzell, E., Delong, E.R., & Cohen, H.J. (1985). Multiple myeloma and family history of cancer: A case-control study. *Cancer, 56,* 2133–2139. doi:10.1002/1097-0142(19851015)56:8<2133::AID-CNCR2820560842>3.0.CO;2-F

Broderick, P., Chubb, D., Johnson, D.C., Weinhold, N., Forsti, A., Lloyd, A., ... Houlston, R.S. (2012). Common variation at 3p22.1 and 7p15.3 influences multiple myeloma risk. *Nature Genetics, 44,* 58–61. doi:10.1038/ng.993

Brown, L.M., Gridley, G., Check, D., & Landgren, O. (2008). Risk of multiple myeloma and monoclonal gammopathy of undetermined significance among white and black male United States veterans with prior autoimmune, infectious, and allergic disorders. *Blood, 111,* 3388–3394. doi:10.1182/blood-2007-10-121285

Brown, L.M., Gridley, G., Pottern, L.M., Baris, D., Swanson, C.A., Silverman, D.T., ... Fraumeni, J.F. (2001). Diet and nutrition as risk factors for multiple myeloma among blacks and whites in the United States. *Cancer Causes and Control, 12,* 117–125. doi:10.1023/A:1008937901586

Chatenoud, L., Tavani, A., La Vecchia, C., Jacobs, D.R., Jr., Negri, E., Levi, F., & Franceschi, S. (1998). Whole grain food intake and cancer risk. *International Journal of Cancer, 77,* 24–28. doi:10.1002/(SICI)1097-0215(19980703)77:1<24::AID-IJC5>3.0.CO;2-1

Demers, P.A., Boffetta, P., Kogevinas, M., Blair, A., Miller, B.A., Robinson, C.F., ... Vainio, H. (1995). Pooled re-analysis of cancer mortality among five cohorts of workers in wood-related industries. *Scandinavian Journal of Work, Environment and Health, 21,* 179–190. doi:10.5271/sjweh.26

Dezube, B.J., Aboulafia, D.M., & Pantanowitz, L. (2004). Plasma cell disorders in HIV-infected patients: From benign gammopathy to multiple myeloma. *AIDS Reader, 14,* 372–374.

Dilworth, D., Liu, L., Stewart, A.K., Berenson, J.R., Lassam, N., & Hogg, D. (2000). Germline CDKN2A mutation implicated in predisposition to multiple myeloma. *Blood, 95,* 1869–1871.

Eriksson, M., & Hallberg, B. (1992). Familial occurrence of hematologic malignancies and other diseases in multiple myeloma: A case-control study. *Cancer Causes and Control, 3,* 63–67. doi:10.1007/BF00051914

Freeman, L.E.B., Bonner, M.R., Blair, A., Hoppin, J.A., Sandler, D.P., Lubin, J.H., ... Alavanja, M.C.R. (2005). Cancer incidence among male pesticide applicators in the Agricultural Health Study cohort exposed to diazinon. *American Journal of Epidemiology, 162,* 1070–1079. doi:10.1093/aje/kwi321

Friedman, G.D., & Herrinton, L.J. (1994). Obesity and multiple myeloma. *Cancer Causes and Control, 5,* 479–483. doi:10.1007/BF01694762

Frisch, M., Biggar, R.J., Engels, E.A., & Goedert, J.J. (2001). Association of cancer with AIDS-related immunosuppression in adults. *JAMA, 285,* 1736–1745. doi:10.1001/jama.285.13.1736

Fritschi, L., Ambrosini, G.L., Kliewer, E.V., & Johnson, K.C. (2004). Dietary fish intake and risk of leukaemia, multiple myeloma, and non-Hodgkin lymphoma. *Cancer Epidemiology, Biomarkers and Prevention, 13,* 532–537.

Frumkin, H. (2003). Agent orange and cancer: An overview for clinicians. *CA: A Cancer Journal for Clinicians, 53,* 245–255. doi:10.3322/canjclin.53.4.245

Gerkes, E.H., de Jong, M.M., Sijmons, R.H., & Vellenga, E. (2007). Familial multiple myeloma: Report on two families and discussion of screening options. *Hereditary Cancer in Clinical Practice, 5,* 72–78. doi:10.1186/1897-4287-5-2-72

Goedert, J.J., Coté, T.R., Virgo, P., Scoppa, S.M., Kingma, D.W., Gail, M.H., ... Biggar, R.J. (1998). Spectrum of AIDS-associated malignant disorders. *Lancet, 351,* 1833–1839. doi:10.1016/S0140-6736(97)09028-4

Gold, L.S., Stewart, P.A., Milliken, K., Purdue, M., Severson, R., Seixas, N., ... De Roos, A.J. (2011). The relationship between multiple myeloma and occupational exposure to six chlorinated solvents. *Occupational and Environmental Medicine, 68,* 391–399. doi:10.1136/oem.2009.054809

Goldin, L.R., & Landgren, O. (2009). Autoimmunity and lymphomagenesis. *International Journal of Cancer, 124,* 1497–1502. doi:10.1002/ijc.24141

Gorey, K.M., & Vena, J.E. (1994). Cancer differentials among US blacks and whites: Quantitative estimates of socioeconomic-related risks. *Journal of the National Medical Association, 86,* 209–215.

Gramenzi, A., Buttino, I., D'Avanzo, B., Negri, E., Franceschi, S., & La Vecchia, C. (1991). Medical history and the risk of multiple myeloma. *British Journal of Haematology, 63,* 769–772.

Greenberg, A.J., Lee, A.M., Serie, D.J., McDonnell, S.K., Cerhan, J.R., Liebow, M., ... Vachon, C.M. (2013). Single nucleotide polymorphism rs1052501 associated with monoclonal gammopathy of undetermined significance and multiple myeloma. *Leukemia, 27,* 515–516. doi:10.1038/leu.2012.232

Greenberg, A.J., Rajkumar, S.V., & Vachon, C.M. (2011). Familial monoclonal gammopathy of undetermined significance and multiple myeloma: Epidemiology, risk factors, and biological characteristics. *Blood, 119,* 5359–5366. doi:10.1182/blood-2011-11-387324

Greenberg, A.J., Vachon, C.M., & Rajkumar, S.V. (2012). Disparities in the prevalence, pathogenesis and progression of monoclonal gammopathy of undetermined significance and multiple myeloma between blacks and whites. *Leukemia, 26,* 609–614. doi:10.1038/leu.2011.368

Greenberg, R.S., Mandel, J.S., Pastides, H., Britton, N.L., Rudenko, L., & Starr, T.B. (2001). A meta-analysis of cohort studies describing mortality and cancer incidence among chemical workers in the United States and Western Europe. *Epidemiology, 12,* 727–740. doi:10.1097/00001648-200111000-00023

Grosbois, B., Jego, P., Attal, M., Payen, C., Rapp, M.J., Fuzibet, J.G., ... Bataille, R. (1999). Familial multiple myeloma: Report of fifteen families. *British Journal of Haematology, 105,* 768–770. doi:10.1046/j.1365-2141.1999.01415.x

Grulich, A.E., Li, Y., McDonald, A., Correll, P.K.L., Law, M.G., & Kaldor, J.M. (2002). Rates of non-AIDS-defining cancers in people with HIV infection before and after AIDS diagnosis. *AIDS, 16,* 1155–1161. doi:10.1097/00002030-200205240-00009

Grulich, A.E., Wan, X., Law, M.G., Coates, M., & Kaldor, J.M. (1999). Risk of cancer in people with AIDS. *AIDS, 13,* 839–843. doi:10.1097/00002030-199905070-00014

Haabeth, O.A.W., Lorvik, K.B., Hammarstrom, C., Donaldson, I.M., Haroldson, G., Bogen, B., & Corthay, A. (2011). Inflammation driven by tumour-specific Th1 cells protects against B-cell cancer. *Nature Communications, 2,* 240. doi:10.1038/ncomms1239

Herrinton, L.J., Weiss, N.S., Koepsell, T.D., Daling, J.R., Taylor, J.W., Lyon, J.L., ... Greenberg, R.S. (1994). Exposure to hair-coloring products and the risk of multiple myeloma. *American Journal of Public Health, 84,* 1142–1144. doi:10.2105/AJPH.84.7.1142

Howlader, N., Noone, A.M., Krapcho, M., Garshell, J., Miller, D., Altekruse, S.F., ... Cronin, K.A. (Eds.). (2015). SEER cancer statistics review, 1975–2012. Retrieved from http://seer.cancer.gov/csr/1975_2012

Hwang, A.E., Ailawadhi, S., Bernal-Mizrachi, L., Zimmerman, T.M., Haiman, C., Van Den Berg, D.J., ... Cozen, W. (2013). Obesity in young adulthood is associated with early onset multiple myeloma in African Americans [Abstract No. 1872]. *Blood, 122.*

Ichimaru, M., Ishimaru, T., Mikami, M., & Matsunaga, M. (1982). Multiple myeloma among atomic bomb survivors in Hiroshima and Nagasaki, 1950–1976: Relationship to radiation dose absorbed by marrow. *Journal of the National Cancer Institute, 69,* 323–328.

Jain, M., Ascensao, J., & Schechter, G.P. (2009). Familial myeloma and monoclonal gammopathy: A report of eight African American families. *American Journal of Hematology, 84,* 34–38. doi:10.1002/ajh.21325

Kachuri, L., Demers, P.A., Blair, A., Spinelli, J.J., Pahwa, M., McLaughlin, J.R., ... Harris, S.A. (2013). Multiple pesticide exposures and the risk of multiple myeloma in Canadian men. *International Journal of Cancer, 133,* 1846–1858. doi:10.1002/ijc.28191

Khuder, S.A., & Mutgi, A.B. (1997). Meta-analyses of multiple myeloma and farming. *American Journal of Industrial Medicine, 32,* 510–516. doi:10.1002/(SICI)1097-0274(199711)32:5<510::AID-AJIM11>3.0.CO;2-5

Konstantinopoulos, P.A., Pantanowitz, L., & Dezube, B.J. (2006). Higher prevalence of monoclonal gammopathy of undetermined significance in African Americans than whites—The unknown role of underlying HIV infection. *Journal of the National Medical Association, 98,* 1860–1861.

Koura, D.T., & Langston, A.A. (2013). Inherited predisposition to multiple myeloma. *Therapeutic Advances in Hematology, 4,* 291–297. doi:10.1177/2040620713485375

Kyle, R.A., & Rajkumar, S.V. (2008). Multiple myeloma. *Blood, 111,* 2962–2972. doi:10.1182/blood-2007-10-078022

Kyle, R.A., Therneau, T.M., Rajkumar, S.V., Larson, D.R., Plevak, M.F., Offord, J.R., ... Melton, J., III. (2006). Prevalence of monoclonal gammopathy of undetermined significance. *New England Journal of Medicine, 354,* 1362–1369. doi:10.1056/NEJMoa054494

Kyle, R.A., Therneau, T.M., Rajkumar, S.V., Offord, J.R., Larson, D.R., Plevak, M.F., & Melton, L.J., III. (2002). A long-term study of prognosis in monoclonal gammopathy of undetermined significance. *New England Journal of Medicine, 346,* 564–569. doi:10.1056/NEJMoa01133202

Landgren, O., Graubard, B.I., Katzmann, J.A., Kyle, R.A., Ahmadizadeh, I., Clark, R., ... Rajkumar, S.V. (2014). Racial disparities in the prevalence of monoclonal gammopathies: A population-based study of 12,482 persons from the National Health and Nutritional Examination Survey. *Leukemia, 28,* 1537–1542. doi:10.1038/leu.2014.34

Landgren, O., Gridley, G., Turesson, I., Caporaso, N.E., Goldin, L.R., Baris, D., ... Linet, M.S. (2006). Risk of monoclonal gammopathy of undetermined significance (MGUS) and subsequent multiple myeloma among African American and white veterans in the United States. *Blood, 107,* 904–906. doi:10.1182/blood-2005-08-3449

Landgren, O., Katzmann, J.A., Hsing, A.W., Pfeiffer, R.M., Kyle, R.A., Yeboah, E.D., ... Rajkumar, S.V. (2007). Prevalence of monoclonal gammopathy of undetermined significance among men in Ghana. *Mayo Clinic Proceedings, 82,* 1468–1473. doi:10.1016/S0025-6196(11)61089-6

Landgren, O., Rajkumar, V., Pfeiffer, R.M., Kyle, R.A., Katzmann, J.A., Dispenzieri, A., ... Signorello, L.B. (2010). Obesity is associated with an increased risk of monoclonal gammopathy of undetermined significance among black and white women. *Blood, 116,* 1056–1059. doi:10.1182/blood-2010-01-262394

Landgren, O., & Weiss, B.M. (2009). Patterns of monoclonal gammopathy of undetermined significance and multiple myeloma in various ethnic/racial groups: Support for genetic factors in pathogenesis. *Leukemia, 23,* 1691–1697. doi:10.1038/leu.2009.123

Lee, W.J., Hoppin, J.A., Blair, A., Lubin, J.H., Dosemeci, M., Sandler, D.P., & Alavanja, M.C.R. (2004). Cancer incidence among pesticide applicators exposed to alachlor in the Agricultural Health Study. *American Journal of Epidemiology, 159,* 373–380. doi:10.1093/aje/kwh040

Leech, S.H., Bryan, C.F., Elston, R.C., Rainey, J., Bickers, J.N., & Pelias, M.Z. (1983). Genetic studies in multiple myeloma: Association with HLA-Cw5. *Cancer, 51,* 1408–1411. doi:10.1002/1097-0142(19830415)51:8<1408::AID-CNCR2820510814>3.0.CO;2-7

Lewis, D.R., Pottern, L.M., Brown, L.L.M., Silverman, D.T., Hayes, R.B., Schoenberg, J.B., ... Hoover, R.N. (1994). Multiple myeloma among Blacks and Whites in the United States: The role of chronic antigenic stimulation. *Cancer Causes and Control, 5,* 529–539. doi:10.1007/BF01831381

Lichtman, M.A. (2010). Obesity and the risk for a hematological malignancy: Leukemia, lymphoma, or myeloma. *Oncologist, 15,* 1083–1101. doi:10.1634/theoncologist.2010-0206

Lynch, H.T., Ferrara, K., Barlogie, B., Coleman, E.A., Lynch, J.F., Weisenburger, D., ... Thome, S. (2008). Familial myeloma. *New England Journal of Medicine, 359,* 152–157. doi:10.1056/NEJMoa0708704

Lynch, H.T., Watson, P., Tarantolo, S., Wiernik, P.H., Quinn-Laquer, B., Bergsagel, K.I., ... Weisenburger, D. (2005). Phenotypic heterogeneity in multiple myeloma families. *Journal of Clinical Oncology, 23,* 685–693. doi:10.1200/JCO.2005.10.126

Morgan, G.J., Johnson, D.C., Weinhold, N., Goldschmidt, H., Landgren, O., Lynch, H.T., ... Houlston, R.S. (2014). Inherited genetic susceptibility to multiple myeloma. *Leukemia, 28,* 518–524. doi:10.1038/leu.2013.344

National Cancer Institute. (2014). A snapshot of multiple myeloma. Retrieved from http://www.cancer.gov/researchandfunding/snapshots/myeloma

Negri, E., La Vecchia, C., Franceschi, S., D'Avanzo, B., & Parazzini, F. (1991). Vegetable and fruit consumption and cancer risk. *International Journal of Cancer, 48,* 350–354. doi:10.1002/ijc.2910480307

Neriishi, K., Nakashima, E., & Suzuki, G. (2003). Monoclonal gammopathy of undetermined significance in atomic bomb survivors: Incidence and transformation to multiple myeloma. *British Journal of Haematology, 121,* 405–410. doi:10.1046/j.1365-2141.2003.04287.x

Ogmundsdottir, H.M., Haraldsdottirm, V., Johannesson, G.M., Olafsdottir, G., Bjarnadottir, K., Sigvaldason, H., & Tulinius, H. (2005). Familiality of benign and malignant paraproteinemias. A population-based cancer-registry study of multiple myeloma families. *Haematologica, 90,* 66–71.

Pan, S.Y., Johnson, K.C., Ugnat, A.M., Wen, S.W., & Mao, Y. (2004). Association of obesity and cancer risk in Canada. *American Journal of Epidemiology, 159,* 259–268. doi:10.1093/aje/kwh041

Parkin, D.M., Bray, F., Ferlay, J., & Pisani, P. (2005). Global cancer statistics, 2002. *CA: A Cancer Journal for Clinicians, 55,* 74–108. doi:10.3322/canjclin.55.2.74

Parkin, D.M., Whelan, S.L., Ferlay, J., Teppo, L., & Thomas, D.B. (2002). Cancer in five continents. *IARC Scientific Publications, VIII*(155), 1–781.

Perrotta, C., Kleefeld, S., Staines, A., Tewari, P., De Roos, A.J., Baris, D., ... Cocco, P. (2013). Multiple myeloma and occupation: A pooled analysis by the International Multiple Myeloma Consortium. *Cancer Epidemiology, 37,* 300–305. doi:10.1016/j.canep.2013.01.008

Preston, D.L., Kusumi, S., Tomonaga, M., Izumi, S., Ron, E., Kuramoto, A., ... Mabuchi, K. (1994). Cancer incidence in atomic bomb survivors. Part III. Leukemia, lymphoma, and multiple myeloma, 1950–1987. *Radiation Research, 137*(Suppl. 2), S68–S97. doi:10.2307/3578893

Rajkumar, S.V., Kyle, R.A., Therneau, T.M., Melton, L.J., III, Bradwell, A.R., Clark, R.J., ... Katzmann, J.A. (2005). Serum free light chain ratio is an independent risk factor for progression in monoclonal gammopathy of undetermined significance. *Blood, 106,* 812–817. doi:10.1182/blood-2005-03-1038

Rand, K.A., Camp, N., Martino, A., Dean, E.W., Serie, D.J., Edlund, C.K., ... Cozen, W. (2013). A meta-analysis of genome-wide association studies of multiple myeloma in cases and controls of European origin identifies a risk locus in 12q23.1 [Abstract No. 3111]. *Blood, 122.*

Rota, M., Porta, L., Pelucchi, C., Negri, E., Bagnardi, V., Bellocco, R., ... La Vecchia, C. (2014). Alcohol drinking and multiple myeloma risk—A systematic review and meta-analysis of the dose-risk relationship. *European Journal of Cancer Prevention, 23,* 113–121. doi:10.1097/CEJ.0000000000000001

Rusiecki, J.A., De Roos, A., Lee, W.J., Dosemeci, M., Lubin, J.H., Hoppin, J.A., ... Alavanja, M.C. (2004). Cancer incidence among pesticide applicators exposed to atrazine in the agricultural health study. *Journal of the National Cancer Institute, 96,* 1375–1382. doi:10.1093/jnci/djh264

Samanic, C., Gridley, G., Chow, W., Lubin, J., & Hoover, R.J.F., Jr. (2004). Obesity and cancer risk among white and black United States veterans. *Cancer Causes and Control, 15,* 35–43. doi:10.1023/B:CACO.0000016573.79453.ba

Semenciw, R.M., Morrison, H.I., Riedel, D., Wilkins, K., Ritter, L., & Mao, Y. (1993). Multiple myeloma mortality and agricultural practices in the prairie provinces of Canada. *Journal of Occupational Medicine, 36,* 557–561. doi:10.1097/00043764-199306000-00010

Sobol, H., Vey, N., Sauvan, R., Philip, N., Noguchi, T., & Eisinger, F. (2002). Familial multiple myeloma: A family study and review of the literature. *Journal of the National Cancer Institute, 94,* 461–462. doi:10.1093/jnci/94.6.461

Struewing, J.P., Hartge, P., Wacholder, S., Baker, S.M., Berlin, M., McAdams, M., ... Tucker, M.A. (1997). The risk of cancer associated with specific mutations of BRCA1 and BRCA2 among Ashkenazi Jews. *New England Journal of Medicine, 336,* 1401–1408. doi:10.1056/NEJM199705153362001

Takkouche, B., Etminan, M., & Montes-Martinez, A. (2005). Personal use of hair dyes and risk of cancer: A meta-analysis. *JAMA, 293,* 2516–2525. doi:10.1001/jama.293.20.2516

Tavani, A., La Vecchia, C., Gallus, S., Lagiou, P., Trichopoulos, D., Levi, F., & Negri, E. (2000). Red meat intake and cancer risk: A study in Italy. *International Journal of Cancer, 86,* 425–428. doi:10.1002/(SICI)1097-0215(20000501)86:3<425::AID-IJC19>3.0.CO;2-S

Tavani, A., Pregnolato, A., Negri, E., Franceschi, S., Serraino, D., Carbone, A., & La Vecchia, C. (1997). Diet and risk of lymphoid neoplasms and soft tissue sarcomas. *Nutrition and Cancer, 27,* 256–260. doi:10.1080/01635589709514535

Tewari, P., Ryan, A.W., Hayden, P.J., Catherwood, M., Drain, S., Staines, A., ... Browne, P.V. (2011). Genetic variation at the 8q24 locus confers risk to multiple myeloma. *British Journal of Haematology, 156,* 129–152. doi:10.111/j.1365-2141.2011.08792.x

Thun, M.J., Altekruse, S.F., Namboodiri, M.M., Calle, E.E., Myers, D.G., & Heath, C.W., Jr. (1994). Hair dye use and risk of fatal cancers in U.S. women. *Journal of the National Cancer Institute, 86,* 210–215. doi:10.1093/jnci/86.3.210

U.S. Department of Veterans Affairs. (2014). Agent Orange. Retrieved from http://www1.va.gov/agentorange

Vangsted, A.J., Nielsen, K.R., Klausen, T.W., Haukaas, E., Tjonneland, A., & Vogel, U. (2012). A functional polymorphism in the promoter region of the IL1B gene is associated with risk of multiple myeloma. *British Journal of Haematology, 158,* 515–518. doi:10.1111/j.1365-2141.2012.09141.x

Waxman, A.J., Mink, P.J., Devesa, S.S., Anderson, W.F., Weiss, B.M., Kristinsson, S.Y., ... Landgren, O. (2010). Racial disparities in incidence and outcome in multiple myeloma: A population-based study. *Blood, 116,* 5501–5506. doi:10.1182/blood-2010-07-298760

Weiss, B.M., Abadie, J., Verma, P., Howard, R.S., & Kuehl, W.M. (2009). A monoclonal gammopathy precedes multiple myeloma in most patients. *Blood, 113,* 5418–5422. doi:10.1182/blood-2008-12-195008

World Cancer Research Fund International. (2014). Worldwide data. Retrieved from http://www.wcrf.org/int/cancer-facts-figures/worldwide-data

CHAPTER 5

High-Dose Therapy and Stem Cell Transplantation

Ima N. Garcia, MSN, RN, ACNP-BC, AOCNP®

Introduction

Over the past 30 years, patients with multiple myeloma have experienced numerous advancements in therapy for the disease. Since the early 1990s, high-dose therapy (HDT) followed by autologous stem cell transplant (ASCT) has remained the standard treatment for patients younger than 65 years of age with newly diagnosed symptomatic multiple myeloma (Faussner & Dempke, 2012). Notwithstanding recent improvements in therapy, multiple myeloma remains incurable with an annual mortality rate of 3 per 100,000 (National Cancer Institute Surveillance, Epidemiology, and End Results Program, 2014). Treatment of multiple myeloma remains difficult, and regrettably, most patients ultimately develop drug resistance and relapse (El-Amm & Tabbara, 2015). Improving survival remains the primary goal of treatment. Uncontrolled studies have shown that, for patients responding to initial induction chemotherapy, ASCT is a safe (less than 5% toxic deaths) and effective consolidation therapy. Most importantly, some studies have suggested that levels of 30%–50% complete response (CR) could be achieved, leading to prolonged remission and overall survival (OS) (Harousseau, 2002).

Over the past decade, novel therapeutic agents, such as thalidomide, bortezomib, lenalidomide, and more recently carfilzomib and pomalidomide, have been used in combination with HDT and ASCT, thus expanding the therapeutic options for patients with multiple myeloma. The use of novel agents has given rise to substantial and profound improvements in median survival time, from three years in the 1960s to mid-1990s to approximately five years from the late 1990s to 2008 (Djulbegovic & Kumar, 2008;

Harousseau, 2010). Clinical management of patients with myeloma is multifaceted and requires a comprehensive approach that integrates healthcare professionals from a variety of clinical settings as well as caregivers and patients. Oncology nurses play an integral role across the treatment continuum for patients undergoing the transplantation process, making their knowledge of transplantation guidelines essential (Faiman, Miceli, Noonan, & Lilleby, 2013).

Evolution of High-Dose Therapy for Multiple Myeloma

Multiple myeloma was first described in the 19th century as *mollities ossium* accompanied by Bence Jones protein in the urine (Kyle & Rajkumar, 2008). The prognosis was fatal, and OS was 7–10 months due to lack of successful treatment at that time. By the 1950s, the first effective treatment for multiple myeloma was established using alkylating agent–based therapy, which improved the OS to 36 months from the time of diagnosis for the approximately 50% of patients who responded to therapy but was associated with an 18% mortality rate in nonresponders (Bergsagel, Sprague, Austin, & Griffith, 1962). Over the past 15 years, many advances in multiple myeloma therapy have further improved OS, and HDT/ASCT has established itself as an accepted treatment for patients with myeloma. This approach has been founded by a number of randomized trials, exhibiting an advantage when compared with conventional chemotherapy in regard to response rate and event-free survival (EFS), and in some trials OS as well (Attal et al., 1996; Child et al., 2003). The preeminence of HDT/ASCT equated with conventional chemotherapy was largely attributed to a superior quality of response, with increased CR or very good partial response (VGPR). Generally with HDT/ASCT, the CR plus VGPR rates were 40%–50%, with a median progression-free survival (PFS) of 24–36 months and a median OS of 5–6 years (Kumar, 2009; Naumann-Winter et al., 2012). Recently, novel agents are challenging HDT/ASCT as a treatment option, and randomized clinical trials currently are being conducted to determine whether novel agents can produce similar or superior results compared to HDT/ASCT (Richardson, 2014).

Stem cell transplantation (SCT) has evolved over the years as a unique treatment modality for various diseases that may benefit from the use of blood and bone marrow hematopoietic stem cells. Blood-derived stem cells result in faster hematologic recovery than marrow stem cells. Additionally, EFS and OS appear to be identical in patients with myeloma who received blood- or marrow-derived stem cells (Singhal, 2002). SCT is classified based on the relationship of the donor to the patient. ASCT uses cells derived from the patient, allogeneic SCT (alloSCT) uses cells derived from a human leukocyte antigen (HLA)–matched sibling or unrelated donor, and syngeneic SCT uses cells from an identical twin. Transplant-eligible patients with multiple myeloma can undergo either a single ASCT, tandem ASCT, myeloablative alloSCT, or nonmyeloablative (mini) alloSCT. Figure 5-1 illustrates the process of SCT.

Transplantation Process

The transplantation sequence is a multistep process that can be dissected into several phases. In general, these phases can be categorized broadly as the pretransplant phase, transplant phase, and post-transplant phase. The pretransplant phase could take weeks to months prior to transplant and involves having induction therapy, patient and caregiver education with the transplant nurse coordinator, and determination of health insurance coverage. The pretransplant phase is also described below in detail during phase 0 and phase 1. The transplant phase could take up to eight weeks. This phase involves the administration of high-dose chemotherapy followed by stem cell reinfusion and engraftment. The details involved in this phase are well described below in phases 2 and 3. The post-transplant phase involves ongoing follow-up with the transplant team as well as coordinated care with community providers. Most transplant centers will require a full post-transplant evaluation or disease restaging to assess the outcomes of the whole transplantation process. The oncology nurse must remember that each phase comprises unique factors and treatment approaches to enhance the overall process. Decades of clinical investigation and practice have given insight

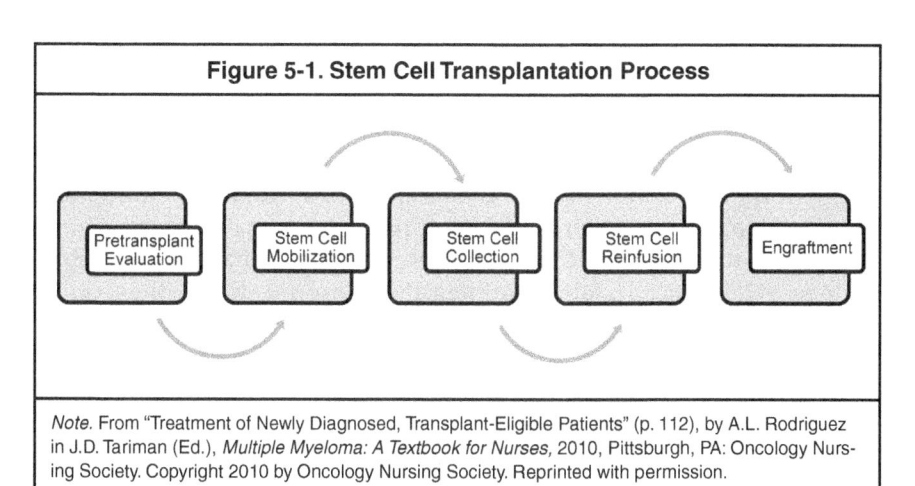

Figure 5-1. Stem Cell Transplantation Process

Pretransplant Evaluation → Stem Cell Mobilization → Stem Cell Collection → Stem Cell Reinfusion → Engraftment

Note. From "Treatment of Newly Diagnosed, Transplant-Eligible Patients" (p. 112), by A.L. Rodriguez in J.D. Tariman (Ed.), *Multiple Myeloma: A Textbook for Nurses,* 2010, Pittsburgh, PA: Oncology Nursing Society. Copyright 2010 by Oncology Nursing Society. Reprinted with permission.

as to when obstacles, side effects, and suitable interventions can occur. Therefore, knowledgeable transplantation teams can foresee patient needs throughout the transplant continuum. Long-term side effects and complications also can occur and require management and intervention from highly specialized stem cell transplant physicians and well-informed transplant nurses (Durie et al., 2006; Faiman et al., 2013; Giralt et al., 2009).

Phase 0: Induction or Initial Treatment

Patients begin induction chemotherapy once a confirmed diagnosis of symptomatic multiple myeloma has been made. Induction therapy goals are to provoke a tumor response and reduce symptoms by diminishing disease burden. Therapy response is organized based on the decrease of myeloma protein from baseline. Achievement of a CR is the preeminent predictor for PFS and occurs when patients attain negative immunofixation of the serum and urine, resolution of plasmacytomas, and decrease of the number of plasma cells in the bone marrow to 5% or less (Faiman et al., 2013). Table 5-1 describes the European Group for Blood and Marrow Transplantation response criteria for evaluating success of treatment (Bladé et al., 1998).

Currently, no general consensus exists with regard to the optimal timing of transplantation (see Figure 5-2). There are many factors to consider for eligibility for transplantation. Among them are age, performance status, cardiac health, pulmonary health, renal insufficiency or failure, myeloma risk features, and socioeconomic factors (Faiman et al., 2013; Miceli et al., 2013). When it comes to the patient's age, chronologic age does not matter as much as physiologic age. Hence, performance status is important. One could be a 75-year-old patient with excellent performance status (Karnofsky Performance Status [KPS] greater than 60% or Eastern Cooperative Oncology Group [ECOG] performance status greater than 3) and could qualify for transplant, whereas a 60-year-old patient with KPS of 50% or ECOG performance status of 4 will be deemed ineligible for transplant. Enrollment in a well-designed clinical trial should also be considered to help ascertain the best induction therapy, transplantation timing, and maintenance therapy. Both cardiac and pulmonary health must be good to excellent to surmount the high-dose chemotherapy that is administered prior to SCT. Typically, adequate lung function with diffuse lung capacity oxygenation greater than 50% and a left ventricular ejection fraction greater than 50% are required for the transplantation process to move forward without any difficulty. Patients with renal insufficiency or failure are not excluded for transplant, but they will require dose adjustment of the conditioning regimen. Lastly, socioeconomic factors such as insurance coverage, caregiver support during and after transplant, and personal phi-

Table 5-1. European Group for Blood and Marrow Transplantation Therapy Response Criteria

Response Criteria[a]	M Protein[b]	Immunofixation Test	Bone Marrow Biopsy[b]	Bone Lytic Lesions[c]	Plasmacytomas
Complete response[a]	Absent in serum and urine	Negative	< 5% plasma cells in bone marrow aspirate	No increase in size or number of lytic bone lesions	Disappearance of soft tissue plasmacytomas
Near complete response	Absent in serum and urine	Positive	< 5% plasma cells in bone marrow aspirate	No increase in size or number of lytic bone lesions	Disappearance of soft tissue plasmacytomas
Partial response[a]	50% reduction in serum and ≥ 90% reduction in urine Reduction in 24-hour urine light-chain excretion by ≥ 90% or to 200 mg	Positive	≥ 50% reduction in plasma cells in bone marrow aspirate	No increase in size or number of lytic bone lesions	≥ 50% reduction in size of soft tissue plasmacytomas
Minimal response[a]	24%–49% reduction in serum 50%–89% reduction in 24-hour urine light chain still exceeding 200 mg/24 hours	Positive	25%–49% reduction in plasma cells in bone marrow aspirate	No increase in size or number of lytic bone lesions	25%–49% reduction in size of soft tissue plasmacytomas
No change	Not meeting criteria of either minimal response or progressive disease				
Plateau	Stable values within 25% above or below value at the time response is assessed, maintained for at least 3 months				

[a] All response criteria components must be met unless otherwise indicated.
[b] Response must be maintained for a minimum of 6 weeks.
[c] Development of a compression fracture does not exclude response.

Note. Based on information from Bladé et al., 1998.

From "Treatment of Newly Diagnosed, Transplant-Eligible Patients" (p. 111), by A.L. Rodriguez in J.D. Tariman (Ed.), *Multiple Myeloma: A Textbook for Nurses*, 2010, Pittsburgh, PA: Oncology Nursing Society. Copyright 2010 by Oncology Nursing Society. Reprinted with permission.

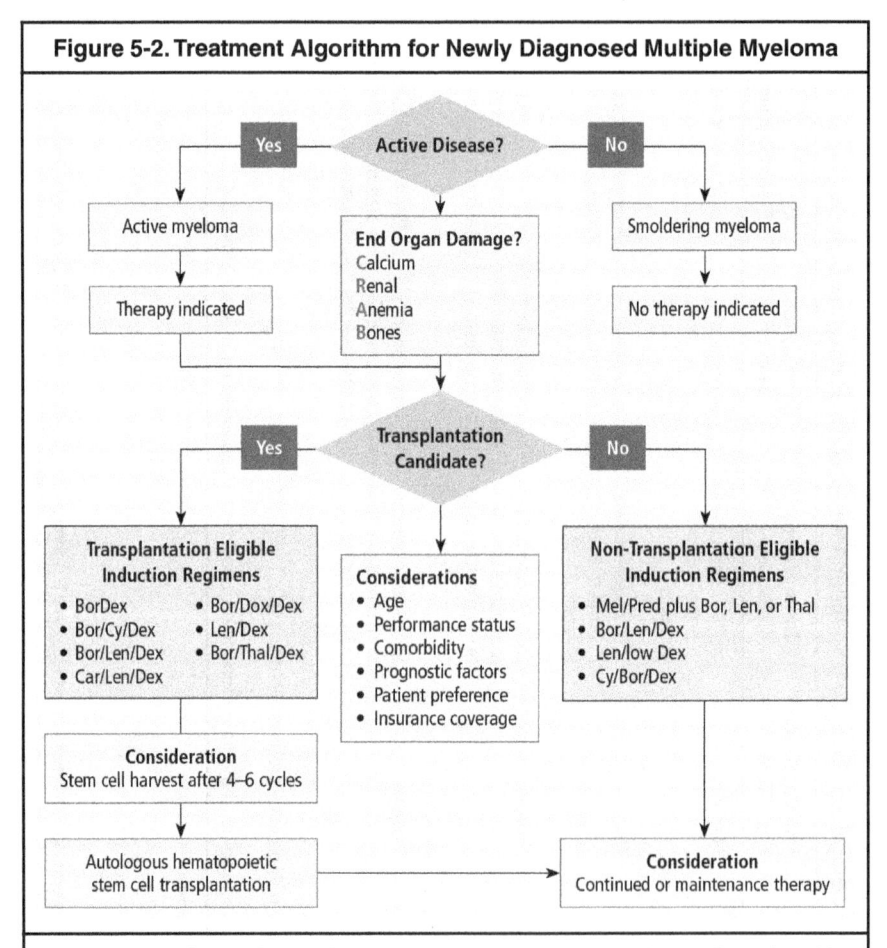

Figure 5-2. Treatment Algorithm for Newly Diagnosed Multiple Myeloma

Active Disease?
- Yes → Active myeloma → Therapy indicated
- No → Smoldering myeloma → No therapy indicated

End Organ Damage?
- Calcium
- Renal
- Anemia
- Bones

Transplantation Candidate?

- **Yes → Transplantation Eligible Induction Regimens**
  - BorDex
  - Bor/Cy/Dex
  - Bor/Len/Dex
  - Car/Len/Dex
  - Bor/Dox/Dex
  - Len/Dex
  - Bor/Thal/Dex

  Consideration: Stem cell harvest after 4–6 cycles
  → Autologous hematopoietic stem cell transplantation

- **Considerations**
  - Age
  - Performance status
  - Comorbidity
  - Prognostic factors
  - Patient preference
  - Insurance coverage

- **No → Non-Transplantation Eligible Induction Regimens**
  - Mel/Pred plus Bor, Len, or Thal
  - Bor/Len/Dex
  - Len/low Dex
  - Cy/Bor/Dex

Consideration: Continued or maintenance therapy

Bor—bortezomib; Car—carfilzomib; Cy—cyclophosphamide; Dex—dexamethasone; Dox—doxorubicin; Len—lenalidomide; Mel—melphalan; Pred—prednisone; Thal—thalidomide

Note. Based on information from Mikhael et al., 2013; National Comprehensive Cancer Network®, 2015.

From "Autologous Hematopoietic Stem Cell Transplantation for Patients With Multiple Myeloma: An Overview for Nurses in Community Practice," by T. Miceli, K. Lilleby, K. Noonan, S. Kurtin, B. Faiman, and P.A. Mangan, 2013, *Clinical Journal of Oncology Nursing, 17*(Suppl. 6), p. 16. Copyright 2013 by Oncology Nursing Society. Adapted with permission.

---

losophy (e.g., acceptance of blood products transfusion) and commitment are equally as important as the other factors in order to have successful SCT.

When proceeding to transplant, it is important to utilize stem cell–sparing induction regimens to ensure an adequate harvest. Table 5-2 outlines common multiple myeloma therapies, side effects, and clinical implications (Faiman et al., 2013; Miceli et al., 2013).

CHAPTER 5. HIGH-DOSE THERAPY AND STEM CELL TRANSPLANTATION   77

Table 5-2. Common Multiple Myeloma Therapies, Side Effects, and Clinical Implications*

Drug, Class, Route	Potential Side Effects and Toxicities	Clinical Implications	Additional Information
Myeloma Therapy Medications			
Bortezomib (Velcade®) Proteasome inhibitor; IV or SC administration	MS, PN, diarrhea or constipation, irritation or erythema at injection site; VZV activation	Monitor CBC, monitor PN symptoms, bowel management; use antiviral prophylaxis.	Used as combination therapy or single agent; consider SC administration to reduce PN
Carfilzomib (Kyprolis®) Proteasome inhibitor; IV administration	Fatigue, anemia, thrombocytopenia, nausea, diarrhea, dyspnea, and fever	Monitor CBC and liver function tests. Prevent tumor lysis syndrome via PO and IV hydration; premedicate with dexamethasone in the first cycle.	Approved for patients who have had two or more prior therapies, including bortezomib and an immunomodulatory agent
Cyclophosphamide Alkylating agent; IV or oral administration	For conventional doses, MS; for high doses, myeloablation, GI disturbance, alopecia, bladder limitation	Encourage frequent urination and increased oral hydration, IV hydration if needed, antiemetics, bowel management.	Used as combination therapy and as part of autologous stem cell mobilization plan
Lenalidomide (Revlimid®) Immunomodulator; oral administration	MS, TEE when combined with steroids, skin rash	Monitor CBC, bowel management; dose adjust for renal impairments; TEE prophylaxis.	Used in combination therapy or as single-agent maintenance; hold for two weeks prior to autologous stem cell collection
Melphalan (Alkeran®) Alkylating agent; IV or oral administration	For conventional doses, MS; for high doses, myeloablation, GI disturbance, and alopecia	Monitor CBC. Conditioning chemotherapy for ASCT	Should be avoided prior to autologous stem cell collection; long-term use can cause myelodysplasia

(Continued on next page)

Table 5-2. Common Multiple Myeloma Therapies, Side Effects, and Clinical Implications* *(Continued)*

Drug, Class, Route	Potential Side Effects and Toxicities	Clinical Implications	Additional Information
Pomalidomide (Pomalyst®) Immunomodulator; oral administration	MS, TEE	Monitor CBC, bowel management, TEE prophylaxis.	Approved for patients who have had 2 or more prior therapies including bortezomib and an immunomodulatory agent
Thalidomide (Thalomid®) Immunomodulator; oral administration	MS, TEE when combined with steroids, PN, constipation	Monitor CBC, bowel management, TEE prophylaxis.	Used in combination with dexamethasone
Supportive Care Medications			
G-CSF/filgrastim (Neupogen®) Cytokine; SC administration	Joint and bone pain; increased white blood cells	Assess and medicate for pain.	Management of neutropenia; autologous stem cell mobilization
Pamidronate (Aredia®) Bisphosphonate; IV administration	Initial phase reaction, hyperalbuminuria, and osteonecrosis of the jaw	Dental evaluation prior to start (if possible), regular dental cleaning; avoid invasive dental procedure while receiving treatment.	Inhibition of bone resorption and associated hypercalcemia. See ASCO and IMWG guidelines for duration of use. May be held during transplantation and resumed post-transplant.
Plerixafor (Mozobil®) Chemokine inhibitor; SC administration	Diarrhea and erythema at injection site	Bowel management	Used in combination with G-CSF for stem cell mobilization

(Continued on next page)

Table 5-2. Common Multiple Myeloma Therapies, Side Effects, and Clinical Implications* (Continued)

Drug, Class, Route	Potential Side Effects and Toxicities	Clinical Implications	Additional Information
Zoledronic acid (Zometa®) Bisphosphonate; IV administration	Initial phase reaction, hyperalbuminuria, and osteonecrosis of the jaw	Dental evaluation prior to start (if possible), regular dental cleaning; avoid invasive dental procedure while receiving treatment.	Inhibition of bone resorption and associated hypercalcemia. See ASCO and IMWG guidelines for duration of use. May be held during transplantation and resumed post-transplant.

* See package insert for a complete listing of possible side effects. Practical use of medications may differ from U.S. Food and Drug Administration–approved indications and is done at the discretion of a licensed provider.

ASCO—American Society of Clinical Oncology; ASCT—autologous stem cell transplant; CBC—complete blood count; G-CSF—granulocyte–colony-stimulating factor; GI—gastrointestinal; IMWG—International Myeloma Working Group; MS—myelosuppression; PN—peripheral neuropathy; SC—subcutaneous; TEE—thromboembolic event; VZV—varicella zoster virus

Note. Based on information from Amgen Inc., 2013; Bertolotti et al., 2008; Bilotti et al., 2011; Celgene Corporation, 2013a, 2013b, 2013c; Genzyme Corporation, 2014; GlaxoSmithKline, 2011; Kumar, 2009; Millennium: The Takeda Oncology Company, 2014; Novartis Pharmaceuticals Corporation, 2012a, 2012b; Onyx Pharmaceuticals, 2012; Roxane Laboratories, Inc., 2013.

From "Autologous Hematopoietic Stem Cell Transplantation for Patients With Multiple Myeloma: An Overview for Nurses in Community Practice," by T. Miceli, K. Lilleby, K. Noonan, S. Kurtin, B. Faiman, and P.A. Mangan, 2013, *Clinical Journal of Oncology Nursing, 17*(Suppl. 6), p. 17. Copyright 2013 by Oncology Nursing Society. Adapted with permission.

Phase 1: Collection Process

Pluripotent hematopoietic stem cells (HSCs) can be obtained from the bone marrow, cord blood, or peripheral blood. Peripheral blood currently is the most utilized source for HSC collection. CD34+ cells are progenitor cells with the capability to differentiate and repopulate myeloid and lymphoid cell lines in the wake of bone marrow ablation post-HDT. Their use has resulted in reduced transfusion needs and brisker engraftment. They are measured in cells per deciliter (cells/dl) to the power of 10^6 (million) based on recipient weight (Faiman et al., 2013; Gertz, Wolf, Micallef, & Gastineau, 2010; Giralt et al., 2009). A minimum of two million CD34+ cells are required to ensure engraftment, but higher yields can facilitate faster marrow recovery (Miceli et al., 2013).

Mobilization

The term *mobilization* describes the process of stimulating the bone marrow to release HSCs into the peripheral blood. This can be accomplished by various methods including the use of cytokine growth factors, such as granulocyte–colony-stimulating factor (G-CSF) (e.g., filgrastim), alone or in combination with chemotherapy or the CXCR4-binding agent plerixafor (Faiman et al., 2013). Plerixafor has been shown to improve cell yield, reduce the number of apheresis sessions, and provide timely engraftment following SCT (Faiman et al., 2013; Giralt et al., 2009). Side effects of cytokine growth factors include leukocytosis, bone pain, myalgias, low-grade fever, and flulike symptoms (Faiman et al., 2013; Gertz et al., 2010; Giralt et al., 2009).

Chemotherapy may be added as an additional treatment option, particularly if optimal response to induction has not been achieved. Several chemotherapeutic regimens can be utilized, but cyclophosphamide is used most frequently. Common side effects of high-dose cyclophosphamide include nausea, alopecia, and myelosuppression. Mucositis and hemorrhagic cystitis are rare with the doses used, but IV hydration is often given and patients are encouraged to increase their fluid intake. Nadir following cyclophosphamide/G-CSF generally occurs in 8–12 days. During this time, patients are encouraged to follow neutropenic precautions and notify their nurse or provider if signs or symptoms of infection develop (Faiman et al., 2013; Gertz et al., 2010; Giralt et al., 2009).

Collection

The timing of stem cell collection is individualized based on the transplantation plan. Cells are collected via apheresis as an outpatient procedure. Once collected, the cells are cryopreserved in a medium of dimethyl sulfoxide (DMSO) to prevent cell lysis and are viable for an indefinite period of time (Faiman et al., 2013).

Phase 2: Pre-Engraftment

The decision to proceed directly to SCT is individualized based on a variety of patient-specific criteria. Transplantation can occur immediately following the mobilization and collection phase or can be deferred until relapse. Patients also may be given time for hematopoietic recovery if chemotherapy was administered for mobilization. Phase 2 (pre-engraftment) commonly occurs within several weeks and includes three parts: conditioning, stem cell infusion, and supportive treatment and side effect management through engraftment (Faiman et al., 2013).

Conditioning

The term *conditioning* refers to the treatment utilized immediately prior to stem cell infusion. The term is commonly used to describe the process of preparing the bone marrow microenvironment to accept the transplanted cells. In general, high-dose melphalan 200 mg/m^2 is the preferred conditioning agent. Total body irradiation is administered less frequently because of increased toxicity with no proven increase in OS. Dose reductions are made in the setting of impaired renal function, advanced age, or increased comorbidity. Stem cell infusion typically occurs 24 hours following melphalan to allow chemotherapy elimination from the body, thus evading the risk of cytotoxicity to newly infused stem cells (Faiman et al., 2013). Figure 5-3 lists several conditioning regimens used for patients with myeloma, but melphalan is the preferred agent.

Figure 5-3. Conditioning Regimens Used in Multiple Myeloma

- Melphalan
- Melphalan/total body irradiation
- Melphalan/methylprednisolone
- Busulfan/cyclophosphamide
- Busulfan/cyclophosphamide/total body irradiation
- Busulfan/cyclophosphamide/thiotepa
- Busulfan/melphalan/thiotepa
- Carmustine/etoposide/melphalan/total body irradiation
- Fludarabine/melphalan
- Fludarabine/total body irradiation
- Fludarabine/total body irradiation/cyclophosphamide
- Fludarabine/alemtuzumab/total body irradiation
- Busulfan/fludarabine/antithymocyte globulin

Note. Based on information from Fermand et al., 2005; Harousseau, 2007; Singhal, 2002.

From "Treatment of Newly Diagnosed, Transplant-Eligible Patients" (p. 118), by A.L. Rodriguez in J.D. Tariman (Ed.), *Multiple Myeloma: A Textbook for Nurses,* 2010, Pittsburgh, PA: Oncology Nursing Society. Copyright 2010 by Oncology Nursing Society. Reprinted with permission.

Stem Cell Infusion

On the day of stem cell infusion, "Day 0", cryopreserved stem cells are thawed and infused via a central venous catheter. Following infusion, the patient will have a distinctive odor related to the preservative DMSO. This odor is excreted from the patient's breath and pores. DMSO has a characteristic odor often described as creamed corn or garlic and typically fades over two to three days. Patients also may taste the DMSO. Several studies have suggested that sucking on hard candy or lemon or orange slices may help to lessen the taste of DMSO. Side effects of DMSO can include nausea, vomiting, hypo- or hypertension, tachy- or bradycardia, and anaphylaxis. Premedications prior to stem cell infusion are variable based on institutional protocol. Vital signs should be monitored frequently, and hydration and emergency medications (e.g., epinephrine) should be available at the bedside (Antin & Raley, 2009; Faiman et al., 2013; Potter, Eisenberg, Cain, & Berry, 2011).

Supportive Therapy

Prior to transplant, patients undergo a thorough medical evaluation to identify any baseline renal, liver, cardiac, and pulmonary dysfunction. However, despite pretransplant testing, end-organ complications may occur during the pre-engraftment phase of the transplant process (Laffan & Biedrzycki, 2006; Pallera & Schwartzberg, 2004). HDT and ASCT are associated with expected side effects including alopecia, gastrointestinal (GI) toxicities, and bone marrow ablation. These side effects occur post-chemotherapy and are a reflection of rapidly dividing cells that are damaged from the effects of HDT. It is important to note that complications of end-organ toxicity and life-threatening side effects may cause mortality not related to relapsed disease. Common complications include infectious issues and pulmonary problems. Table 5-3 describes an overview of common side effects associated with multiple myeloma therapies, clinical findings, and management strategies.

Alopecia commonly occurs days to weeks following transplantation. Psychosocial support and counseling regarding hair loss are essential for both men and women (Hesketh et al., 2004). Use of a wig or other hair accessories may be comforting and can provide safety and warmth. The expense of a wig may be covered by insurance if ordered as a "hair or cranial prosthetic" (Faiman et al., 2013).

GI toxicity may include mucositis, esophagitis, nausea, vomiting, and diarrhea. Antiemetic therapy, hydration, and pain medication often are necessary for symptom management (Antin & Raley, 2009; Rodriguez, 2010). Patients who experience GI toxicities may develop weight loss, anorexia, dehydration, and infection (Pallera & Schwartzberg, 2004; Rodriguez, 2010). Mucositis related to melphalan administration also is a common side effect. A study found that holding ice chips in the pock-

Table 5-3. Post-Transplantation Symptoms, Clinical Findings, and Management Strategies

Symptom	Clinical Findings and Risk Factors	Management Strategies
Anorexia	Weight loss, taste changes, change in performance status, fatigue, nausea and vomiting, diarrhea	Review medications for possible source. Medical nutritional therapies: oral nutritional supplements, IV hydration. Small, frequent meals, calorie counts, weekly weight, nutrition consult. Reinforce improvement with time. Adjust medications as needed. Treat underlying cause (e.g., medication for nausea and vomiting).
Anxiety and depression	Fatigue, exhaustion, difficulty sleeping, difficulty concentrating, restlessness, irritability and impatience, recurrent thoughts of diagnosis and treatment, anorexia	Listen to and validate concerns. Refer to social services, psychiatry, and support groups. Pharmacologic: antianxiety medications, antidepressants. Complementary and alternative medicine therapy: relaxation therapy, mild exercise such as walking.
Diarrhea	Increased frequency of bowel movements, abdominal cramps, dehydration, decrease in weight	Review medications for possible source (e.g., antibiotics, narcotic withdrawal). Evaluate electrolytes. Assess stool sample for enteric pathogens (e.g., *Clostridium difficile*). Administer antidiarrheal medication. Ensure appropriate fluid and electrolyte replacement. Adjust diet for food sensitivities: milk products, certain spicy foods, nutritional supplements, fatty foods, chocolate. Provide antibiotics as needed; adjust medications as needed.
Fatigue	Decrease in energy, inability to complete tasks, insomnia or hypersomnia, not feeling rested after sleeping at night, generalized weakness	Review medications that may cause fatigue. Assess for anemia. Encourage mild exercise such as walking. Potentially decrease or discontinue medications that cause fatigue. Counsel patient on sleep hygiene, such as minimizing napping or staying in bed throughout the day. Provide ESAs if indicated and after obtaining written consent. Administer red blood cell transfusion, if needed.

(Continued on next page)

Table 5-3. Post-Transplantation Symptoms, Clinical Findings, and Management Strategies *(Continued)*

Symptom	Clinical Findings and Risk Factors	Management Strategies
Fever	Diarrhea, muscle weakness, fatigue, confusion, seizures	Obtain panculture, chest x-ray, and CBC with differential and platelets. Administer prophylactic antibiotics if neutropenic; therapeutic antibiotics if culture positive. Provide acetaminophen, IV hydration, and symptom management. Monitor for fever greater than 101.3°F (or lower temperature if patient is not feeling well), blood pressure declining from baseline, and tachycardia.
Nausea and vomiting	Anorexia, nausea and vomiting, weight loss, diminished skin turgor	Quantify episodes of emesis. Assess fluid and electrolyte status. Review medications for antiemetics and medications that may cause nausea and vomiting. Adjust medications if possible and as needed. Provide IV or oral hydration and replace electrolytes as needed.
Pain	New or existing pain symptoms, current pain medication, pain related to infection, symptoms of depression or anxiety	Provide appropriate pain medication regimen: long-acting pain medication together with breakthrough pain medication, doses titrated to effectiveness. Consider imaging for source of new or worsening pain. Consult with appropriate specialty, if indicated.
Peripheral neuropathy	Paresthesias, impaired proprioception, pain, sensory deficits; patients at increased risk: those with a history of diabetes, alcohol use, vitamin B_{12} deficiency, paraneoplastic syndrome, vascular insufficiency	Obtain baseline assessment of peripheral neuropathy, description of peripheral neuropathy symptoms, previous chemotherapy, current medications; neurologic examination including sensory and motor use. Perform safety evaluation and nutritional assessment. Treatment of neuropathic pain: medications, acupuncture, massage, medications. Promote safety with use of assistive devices: cane, orthotics, wheelchair. Recommend physical therapy and activity; massage.

(Continued on next page)

Table 5-3. Post-Transplantation Symptoms, Clinical Findings, and Management Strategies *(Continued)*

Symptom	Clinical Findings and Risk Factors	Management Strategies
Thrombosis (DVT or PE)	Painful, swollen, and erythematous extremity (most often lower extremity), shortness of breath, tachycardia, chest pain, HTN; patients at increased risk: those with obesity, diabetes, cardiovascular disease, HTN, hyperlipidemia, immunomodulatory agents with concurrent high-dose steroids, anthracyclines, ESAs, hospitalizations, and immobility	Prevention: thromboprophylaxis for all patients at risk. Full therapeutic anticoagulation for any patients with more than two risk factors. If DVT or PE is suspected: Doppler ultrasound of suspected extremity. High-resolution chest CT with PE protocol if PE is suspected. Medication to treat thrombosis: low-molecular-weight heparin, warfarin, and alternative anticoagulants. Consult with coagulation specialist if appropriate.

CBC—complete blood count; CT—computed tomography; DVT—deep vein thrombosis; ESA—erythropoiesis-stimulating agent; HTN—hypertension; PE—pulmonary embolism

Note. Based on information from Antin & Raley, 2008; Irwin & Johnson, 2014; Rodriguez, 2010.

ets of one's cheeks versus swishing saline prior to and for two hours following melphalan infusion reduced the severity and duration of mucositis by decreasing the circulation of the chemotherapy to the oral tissues. These findings were significant in that the incidence of grade 3–4 mucositis was only 14% in the ice chip group compared to 74% in the saline group (Lilleby et al., 2006).

GI toxicities can be the consequence of more than one condition. Careful consideration must be given when developing strategies for symptom management. For example, patients may develop pain related to oral mucositis. Appropriate interventions may include oral care and pain management. Medications such as narcotics commonly are used to control pain but can potentially cause nausea and constipation. This may create a clinical challenge for nursing because the goal of supportive care is not only to alleviate symptoms but also to prevent further GI problems such as ileus, anorexia, and infection (Cooke, Grant, & Gemmill, 2012). Anorexia and the inability to maintain oral intake as a result of GI toxicity may require IV hydration as well as scheduled administration of antiemetics and pain medications. In some instances, patients may be required to remain on "nothing by mouth" status for several days and may require hyperalimentation. Supportive care guidelines vary with each transplant center, and oncology nurses must refer to their individual institutional policies and procedures.

When marrow ablation occurs, the period of profound pancytopenia lasts for approximately 10–14 days. Anemia and thrombocytopenia are managed by transfusion support based on institutional guidelines. It is well documented that transplant patients receiving HDT develop severe neutropenia, thus putting them at risk for infection and sepsis. Infection risk varies based on the type of transplant, source of hematopoietic cells, underlying disease, disease status, conditioning regimen, prior infections, and environmental exposure to microorganisms (Bevans et al., 2009). Prophylaxis with antibacterials, antivirals, and antifungals is given routinely in the setting of anticipated neutropenia and therapeutically for febrile neutropenia or occult infection. Common causes of infection include use of central venous catheters, GI infections such as *Clostridium difficile*, and skin sources. However, enteric organisms (e.g., *Escherichia coli*) and opportunistic infections (e.g., *Pneumocystis jiroveci*) also can occur during this time (Pallera & Schwartzberg, 2004). In general, causative bacterial organisms commonly seen in transplant recipients during the pre-engraftment period include *Streptococcus aureus*, coagulase-negative *Staphylococcus*, *Enterococcus*, *Acinetobacter*, *Klebsiella*, *Pseudomonas*, *Escherichia coli*, and *Lactobacillus*. Among the viruses, the common causative agents include herpes simplex, respiratory syncytial virus, rhinovirus, parainfluenza, and cytomegalovirus. Fungal infections primarily are caused by *Aspergillus* and *Candida*. Surveillance for all these types of infections is paramount. Nose/throat and stool cultures prior to admission are becoming standard of care to identify bacterial colonization, and in some cases, Galactomannan assay test will be warranted to identify invasive *Aspergillus*.

Renal failure can occur at any time throughout the transplant continuum. When renal insufficiency arises prior to stem cell engraftment, the reason can be multifactorial. The cause of renal failure often is linked to nephrotoxic medications such as antibiotics, antihypertensives, chemotherapy, or antifungal agents. Acute renal failure from tubular necrosis may also develop. Dehydration resulting from diarrhea, nausea and vomiting, or anorexia also can cause impaired renal function. Other sources of renal problems in the early phase of transplant include sepsis and relapsed disease (Pallera & Schwartzberg, 2004).

Pulmonary complications occur in 30%–60% of SCT recipients and often are caused by chemotherapy agents in the early phase of transplant. Pre-engraftment pulmonary complications include pulmonary edema, bronchiolitis obliterans, and pneumonia (Blombery et al., 2011). Diffuse alveolar hemorrhage (DAH) is characterized by multilobular culture–negative lung injury. An estimated 5% of all SCT recipients develop DAH, with an estimated mortality rate of 30%–60%. Presenting symptoms include acute shortness of breath, hemoptysis, fever, chest pain, and cough. Risk factors include older age, total body irradiation, severe mucositis, renal insuffciency, and white blood cell recovery. Identifying bloody return on bronchoalveolar lavage makes the definitive diagnosis of DAH. Early diagnosis is imperative, and treatment consists of corticosteroids and supportive care (Lara & Schwarz, 2010; Pallera & Schwartzberg, 2004).

Phase 3: Engraftment

The term *engraftment*, or blood count recovery, describes the time it takes for HSCs to migrate from the peripheral blood to the bone marrow and begin to grow. Engraftment is achieved when the absolute neutrophil count (ANC) is greater than 500 cells/mm^3 for three consecutive days or greater than 1,000 cells/mm^3 for one day, and platelets remain greater than 20,000 cells/mm^3, independent of platelet transfusions, for at least seven days (DiPersio et al., 2009). Approximately three weeks (day +17 to +25) following infusion of HSCs, most acute toxicities, including myelosuppression, have resolved (Russell et al., 2013). Once the patient has no evidence of active infection and has demonstrated engraftment and the ability to maintain oral hydration and nutritional status, arrangements can be made for discharge.

Types of Autologous Transplantation and Novel Therapies

Single Autologous Hematopoietic Cell Transplant

HDT followed by ASCT as a treatment modality for patients with multiple myeloma was studied in several nonrandomized and randomized clinical trials beginning in the 1990s (Attal et al., 1996; Bladé et al., 2000; Child et al., 2003; Palumbo et al., 2004), comparing conventional chemotherapy with HDT followed by ASCT. These studies demonstrated the superiority of HDT with ASCT in terms of response rates and EFS, but not all studies demonstrated an OS advantage. A study by Fermand et al. (2005) with a median follow-up time of approximately 10 years did not provide evidence for superiority of HDT over conventional chemotherapy in OS of patients ages 55–65 with symptomatic newly diagnosed multiple myeloma but confirmed benefits of HDT in terms of EFS and time without symptoms, treatments, and treatment toxicities (known as *TwiSTT*). Similarly, long-term results of the prospective randomized clinical trial from the Spanish group PETHEMA showed a significant increase in CR rate but no significant impact on PFS or OS (Bladé et al., 2005). Additionally, Moreau et al. (2002) and Barlogie, Kyle, et al. (2006) also reported similar findings in terms of no OS advantage. Moreover, a systematic review and meta-analysis of randomized trials confirmed PFS benefit but not OS benefit for HDT with ASCT early in patients with multiple myeloma (Koreth et al., 2007). Despite no significant benefit to OS, the ability of HDT to overcome tumor resistance, demonstrated by superior response in CR rates ranging from 25% to 50% and EFS advantage, has established HDT followed by ASCT as the standard form of management after induction therapy for newly diagnosed patients with symptomatic multiple myeloma (Cavo et al., 2011; Fermand et al., 2005; National Comprehensive Cancer Network®, 2015).

Induction therapy preceding SCT, including thalidomide and novel agents bortezomib and lenalidomide combined with corticosteroids, alkylators, and anthracyclines, demonstrated very high response rates and CR rates before and after ASCT with a positive impact on PFS (Bensinger, 2009; Palumbo & Rajkumar, 2009). The various combination regimens used for induction include thalidomide/dexamethasone (Thal/Dex) and novel agents bortezomib/dexamethasone (Bort/Dex) or lenalidomide/dexamethasone (Rev/Dex) (Palumbo & Rajkumar, 2009). The preferred conditioning regimen is high-dose melphalan at 200 mg/m^2 (Faiman et al., 2013).

Tandem Autologous Hematopoietic Stem Cell Transplant

To further increase cytotoxic dose intensity, the value of an even more assertive approach with tandem ASCT was explored in several pilot studies. Following demonstration that such a procedure was feasible and effective, five randomized trials were conducted to investigate the question of single versus tandem ASCT as up-front therapy for multiple myeloma. Results of these trials were contradictory, most likely because of heterogeneity across different trials with respect to their structural and methodological characteristics. Tandem ASCT has been widely advocated by Barlogie and colleagues because of its superior outcome, although the patients were not randomized in a clinical trial (Barlogie et al., 1997). In summary, tandem ASCT improved CR rates and PFS compared with single ASCT in most of the studies, but improvement in OS was not consistently shown (Cherry, Korde, Kwok, Roschewski, & Landgren, 2013; Kumar, Kharfan-Dabala, Glasmacher, & Djulbegovic, 2009). Furthermore, only patients who were not at least in VGPR after one ASCT appeared to benefit from the second (Attal et al., 2003). As a final point, patients with poor-risk cytogenetics continued to do poorly despite receiving tandem HDT/ASCT. With the recent integration of novel agents into the transplantation paradigm, the value of single versus tandem transplants still continues to be uncertain, and prospective randomized clinical trials are warranted. Two such studies currently are in progress in Europe and the United States (Cherry et al., 2013).

Novel Agents as First-Line Therapy in Transplant-Eligible Patients

Prior to the development of novel therapies, the prospect of attaining CR for transplant-eligible patients with multiple myeloma predominantly treated with conventional induction regimens was less than 5% (Cherry et al., 2013). The aim of induction therapy preceding ASCT is (a) reduction of tumor burden and increased post-ASCT CR/VGPR rate, (b) reversal of organ damage, and (c) diminution of plasma cell bone marrow infiltration (Harousseau, 2010).

Before the introduction of the proteasome inhibitor (PI) bortezomib and immunomodulatory agents (IMiDs) thalidomide and lenalidomide, the standard induction was dexamethasone based, either as a single agent or used in combination with vincristine and doxorubicin (VAD). Although high-dose dexamethasone provoked adverse events, these regimens were chosen over melphalan/prednisone-based regimens because of the better quality of stem cell collection. Nonetheless, the CR/VGPR rates after three to four cycles remained low (less than 10% CR and less than 20% CR plus VGPR) (Barlogie, 2014). In this age of novel agents, management differs contingent on whether the patient is ASCT eligible. Age greater than 65, poor performance status (ECOG performance status 3–4), and organ dysfunction (significant liver disease, renal disease unless on stable chronic dialysis and/or New York Heart Association class III–IV) renders patients inappropriate for such intensive therapy (Harousseau, 2010).

In a meta-analysis of nine randomized trials, findings showed a PFS advantage with up-front ASCT in comparison with conventional chemotherapy combinations (Cavo et al., 2013). Three randomized studies revealed that OS was comparable whether ASCT was performed early or as salvage therapy at relapse. Remarkably, in one trial, early ASCT improved median EFS (39 versus 13 months), along with the average time without symptoms (27.8 versus 22.3 months) compared with late ASCT, but OS survival was unchanged (64.6 versus 64 months). The early approach also was correlated with a lower relapse rate, decreased treatment-related toxicities, and termination. An additional trial identified no significant PFS improvement with early ASCT (42 versus 33 months; p = 0.57) and proposed that the largest benefit from early ASCT was among patients with disease refractory to induction therapy (Cavo et al., 2013).

The novel agents thalidomide, bortezomib, and lenalidomide have been effectively intermixed with one another or with cytotoxic drugs to form various doublet, triplet, and quadruplet combinations that have been extensively studied as induction therapy before ASCT. All trials evaluating combinations of dexamethasone and thalidomide or bortezomib to high-dose dexamethasone alone or VAD as induction regimens have shown a superiority of the novel agents in terms of increased overall response rate (ORR), including CR, emphasizing that there is no longer a role for VAD as standard induction therapy prior to HDT/ASCT (Cavo et al., 2013; Cherry et al., 2013).

With thalidomide/dexamethasone (TD), while the postinduction ORR was superior to dexamethasone alone or to VAD, the postinduction CR or the post-HDT/ASCT CR plus VGPR rate was not significantly increased. In contrast, with bortezomib/dexamethasone (VD), the CR plus VGPR rate is significantly improved compared with VAD, both pre- and post-HDT/ASCT. As reported by Cavo et al. (2013), one randomized study has investigated the response rate following four cycles of lenalidomide/dexamethasone as induction therapy. Herein, CR plus VGPR rate is improved with lenalidomide plus high-dose dexamethasone compared with low-dose dexamethasone. Lenalidomide/dexamethasone is yet to be examined with other induction regimens in the setting of HDT/ASCT (Cavo et al., 2013).

The inclusion of cytotoxic drugs such as doxorubicin or cyclophosphamide with either thalidomide (TAD, CTD) or bortezomib (PAD, CyBorD) improved response rates. The TAD regimen extended PFS when compared to VAD (34 versus 22 months; $p < 0.001$), while the PFS generated by CTD was comparable to cyclophosphamide-VAD (median, 27 versus 25 months; $p = 0.59$). The regimen of CyBorD led to 70% CR/near complete response (nCR) rates post-ASCT. The grouping of PAD significantly enhanced PFS compared with VAD (35 to 28 months; $p = 0.002$). The combination of bortezomib and IMiDs has displayed similar outcomes. Bortezomib-thalidomide-dexamethasone (BTD) was preferable to TD in view of a superior CR/nCR rate achieved with BTD induction compared with TD (55% versus 41%; $p \leq 0.002$) as well as three-year PFS (68% versus 56%; $p < 0.006$) (Cavo et al., 2013).

Because of these encouraging results, a triple combination that includes corticosteroids joined with a PI and/or an IMiD, and/or a cytotoxic agent (cyclophosphamide or doxorubicin) currently is considered the standard of care for induction for ASCT. ASCT using high-dose melphalan as a preparatory regimen is congruent with novel agents and augments the rate of CR and VGPR, even in the setting of high tumor cell mass reduction influenced by modern induction treatments. In numerous phase III studies, the benefit attained by novel agents assimilated into the ASCT regimen in terms of improved first-rate responses translated into protracted PFS and, notwithstanding less frequently, OS. Attainment of traditionally defined CR following induction therapy and ASCT is correlated with better outcomes and signifies a key culmination of existing treatment approaches combining up-front ASCT. Conversely, improving the depth of response to the point of indiscernible minimal residual disease and preserving a lasting CR are more durable forecasters of promising long-standing outcomes than achievement of CR as such (Cherry et al., 2013).

In general, stem cell mobilization and collection are not adversely affected by thalidomide treatment. However, lower stem cell yields have been reported in patients receiving lenalidomide-containing induction therapy. It has been suggested that stem cell collection should be pursued within six months of initiating lenalidomide, or following cyclophosphamide plus G-CSF mobilization, for which no impairment was observed. Also, the use of novel stem cell mobilizers like plerixafor appears to overcome the lower stem cell yield observed after lenalidomide therapy. Bortezomib does not exhibit long-term myelotoxic characteristics and does not negatively affect cell yield or stem cell mobilization, therefore allowing for adequate collection of peripheral blood stem cells. Alkylating agents such as melphalan should be avoided because they are damaging to stem cells and will make it difficult to collect stem cells for a future transplant (Al-Farsi, 2013; Harousseau, 2010).

The concept of applying all active therapeutic agents in Total Therapy (TT) clinical trials for newly diagnosed multiple myeloma was pursued with the intent of developing curative treatment. The results of TT1 (n = 231), TT2 (n = 668), and TT3 (n = 303) have been reported. All three protocols used melphalan (200 mg/m^2)-based tandem transplants. TT1 was a phase II trial that used three cycles of VAD, high-dose cyclophosphamide for stem cell mobilization, and etoposide, dexamethasone, cytarabine, cisplatin, and interferon-α2b as maintenance therapy until relapse or intolerance (Zangari et al., 2008). In TT2, a phase III trial, patients were randomized to an experimental arm with thalidomide added from the outset and continuing throughout consolidation and maintenance (Barlogie, Tricot, et al., 2006). Induction consisted of VAD followed by DCEP (dexamethasone and four-day continuous infusions of cyclophosphamide, etoposide, and cisplatin), cyclophosphamide, doxorubicin, dexamethasone with collection of peripheral blood stem cells, and a further cycle of DCEP. Consolidation varied and eventually utilized DPACE (dexamethasone and four-day continuous infusions of cisplatin, doxorubicin, cyclophosphamide, and etoposide) quarterly for one year. Maintenance therapy consisted of dexamethasone pulsing in year one with interferon-α2b, which was continued indefinitely until recurrence or intolerance. TT3 was a phase II trial that utilized two cycles of VTD-PACE (bortezomib, thalidomide, and dexamethasone and four-day continuous infusions of cisplatin, doxorubicin, cyclophosphamide, and etoposide) as induction before and consolidation therapy following melphalan-based tandem ASCT, which was followed by three years of maintenance with VTD in year one and TD in years two and three. An update with median follow-up times of 17.1, 8.7, and 5.5 years, respectively, revealed that OS, PFS, and CR duration all improved with the transitions from TT1 to TT2 to TT3 (Barlogie et al., 2007). Improvement also was apparent in time to progression (TTP) estimates, four-year conditional survival data, and cumulative relative survival. Interval-specific relative survival normalized progressively sooner, reaching near-normal levels with TT3 in patients who achieved a CR. The authors concluded that a strategy utilizing all myeloma-effective agents up front appeared to be effective at preventing the outgrowth of resistant tumor cells that constitute ongoing relapses (Usmani et al., 2013).

More recently, Nair et al. (2010) published the results of TT3 in gene expression profiling (GEP) when compared to a successor trial 2006-66 with bortezomib/lenalidomide/dexamethasone maintenance. Results revealed superior outcomes, especially in GEP-defined low-risk multiple myeloma, compared with its predecessor TT2. In further analyses examining the timeliness of completion of intended protocol steps, the authors concluded that the improved results in TT3 versus TT2 were attributable to the integration of bortezomib up front in TT3 (Pineda-Roman et al., 2008). The trial 2006-66 was conducted to validate these results and bortezomib pharmacogenomics data. One hundred seventy-seven patients were enrolled. The trials were identical in design, except that the maintenance phases in 2006-66 included three years, rather than one year, of bortezomib and used lenalidomide instead of thalidomide (Nair et al., 2010). Clinical outcomes in the two studies were comparable except for a higher incidence of several adverse features in 2006-66: albumin less than 3.5 g/dl (45% versus 26%, $p < 0.001$) and beta-2 microglobulin ($\beta 2M$) greater than or equal to 3.5 mg/L (57% versus 45%, $p = 0.12$), resulting in higher incidence of International Staging System (ISS) stages 2 and 3 (70% versus 55%, $p < 0.001$). GEP-defined high risk also was more frequent in 2006-66 (22% versus 15%, $p = 0.038$), and GEP-defined CD-1 molecular subgroup also was overrepresented in 2006-66 (11% versus 5%, $p = 0.037$), whereas myeloid designation was underrepresented (3% versus 14%, $p < 0.001$). The results revealed, with the exception of faster CR onset in 2006-66, similar Kaplan-Meier plots for OS, EFS, and CR duration (Nair et al., 2010).

Carfilzomib as an Induction Agent

The PI carfilzomib is a tetrapeptide epoxyketone-based inhibitor of the chymotrypsin-like activity of the 20S proteasome. It is more selective and associated with fewer side effects, including less neuropathy and less myelosuppression, than bortezomib. Unlike bortezomib, carfilzomib is an irreversible PI (El-Amm & Tabbara, 2015).

The combination of carfilzomib, thalidomide, and dexamethasone was studied in the frontline setting of transplant-eligible patients. The updated results of the first 40 enrolled patients in this phase II trial were presented at the 2012 American Society of Hematology annual meeting. An ORR was achieved in 68% of the patients after one cycle. PFS was 97% at 12 months, and OS was 100% at a median follow-up of 10.4 months. Responses occurred across ISS stages and in both standard-risk and high-risk subgroups, and stem cell harvest was not affected (El-Amm & Tabbara, 2015).

El-Amm and Tabbara (2015) reported on the results of a phase II dose expansion trial of cyclophosphamide, carfilzomib, thalidomide, and dexamethasone (CYCLONE) in patients with newly diagnosed multiple myeloma intended for ASCT (Mikhael et al., 2012). The trial accrued 38 patients, and results of the 27 patients who completed therapy with dose level 0 (20 mg/m^2 for cycle 1 followed by 27 mg/m^2 for the following cycles) were presented. The best ORR during four cycles of CYCLONE was 96% (CR 29%, VGPR 46%, and PR 21%). Participants experienced manageable toxicities with only grade 1 neuropathy and minimal cardiac and pulmonary toxicities. Ongoing trials of carfilzomib in the first-line setting will help to answer the question as to whether this second-generation novel agent will show superiority over bortezomib and lenalidomide. The low incidence of peripheral neuropathy and decreased hematologic side effects, as well as its efficacy, make carfilzomib a potential future first-line agent in transplant-eligible patients (El-Amm & Tabbara, 2015).

Transplantation in Patients With Relapsed/Refractory Myeloma

Treatment of relapsed/refractory multiple myeloma with ASCT or alloSCT has been investigated in a number of studies. Second ASCT generally is regarded as a suitable possibility in selected patients. Its success seems to be guided by the success of the previous transplant, the number of prior therapies, the extent of previous toxicities, age, and performance status, as well as the interval between the first and second transplant (Al-Farsi, 2013; Attal et al., 2003). Usually, the longer the interval between the first ASCT and disease relapse, the better the outcome after the salvage second ASCT. It is approximated that the use of novel therapeutics has increased the median OS by 50% (Al-Farsi, 2013; Harousseau, 2010). While these agents and ASCT have clearly improved response rates, their use in the induction therapy setting has created a new set of challenges when determining how to manage patients who relapse following exposure to one or more of these agents during their initial therapy (Al-Farsi, 2013; Harousseau, 2010).

The addition of a second ASCT could be considered in the patient who achieved a CR following ASCT and maintained disease-free survival for approximately three years. Existing data on second ASCT for relapsed patients imply that a subsequent ASCT is relatively well tolerated, with a 110-day mortality of 2%–8%. Of late, studies of second, salvage transplants include a considerable percentage of patients who have received thalidomide, lenalidomide, or bortezomib during induction. The ORR in studies completed in recent years ranges from 55% to 69%. Due to lack of significant numbers of patients enrolled in these studies, it has been challenging to identify key factors in selecting ideal candidates to undergo a repeat ASCT. In spite of this, one small study proposed that a relapse-free survival of greater than 18 months following the first ASCT is the most reliable predictor of clinical outcome after a second ASCT. Although there are no official recommendations, the prevailing school of thought is that a salvage transplant with the goal of producing long-term remission should be offered only to those patients who achieved a durable response of 18–24 months in the wake of their first ASCT (Al-Farsi, 2013; Harousseau, 2010).

Moreover, the use of alloSCT has been investigated in a number of recent studies and also may be reasonable in the relapsed/refractory setting. It has been suggested that alloSCT may be effective in patients with high-risk disease, but that currently remains an investigational approach with some studies showing no overall benefit (Al-Farsi, 2013). Other studies suggest the role of alloSCT may be a curative therapy in 10%–20% of patients in the relapsed refractory setting (Efebera et al., 2010). This is due to a tumor-free graft and improved survival associated with an immunologically mediated graft-versus-myeloma (GVM) effect similar to the graft-versus-leukemia effect (Mehta & Singhal, 1998). With the use of reduced-intensity conditioning (RIC) regimens, more patients have received this treatment modality as upfront therapy, at relapse, or as a tandem following ASCT. However, a significant portion of patients experience treatment-related morbidities, including infection and chronic graft-versus-host disease (GVHD) (Kuruvilla et al., 2007). Unfortunately, the majority of patients might not be eligible because of advanced age, comorbidities, and lack of available HLA-matched donors (Al-Farsi, 2013). Finally, the prospective data for salvage alloSCT in the era of novel agents are limited and, until its safety and efficacy are established, salvage ASCT only should be used in the context of a clinical trial (National Comprehensive Cancer Network, 2015).

Although matched related alloSCT has demonstrated reduced relapse rates and improved survival, only 25%–30% of patients have a matched sibling donor (Ballen et al., 2005). Another option is SCT using matched unrelated donors. The results of a study utilizing myeloablative SCT with matched unrelated donors demonstrated poor survival with a five-year OS of only 9% with high treatment-related mortality (TRM) of 42% resulting from infection, GVHD, and other toxicities (Ballen et al., 2005). However, when nonmyeloablative unrelated donor transplantation is used following cytoreductive ASCT, responses are significantly better. Georges et al. (2007) conducted a study to determine the long-term outcomes of unrelated donor nonmyeloablative SCT in patients with poor-risk multiple myeloma. Investigators concluded that unrelated SCT is an effective treatment approach with low nonrelapse mortality, high complete remission rates, and prolonged disease-free survival. A total of 24 patients were enrolled with 17 patients (71%) having chemotherapy-refractory disease and 14 (58%) experiencing disease relapse or progression after previous autologous transplantation. Thirteen patients underwent planned autologous transplantation followed with unrelated transplantation, and 11 patients proceeded directly to unrelated transplantation. All 24 patients were treated with fludarabine (90 mg/m^2) and

2 Gy of total body irradiation (TBI) before HLA-matched unrelated SCT. At three years, OS and PFS rates were 61% and 33%, respectively. Patients receiving tandem autologous unrelated SCT had superior OS at 77% and PFS 51% compared to only 44% OS and 11% PFS in patients proceeding directly to unrelated donor transplantation (PFS p = 0.03).

Nonmyeloablative or Reduced-Intensity Allogeneic Stem Cell Transplantation

Because of the high toxicity associated with myeloablative alloSCT, nonmyeloablative, or RIC, alloSCT has been investigated. The rationale is to exploit the sensitivity of the myeloma cell to irradiation and alkylating agents and the ability of the newly transplanted immunocompetent cells to mount a GVM effect (Hunter et al., 2005). The goal is to utilize the antitumor effect of the GVM reaction while reducing the treatment-related complications of high-dose conditioning by inducing maximum cytoreduction. Common regimens include high-dose chemotherapy (usually high-dose melphalan) with ASCT support followed by consolidation with RIC alloSCT (Bjorkstrand, 2005). Figure 5-3 lists various RIC regimens.

Bruno et al. (2007) studied the outcomes of tandem transplant protocols requiring an initial ASCT followed by a second ASCT or an allograft from an HLA-identical sibling. A total of 58 patients completed the autograft-allograft treatment and 46 patients completed the double-autologous transplant regimen from September 1998 through July 2004. Patients with HLA-identical siblings received nonmyeloablative TBI and sibling stem cells; patients without HLA-identical siblings received two consecutive doses of myeloablative melphalan followed by ASCT. After a median follow-up of 45 months (range 2–90 months), patients with HLA-matched siblings demonstrated 80 months median OS and 54 months EFS compared to 54 months median OS and 29 months EFS in the double ASCT group. Interestingly, the TRM did not differ significantly between the two groups. The disease-related mortality was significantly higher in the double ASCT group (43% versus 7%, p < 0.001). The recipients of auto-allograft tandem transplantation appear to have superior OS and EFS (Bruno et al., 2007; Carella et al., 2004). The superiority of RIC alloSCT is similarly highlighted in a study by the PETHEMA/GEM group (Rosiñol et al., 2008) and one by the Gruppo Italiano Trapianti di Midollo (Bruno et al., 2007). The tandem transplant approach with nonmyeloablative allografting allows prolonged survival and long-term disease control in patients. Dose-reduced–intensity conditioning regimen for alloSCT reduced TRM to 10%–20% with approximately 40%–50% CR rates (Bladé & Rosiñol, 2009).

Efebera et al. (2010) reported the results of 51 patients with heavily pretreated, relapsed multiple myeloma who received RIC alloSCT from a matched related or unrelated donor between 1996 and 2006. Patients aged 18–70 with a performance status of 0 or 1, adequate organ function, and no uncontrolled infections were eligible to participate. Donor bone marrow or G-CSF–primed peripheral blood progenitor cells were collected using standard mobilization protocols and apheresis techniques. Bone marrow from unrelated donors was obtained from the National Marrow Donor Program according to standard guidelines. The RIC regimen consisted of fludarabine (90–120 mg/m^2). Patients who received unrelated donor cells also received antithymocyte globulin as part of their conditioning regimen. GVHD prophylaxis consisted of a combination of tacrolimus and methotrexate. Filgrastim 5 mcg/kg was administered subcutaneously daily from seven days after alloSCT until the recovery of ANC to greater than 1.5×10^9/L for three days. Overall, 12 patients achieved a CR and 26 patients (51%) achieved a PR, with an ORR of 74% following RIC alloSCT. Three patients (6%) had minimal response (less than 50%) and four patients (8%) had stable disease. Two out of three patients with a VGPR pretransplant achieved a CR. Of the 23 patients in PR prior to alloSCT, 4 (17%) achieved a CR, 1 developed PD, and the rest remained in PR; of the 14 patients in SD prior to alloSCT, 3 (21%) achieved a CR and 7 (50%) achieved a PR/VGPR; and of the 8 patients with PD at alloSCT, 1 achieved a CR and 3 achieved a PR, with an ORR of 50% in this group. Seven patients, who received alloSCT from a matched related donor, received a total of 12 donor lymphocyte infusions (DLI) for persistent disease (PD) or relapse after alloSCT. One patient with PD obtained a CR, and one with PD achieved VGPR after one DLI, with the rest having no response. The cumulative incidence of grade II–IV GVHD was 27%. Grade II acute GVHD was seen in 16%, while grade III–IV acute GVHD was seen in 11%. Cumulative incidence of chronic GVHD was 47% with limited chronic GVHD in 23% of patients. Of note, the use of unrelated donor or peripheral blood stem cells as the graft source did not increase the incidence of acute or chronic GVHD. Day 100 TRM was 12%, and one-year TRM was 25%. The most common causes of death were recurrent disease (22 patients; 43%), acute or chronic GVHD (10 patients; 20%), and opportunistic infections (3 patients; 6%). Median follow-up for surviving patients was 27 months. Twenty-five patients (49%) had relapsed at two years. Seven patients received a total of 12 DLI. The use of DLI did not contribute to an improvement in PFS and OS on multivariate and univariate analyses. The investigators believe this is perhaps because of the small number of patients who underwent DLI. The two-year PFS and OS were 19% and 32%, respectively. On univariate analyses, a lower β2M (less than 3.3) and a prior ASCT predicted longer PFS and OS. These two factors also emerged as predictors of longer PFS and OS in a multivariate analysis. Age, immunoglobulin subtype, serum lactate dehydrogenase, serum albumin, stem cell source, donor type, use of DLI, interval between diagnosis and alloSCT, or interval between ASCT and alloSCT did not emerge as statistically significant predictors of outcome (Efebera et al., 2010).

Transplantation in Older Adults

The role of transplantation in older adults has yet to be defined. Factoring in improved life expectancy of the general population and increased performance status of patients older than 65 years, the treatment model of multiple myeloma is being reevaluated (Lahuerta et al., 2003). Inconsistent data with an approach utilizing dose-reduced melphalan (100 mg/m^2) as conditioning for ASCT (MEL100-ASCT) have been reported. One study revealed that MEL100-ASCT was equivalent to melphalan and prednisone (MP) in patients ages 65–75. In another study, MEL100-ASCT was superior to MP in patients 65–75 years of age (Giralt et al., 2009).

A phase II study investigated the safety and efficacy of a sequential approach including a three-drug bortezomib-based induction, intermediate-dose melphalan (MEL100), and ASCT, followed by lenalidomide-based consolidation-maintenance treatment in older adults eligible for transplantation. Newly diagnosed patients with multiple myeloma 65–75 years of age (N = 102) received four cycles of bortezomib-pegylated liposomal doxorubicin-dexamethasone, tandem melphalan (100 mg/m^2) followed by ASCT (MEL100-ASCT), four cycles of lenalidomide-prednisone (LP) consolidation, and lenalidomide (L) maintenance until disease progression. The CR rate was 33% after MEL100-ASCT, 48% after LP, and 53% after L maintenance. After a median follow-up of 66 months, median TTP was 55 months and median PFS was 48 months. Median OS was not reported; five-year OS was 63%. In patients who achieved CR, median TTP was 70 months and five-year OS was 83%. Median survival from relapse was 28 months. Eight deaths occurred related to adverse events reported during induction or transplantation. The rate of death was higher in patients age 70 or older when compared to younger patients (5/26 versus 3/76, p = 0.024). These favorable outcomes may represent a reasonable treatment option for older adult patients without comorbidities and excellent performance status (Gay et al., 2013).

Late Effects of Stem Cell Transplantation

Improvements in SCT science and progress in supportive care have enhanced long-term survival. However, survivors are at risk for developing delayed complications resulting from pre-, peri-, and post-transplant exposures. These complications may lead to significant morbidity and mortality and reduced quality of life (Majhail et al., 2012).

Late complications of HDT and SCT can be wide ranging and difficult to manage. Every organ system is potentially affected, and long-term follow-up guidelines are in place for screening and prevention of delayed transplant complications. Examples of these include infection as well as respiratory, ocular, oral, hepatic, renal, skeletal, neurologic, cardiac, and vascular problems (Majhail et al., 2012). Secondary primary malignancies also are a late complication for the transplant recipient (Faiman et al., 2013; Majhail et al., 2012). Risk factors associated with the development of secondary malignancies include TBI, primary disease, male sex, and pretransplant therapy. Although many late complications are associated with allogeneic recipients such as chronic GVHD, it is important to recognize that autologous transplant recipients also are at risk for late complications as well (Majhail et al., 2012) (see Figure 5-4).

The risk of infection in transplant recipients is estimated to be 20 times higher than that reported in the general population for months to years following transplantation. Common bacterial infections include pneumococcal, streptococcal, and haemophilus organisms. Common viral infections include cytomegalovirus and reactivation of *Varicella zoster*. Hepatitis B or C also can occur (Savani, Griffith, Jagasia, & Lee, 2011).

In addition, patients are prone to developing cardiovascular disease including dyslipidemia, hypertension, diabetes, and kidney disease. The incidence of cardiovascular disease increases after transplantation and is presumed to be attributed to GVHD, use of immunosuppressant agents, and the cumulative effects of chemotherapy. Other cardiovascular complications include cardiomyopathies, arrhythmias, or valvular dysfunction (Majhail et al., 2012; Savani et al., 2011).

Although guidelines for long-term complications are available, barriers for implementation exist. Insurance coverage, insufficient reimbursement for screening, insufficient knowledge, and suboptimal communication regarding guidelines are examples for reasons for guideline noncompliance (Faiman et al., 2013).

Post-Transplantation Needs

Following completion of SCT, patients often describe a "let down" feeling. They may feel unprepared for and overwhelmed about "the next step" as they realize that transplant events are coming to an end. The psychological impact of post-transplantation should be addressed. Recovery may be associated with physical setbacks as well as financial and emotional strain for patients and caregivers. Rates of depression following SCT are estimated to

Figure 5-4. Special Interest: HSCT, Allogeneic HSCT, and Acute GVHD

Allogeneic HSCT uses HDC similar to autologous HSCT, but instead uses HSCs from a donor. The donor cells are used to reconstitute the bone marrow function after HDC while producing a new immune system in the recipient. The new immune function can provide a graft-versus-tumor benefit, but is associated with high treatment-related mortality from intensive conditioning regimens, infection associated with immunosuppression, and GVHD.

Acute GVHD is a major complication of allogeneic HSCT associated with significant morbidity and mortality. GVHD occurs when donor-derived cells recognize recipient tissue as foreign and mount an immune attack against the patient's own tissues, which occurs in 40%–60% of patients undergoing allogeneic HSCT. Although GVHD is a complication of transplantation, it also is considered a treatment for multiple myeloma. As GVHD occurs, graft-versus-myeloma causes an antitumor effect mediated by the donor graft.

Clinical manifestations of acute GVHD can be seen in the immune system, skin, gut, and liver. Transplantation recipients with acute GVHD may present with rash (81%), gut (54%), and liver (50%) symptoms. Acute GVHD has a significant impact on the immune system. Immune reconstitution is an integral part in the prevention of opportunistic infections, and infection is the most frequent cause of death in transplantation recipients who experience acute GVHD. Not only does prolonged myelosuppression occur in these patients, thymic involution and hypogammaglobulinemia further weaken the immune system.

A skin rash often is the initial symptom associated with acute GVHD. The rash typically is described as maculopapular, and often begins in the anterior or posterior torso, neck, palmar and plantar surfaces, and ears. The typical rash can range from a sunburn-like appearance to desquamating and peeling skin.

The symptoms of gastrointestinal acute GVHD include nausea, emesis, diarrhea, abdominal cramping, and pain. Hematochezia, ileus, and anorexia are other notable side effects associated with acute GVHD.

Liver acute GVHD is caused by damage to the bile canaliculi, which can cause cholestasis with hyperbilirubinemia and elevated alkaline phosphatase. The severity of liver acute GVHD is based on the serum bilirubin.

Ruling out other causes of organ dysfunction, such as drug toxicity (skin, gut, liver), viral infection (gut, liver), and sinusoidal obstructive syndrome (liver), is important. Prevention of acute GVHD begins with donor selection and continues with immunosuppressive medication to decrease T-cell activation and proliferation.

Common medications used in the prevention and treatment of GVHD include cyclosporine, methotrexate, mycophenolate mofetil, steroids, sirolimus, and tacrolimus. In addition, bortezomib is an experimental medication for this use.

GVHD—graft-versus-host disease; HDC—high-dose chemotherapy; HSC—hematopoietic stem cell; HSCT—hematopoietic stem cell transplantation

Note. Based on information from Antin & Raley, 2009; El-Cheikh et al., 2013; Koreth et al., 2012; Laffan & Biedrzycki, 2006; Lokhorst et al., 2010; Martin et al., 1990; Mattson, 2007; Pallera & Schwartzberg, 2004; Sung & Chao, 2013.

From "Clinical Updates in Blood and Marrow Transplantation in Multiple Myeloma," by B. Faiman, T. Miceli, K. Noonan, and K. Lilleby, 2013, *Clinical Journal of Oncology Nursing, 17*(Suppl. 6), p. 35. Copyright 2013 by Oncology Nursing Society. Reprinted with permission.

range from 25%–50% (Cooke, Grant, & Gemmill, 2012; Miceli et al., 2013). Depression may have an adverse effect on physical health, may increase symptom-related fatigue and distress, and has been associated with a higher incidence of suicide. Early symptom detection and prompt intervention are vital for overall patient well-being. In some instances, referrals to psychiatry or social services or prescribing of antidepressant medications may be warranted. Caregivers and family members should be educated on the incidence, signs and symptoms, and transplant team contact information should indications of post-transplant depression arise (Cooke et al., 2012; Miceli et al., 2013).

Immunizations

The transplantation process results in a loss of T and B lymphocytes, thus causing loss of immune memory. Immune memory is shaped by the culmination of exposure to infectious agents, environmental antigens, and vaccines during the course of a lifetime. For this reason, patients will require reimmunization post-transplantation (Miceli et al., 2013; Stadtmauer et al., 2011).

Guidelines for post-transplantation immunizations vary by institution. Based on the Centers for Disease Control and Prevention and Advisory Committee on Immune Practices (2011) recommendations, non-live vaccines may be administered as early as three months post-transplantation. Live-attenuated vaccines may be administered two years following transplantation in immune-competent individuals (Kroger, Sumaya, Pickering, & Atkinson, 2011; Tomblyn et al., 2009). An example of a post-transplantation immunization schedule can be found in Table 5-4.

Maintenance Therapy

Maintenance therapy is given for a prolonged period of time with the purpose of extending the duration of response by controlling the malignant clone, thus extending PFS and OS while maintaining a good quality of life (Sahebi et al., 2006). This notion had been established in the past with interferon alpha, but the advantage was not deemed sufficient to warrant the costs and toxicities linked to prolonged administration. In the setting of HDT/ASCT, interferon-based maintenance is associated with minimal improvements in clinical outcomes but is poorly tolerated. Progress has been made in myeloma therapy since the introduction of IMiDs. These novel agents recently have become the focal point of interest for maintenance therapy (Badros, 2010).

The use of thalidomide was investigated in maintenance studies because of its lack of severe hematologic toxicity and its oral formulation. A meta-analysis of six thalidomide maintenance trials (Sahebi et al., 2012) con-

Table 5-4. Post-Transplantation Immunization Schedule

Organism	Vaccine	Time Post-HSCT to Initiate Vaccine	Dose and Route	Comments
Inactivated Vaccines				
Pneumococcus	PCV7/PPSV23	3–6 months	0.5 ml IM or SC	Can be given 6 months post-transplantation
Pertussis, tetanus, diphtheria	DTAP	6–12 months	0.5 ml IM	Can be given 6 months post-transplantation
Haemophilus influenzae type B	HIB	6–12 months	0.5 ml IM	Can be given 6 months post-transplantation
Hepatitis B	–	6–12 months	0.5 ml IM	Administer to patients who are hepatitis B virus negative.
Meningococcus	–	6–12 months	0.5 ml SC	Recommended in areas with an increase in meningococcus
Influenza	–	4–6 months	0.5 ml IM (the nasal version is live and, therefore, not recommended)	Give annually as available in the autumn months. May administer 4 months post-transplantation; however, two doses of the vaccine are suggested.
Live Virus Vaccines				
Measles, mumps, and rubella	MMR	24 months	0.5 ml SC	MMR should not be given if the patient is immunosuppressed.
Varicella zoster virus (shingles)	Zoster vaccine	Not currently recommended. Clinical trials are ongoing.	–	Not currently recommended; inactivated version is under investigation. Prevention with antiviral medication is recommended.

HSCT—hematopoietic stem cell transplantation; IM—intramuscular; SC—subcutaneous

Note. Based on information from Cordonnier et al., 2010; Kroger et al., 2011; Ljungman et al., 2009; Tomblyn et al., 2009.

From "Autologous Hematopoietic Stem Cell Transplantation for Patients With Multiple Myeloma: An Overview for Nurses in Community Practice," by T. Miceli, K. Lilleby, K. Noonan, S. Kurtin, B. Faiman, and P.A. Mangan, 2013, Clinical Journal of Oncology Nursing, 17(Suppl. 6), p. 21. Copyright 2013 by Oncology Nursing Society. Reprinted with permission.

firmed the improvement of both PFS (hazard ratio [HR] = 0.65, p < 0.01) and a trend toward significant improvement in OS (HR = 0.83, p < 0.07). The OS improvement was more pronounced in subgroups using corticosteroids with thalidomide as maintenance (HR = 0.70, p = 0.02). There was increased incidence of venous thrombosis (risk difference, 0.024; p < 0.05) and peripheral neuropathy associated with thalidomide maintenance. The adverse effects of thalidomide restricted long-term use, with the median interval of thalidomide maintenance averaging 7–24 months (Sahebi et al., 2006). Morgan et al. (2013) also conducted a meta-analysis on thalidomide maintenance in transplant and nontransplant patients with multiple myeloma and found no OS advantage. Consequently, although post-ASCT treatment with thalidomide seems to improve outcomes, its use has not been approved in this indication. Furthermore, a number of questions remain related to the recommended daily dose and optimal duration of maintenance therapy.

Toxicities associated with thalidomide's side effects prompted the pursuit of an agent with comparable or superior efficacy and less toxicity. Lenalidomide seems to be an excellent drug for long-term maintenance therapy because of its oral formulation, absence of neurologic toxicities, and dual mechanism of action (Cherry et al., 2013). Of late, three large phase III trials evaluating lenalidomide maintenance compared to placebo found PFS benefits for both ASCT-eligible and ASCT-ineligible patients. Randomized studies (from the Cancer and Leukemia Group B [CALGB] and from the Intergroupe Francophone du Myélome [IFM]) examined low-dose lenalidomide or placebo until progression as post-HDT/ASCT maintenance therapy. Study designs were similar, with the exception that in the IFM study all patients obtained consolidation with full-dose lenalidomide following ASCT. Outcomes in these studies suggest lenalidomide maintenance considerably improved PFS or TTP. Until now this benefit has not consistently translated into prolonged OS. A critical finding from these studies is that lenalidomide looks as if it prolongs PFS across all prognostic subgroups using type of induction treatment and status at transplantation, β2M level, and chromosome 13 deletion by fluorescence in situ hybridization (Cherry et al., 2013). Largely, grade 3–4 adverse events were related to neutropenia and infection as well as a higher incidence of second primary cancers (7%–8%) in the lenalidomide arm. Given reports of a survival benefit with lenalidomide maintenance in the CALGB study, the significance of these findings is not entirely clear (Al-Farsi, 2013). The U.S. Food and Drug Administration (2012) has encouraged providers to evaluate the advantages of lenalidomide therapy against the risk of second primary malignancies and to observe patients closely.

One phase III randomized trial interrogates the role of bortezomib maintenance in the transplant setting. Patients who were randomly assigned to PAD or VAD induction followed by ASCT received bortezomib or thalidomide as maintenance therapy, respectively. Bortezomib maintenance considerably improved CR/nCR, from 31% to 49%, and reduced the risk of progression (p = 0.04). With bortezomib maintenance, the outcomes showed improved CR and superior PFS and OS. The incidence of grade 3–4 peripheral neuropathy was 5%, and grade 3–4 infections were 24%. The median time on therapy was approximately two years in the bortezomib group and one year in the thalidomide group (Sonneveld et al., 2012). Uy and colleagues also have used bortezomib as a pretransplant induction therapy followed by post-transplant bortezomib therapy (Uy et al., 2009).

In a phase II study, lenalidomide (25 mg/day for 21 days) was combined with standard-dose, twice-weekly bortezomib and dexamethasone to form a triplet regimen (RVD) that was given as induction therapy prior to consolidation and after a single ASCT. The primary study endpoint evaluated best overall response achieved after two three-week cycles of RVD consolidation. The rate of CR, including stringent CR, observed among 31 patients who were enrolled was 42% after ASCT and 48% after RVD consolidation. Overall, consolidation therapy improved responses in 26% of patients, but only one patient had undetectable minimal residual disease assessed by flow cytometry (Cherry et al., 2013). Similarly, bortezomib has been combined with thalidomide and dexamethasone for maintenance use following single ASCT. Researchers reported significant improvement in CR following maintenance (32% versus 53%) with no significant peripheral neuropathy (Sahebi et al., 2012).

Conclusion

Currently, high-dose chemotherapy followed by ASCT is considered to be standard first-line consolidation therapy in multiple myeloma. In 2000, only two classes of anticancer drugs were active in myeloma: alkylating agents, including high-dose melphalan, and corticosteroids, including high-dose dexamethasone. The improved understanding of myeloma cell biology and advancement in translational research brought about a new era of therapeutic approaches for patients with myeloma (Giralt et al., 2009). IMiDs and PIs have now been added to the arsenal. Despite the improvements reported with conventional chemotherapy plus novel agents, ASCT remains a necessary component of therapy to attain CR and consequently superior PFS (Cavo et al., 2013). The precipitous development of these promising agents with diverse mechanisms of action poses questions on (a) the optimal induction treatment and sequencing of agents in newly diagnosed symptomatic myeloma and (b) whether an aggressive approach with HDT/ASCT is still necessary, or at least in which patients (Al-Farsi, 2013). In spite of positive developments in myeloma therapy and improved responses reported in clinical trials, the influence of novel agents in an unselected population needs to be established.

Even with the very high response rates reported with various induction regimens, consolidation with high-dose chemotherapy, and ASCT, followed by a variety of maintenance regimens, the sizeable majority of patients with myeloma eventually will relapse and become refractory to treatment. Additional studies are warranted to further investigate the role of transplantation, consolidation, and maintenance therapy. By optimizing the advantages of the detection of new targets, emerging targeted therapies, and evidence-based combination therapies, the eradication of resistant myeloma clones becomes feasible, potentially leading to a cure for the disease.

Survivors of SCT are prone to develop complications throughout their lifetime. Recognition and management of side effects and long-term and short-term problems are essential elements of the transplant process. Nurses require sufficient education and training to develop the knowledge and skills necessary to detect impending complications and carry out approaches to manage both short- and long-term challenges. Oncology nurses should strive to maintain expert knowledge of the changing paradigms in the treatment of multiple myeloma to perform comprehensive assessments and provide individualized care planning and patient education, thus leading to improved overall survival outcomes and enhanced quality of life for patients with myeloma.

The author would like to acknowledge Anna Liza Rodriguez, RN, MSN, MHA, OCN®, for her contribution to this chapter that remains unchanged from the first edition of this book.

References

Al-Farsi, K. (2013). Multiple myeloma: An update. *Oman Medical Journal, 28,* 3–11. doi:10.5001/omj.2013.02

Amgen Inc. (2013). *Neupogen® (filgrastim)* [Package insert]. Retrieved from http://pi.amgen.com/united_states/neupogen/neupogen_pi_hcp_english.pdf

Antin, J.H., & Raley, D.Y. (2009). Stem cell sources. In J.H. Antin & D.Y. Raley (Eds.), *Manual of stem cell and bone marrow transplantation* (pp. 9–15). New York, NY: Cambridge University Press. doi:10.1017/CBO9780511575785.005

Attal, M., Harousseau, J.L., Facon, T., Guilhot, F., Doyen, C., Fuzibet, J.G., ... Bataille, R. (2003). Single versus double autologous stem-cell transplantation for multiple myeloma. *New England Journal of Medicine, 349,* 2495–2502. doi:10.1056/NEJMoa032290

Attal, M., Harousseau, J.L., Stoppa, A.M., Sotto, J.J., Fuzibet, J.G., Rossi, J.F., ... Bataille, R. (1996). A prospective randomized trial of autologous bone marrow transplantation and chemotherapy in multiple myeloma. *New England Journal of Medicine, 335,* 91–97. doi:10.1056/NEJM199607113350204

Badros, A.Z. (2010). The role of maintenance therapy in the treatment of multiple myeloma. *Journal of the National Comprehensive Cancer Network, 8*(Suppl. 1), S21–S27.

Ballen, K.K., King, R., Carston, M., Kollman, C., Nelson, G., Lim, S., ... Vesole, D.H. (2005). Outcome of unrelated transplants in patients with multiple myeloma. *Bone Marrow Transplantation, 35,* 675–681. doi:10.1038/sj.bmt.1704868

Barlogie, B. (2014). A randomized phase III trial of CC–5013 (lenalidomide, NSC-703813) and low dose dexamethasone (LLD) versus bortezomib (PS-341, NSC-681239), lenalidomide and low dose dexamethasone (BLLD) for induction, in patients with previously untreated multiple myeloma without an intent for immediate autologous stem cell transplant. Retrieved from http://myeloma.uams.edu/treating-myeloma-2/multiple-myeloma-clinical-trials-and-research/untreated-myeloma-without-intent-for-autologous-transplant

Barlogie, B., Anaissie, E., van Rhee, F., Haessler, J., Hollmig, K., Pineda-Roman, M., ... Mohiuddin, A. (2007). Incorporating bortezomib into upfront treatment for multiple myeloma: Early results of total therapy 3. *British Journal of Haematology, 138,* 176–185. doi:10.1111/j.1365-2141.2007.06639.x

Barlogie, B., Jagannath, S., Vesole, D.H., Naucke, S., Cheson, B., Mattox, S., ... Tricot, G. (1997). Superiority of tandem autologous transplantation over standard therapy for previously untreated multiple myeloma. *Blood, 89,* 789–793.

Barlogie, B., Kyle, R.A., Anderson, K.C., Greipp, P.R., Lazarus, H.M., Hurd, D.D., ... Crowley, J.C. (2006). Standard chemotherapy compared with high-dose chemoradiotherapy for multiple myeloma: Final results of the phase III US Intergroup Trial S4321. *Journal of Clinical Oncology, 24,* 929–936. doi:10.1200/JCO.2005.04.5807

Barlogie, B., Tricot, G., Anaissie, E., Shaughnessy, J., Rasmussen, E., van Rhee, F., ... Crowley, J. (2006). Thalidomide and hematopoietic-cell transplantation for multiple myeloma. *New England Journal of Medicine, 354,* 1021–1030. doi:10.1056/NEJMoa053583

Bensinger, W.I. (2009). Role of autologous and allogeneic stem cell transplantation in myeloma. *Leukemia, 23,* 442–448. doi:10.1038/leu.2008.396

Bergsagel, D.E., Sprague, C.C., Austin, C., & Griffith, K.M. (1962). Evaluation of new chemotherapeutic agents in the treatment of multiple myeloma. IV. L-Phenylalanine mustard (NSC-8806). *Cancer Chemotherapy Reports, 21,* 87–99.

Bertolotti, P., Bilotti, E., Colson, K., Curran, K., Doss, D., Faiman, B., ... Westphal, J. (2008). Management of side effects of novel therapies for multiple myeloma: Consensus statements developed by the International Myeloma Foundation's Nurse Leadership Board. *Clinical Journal of Oncology Nursing, 12*(Suppl. 3), 9–12. doi:10.1188/08.CJON.S1.9-12

Bevans, M., Tierney, D.K., Bruch, C., Burgunder, M., Castro, K., Ford, R., ... Schmit-Pokorny, K. (2009). Hematopoietic stem cell transplantation nursing: A practice variation study [Online exclusive]. *Oncology Nursing Forum, 36,* E317–E325. doi:10.1188/09.ONF.E317-E325

Bjorkstrand, B. (2005). Stem cell transplantation in multiple myeloma. *Hematology, 10*(Suppl. 1), 26–28. doi:10.1080/10245330512331389809

Bilotti, E., Gleason, C.L., McNeill, A., & the IMF Nurse Leadership Board. (2011). Routine health maintenance in patients living with multiple myeloma: Survivorship care plan of the International Myeloma Foundation Nurse Leadership Board. *Clinical Journal of Oncology Nursing, 15*(Suppl. 1), 25–40. doi:10.1188/11.S1.CJON.25-40

Bladé, J., Esteve, J., Rives, S., Martínez, C., Rovira, M., Urbano-Ispizua, A., ... Montserrat, E. (2000). High-dose therapy autotransplantation/intensification vs continued standard chemotherapy in multiple myeloma in first remission. Results of a non-randomized study from a single institution. *Bone Marrow Transplantation, 26,* 845–849. doi:10.1038/sj.bmt.1702622

Bladé, J., & Rosiñol, L. (2009). Changing paradigms in the treatment of multiple myeloma. *Haematologica, 94,* 163–166. doi:10.3324/haematol.2008.002766

Bladé, J., Rosiñol, L., Sureda, A., Ribera, J.M., Díaz-Mediavilla, J., Garcia-Laraña, J., ... San Miguel, J. (2005). High-dose intensification compared with continued standard chemotherapy in multiple myeloma patients responding to the initial chemotherapy: Long-term results from a prospective randomized trial from the Spanish cooperative group PETH-EMA. *Blood, 106,* 3755–3759. doi:10.1182/blood-2005-03-1301

Bladé, J., Samson, D., Reece, D., Apperley, J., Björkstrand, B., Gahrton, G., ... Vesole, D. (1998). Criteria for evaluating disease response and progression in patients with multiple myeloma treated by high-dose therapy and haemopoietic stem cell transplantation. European Group for Blood and Marrow Transplant. *British Journal of Haematology, 102,* 1115–1123. doi:10.1046/j.1365-2141.1998.00930.x

Blombery, P., Prince, H.M., Worth, L.J., Main, J., Yang, M., Wood, E.M., ... Westerman, D.A. (2011). Prophylactic intravenous immunoglobulin during autologous haemopoietic stem cell transplantation for multiple myeloma is not associated with reduced infectious complications. *Annals of Hematology, 90,* 1167–1172. doi:10.1007/s00277-011-1275-3

Bruno, B., Rotta, M., Patriarca, F., Mordini, N., Allione, B., Carnevale-Schianca, F., ... Boccadoro, M. (2007). A comparison of allografting with autografting for newly diagnosed myeloma. *New England Journal of Medicine, 356,* 1110–1120. doi:10.1056/NEJMoa065464

Carella, A.M., Beltrami, G., Corsetti, M.T., Scalzulli, P., Carella, A.M., & Musto, P. (2004). A reduced intensity conditioning regimen for allografting following autografting is feasible and has strong anti-myeloma activity. *Haematologica, 89,* 1534–1536.

Cavo, M., Brioli, A., Tacchetti, P., Zannetti, B.A., Mancuso, K., & Zamagni, E. (2013). Role of consolidation therapy in transplant eligible multiple myeloma patients. *Seminars in Oncology, 40,* 610–617. doi:10.1053/j.seminoncol.2013.07.001

Cavo, M., Rajkumar, S.V., Palumbo, A., Moreau, P., Orlowski, R., Bladé, J., ... Lonial, S. (2011). International myeloma working group consensus approach to the treatment of multiple myeloma patients who are candidates for autologous stem transplantation. *Blood, 117,* 6063–6073. doi:10.1182/blood-2011-02-297325

Celgene Corporation. (2013a). *Pomalyst® (pomalidomide)* [Package insert]. Retrieved from http://www.pomalyst.com/docs/prescribing_information.pdf

Celgene Corporation. (2013b). *Revlimid® (lenalidomide)* [Package insert]. Retrieved from http://www.revlimid.com/pdf/MCL_PI.pdf

Celgene Corporation. (2013c). *Thalomid® (thalidomide)* [Package insert]. Retrieved from http://www.thalomid.com/pdf/Thalomid_PI.pdf

Centers for Disease Control and Prevention and Advisory Committee on Immune Practices. (2011). Vaccination of hematopoietic stem cell transplant (HSCT) recipients. Retrieved from http://www.cdc.gov/vaccines/pubs/hemato-cell-transplts.htm

Cherry, B., Korde, N., Kwok, M., Roschewski, M., & Landgren, O. (2013). Evolving therapeutic paradigms for multiple myeloma: Back to the future. *Leukemia and Lymphoma, 54,* 451–463. doi:10.3109/10428194.2012.717277

Child, J.A., Morgan, G.J., Davies, F.E., Owen, R.G., Bell, S.E., Hawkins, K., ... Selby, P.J. (2003). High-dose chemotherapy with hematopoietic stem cell rescue for multiple myeloma. *New England Journal of Medicine, 348,* 1875–1883. doi:10.1056/NEJMoa022340

Cooke, L., Grant, M., & Gemmill, R. (2012). Discharge needs of allogeneic transplantation recipients [Online exclusive]. *Clinical Journal of Oncology Nursing, 16,* E142–E149. doi:10.1188/12.CJON.E142-E149

Cordonnier, C., Labopin, M., Chesnel, V., Ribaud, P., De La Cámara, R., ... Ljungman, P. (2010). Immune response to the 23-valent polysaccharide pneumococcal vaccine after the 7-valent conjugate vaccine in allogeneic stem cell transplant recipients: Results from the EBMT IDWOPO1 trial. *Vaccine, 28,* 2730–2734. doi:10.1016/j.vaccine.2010.01.025

DiPersio, J.F., Stadtmauer, E.A., Nademanee, A., Micallef, I.N., Stiff, P.J., Kaufman, J.L., ... Calandra, G. (2009). Plerixafor and G-CSF versus placebo and G-CSF to mobilize hematopoietic stem cells for autologous stem cell transplantation in patients with multiple myeloma. *Blood, 113,* 5720–5726. doi:10.1182/blood-2008-08-174946

Djulbegovic, B., & Kumar, A. (2008). Multiple myeloma: Detecting the effects of new treatments. *Lancet. 371,* 1642–1644. doi:10.1016/S0140-6736(08)60704-7

CHAPTER 5. HIGH-DOSE THERAPY AND STEM CELL TRANSPLANTATION

Durie, B.G., Harousseau, J.L., Miguel, J.S., Bladé, J., Barlogie, B., Anderson, K., ... Rajkumar, S.V. (2006). International uniform response criteria for multiple myeloma. *Leukemia, 20,* 1467–1473. doi:10.1038/sj.leu.2404284

Efebera, Y.A., Qureshi, S.R., Cole, S.M., Salbia, R., Pelosini, M., Patel, R., ... Qazilbash, M.H. (2010). Reduced-intensity allogeneic hematopoietic stem cell transplantation for relapsed multiple myeloma. *Biology of Blood and Marrow Transplantation, 16,* 1122–1129. doi:10.1016/j.bbmt.2010.02.015

El-Amm, J., & Tabbara, I.A. (2015). Emerging therapies in multiple myeloma. *American Journal of Clinical Oncology, 38,* 315–321. doi:10.1097/COC.0b013e3182a4676b

El-Cheikh, J., Crocchiolo, R., Furst, S., Stoppa, A.M., Ladaique, P., Faucher, C., ... Blaise, D. (2013). Long-term outcome after allogeneic stem cell transplantation with reduced-intensity conditioning in patients with multiple myeloma. *American Journal of Hematology, 88,* 370–374. doi:10.1002/ajh.23412

Faiman, B., Miceli, T., Noonan, K., & Lilleby, K. (2013). Clinical updates in blood and marrow transplantation in multiple myeloma. *Clinical Journal of Oncology Nursing, 17*(Suppl. 6), 33–41. doi:10.1188/13.CJON.S2.33-41

Faussner, F., & Dempke, W. (2012). Multiple myeloma: Myeloablative therapy with autologous stem cell support versus chemotherapy: A meta-analysis. *Anticancer Research, 32,* 2103–2110.

Fermand, J.P., Katsahian, S., Divine, M., Leblond, V., Dreyfus, F., Macro, M., ... Ravaud, P. (2005). High-dose therapy and autologous blood stem cell transplantation compared with conventional treatment in myeloma patients aged 55 to 65 years. Long-term results of a randomized control trial from the group Myelome-Autogreffe. *Journal of Clinical Oncology, 23,* 9227–9233. doi:10.1200/JCO.2005.03.0551

Gay, F., Magarotto, V., Crippa, C., Pescosta, N., Guglielmelli, F., Cavallo, S., ... Palumbo, A. (2013). Bortezomib induction, reduced-intensity transplantation and lenalidomide consolidation-maintenance for myeloma: Updated results. *Blood, 122,* 1376–1383. doi:10.1182/blood-2013-02-483073

Genzyme Corporation. (2014). *Mozobil® (plerixafor injection)* [Package insert]. Retrieved from http://www.mozobil.com/document/Package_Insert.pdf

Georges, G., Maris, M., Maloney, D.G., Sandmaier, B.M., Sorror, M.L., Shizuru, J.A., ... Storb, R. (2007). Nonmyeloablative unrelated donor hematopoietic cell transplantation for the treatment of patients with poor-risk, relapsed, or refractory multiple myeloma. *Biology of Blood and Marrow Transplantation, 13,* 423–432. doi:10.1016/j.bbmt.2006.11.011

Gertz, M.A., Wolf, R.C., Micallef, I.N., & Gastineau, D.A. (2010). Clinical impact and resource utilization after stem cell mobilization failure in patients with multiple myeloma and lymphoma. *Bone Marrow Transplantation, 45,* 1396–1403. doi:10.1038/bmt.2009.370

Giralt, S., Vesole, D.H., Somlo, G., Krishnan, A., Stadtmauer, E., McCarthy, P., & Pasquini, M.C. (2009). Re: Tandem vs single autologous hematopoietic cell transplantation for the treatment of multiple myeloma: A systematic review and meta-analysis. *Journal of the National Cancer Institute, 101,* 964. doi:10.1093/jnci/djp126

GlaxoSmithKline. (2011). *Alkeran® (melphalan hydrochloride)* [Package insert]. Retrieved from http://www.accessdata.fda.gov/drugsatfda_docs/label/2011/014691s029lbl.pdf

Harousseau, J.L. (2002). High-dose therapy in multiple myeloma. *Annals of Oncology, 13*(Suppl. 4), 49–54. doi:10.1093/annonc/mdf638

Harousseau, J.L. (2007). The allogeneic dilemma. *Bone Marrow Transplantation, 40,* 1123–1128. doi:10.1038/sj.bmt.1705810

Harousseau, J.L. (2010). Ten years of improvement in the management of multiple myeloma: 2000–2010. *Clinical Lymphoma Myeloma and Leukemia, 10,* 424–442. doi:10.3816/CLML.2010.n.076

Hesketh, P.J., Batchelor, D., Golant, M., Lyman, G.H., Rhodes, N., & Yardley, D. (2004). Chemotherapy-induced alopecia: Psychosocial impact and therapeutic approaches. *Supportive Care in Cancer, 12,* 543–549. doi:10.1007/s00520-003-0562-5

Hunter, H.M., Peggs, K., Powles, R., Rahemtulla, A., Mahendra, P., Cavenagh, J., ... Russell, N.H. (2005). Analysis of outcome following allogeneic haematopoietic stem cell transplantation for myeloma using myeloablative conditioning—Evidence for a superior outcome using melphalan combined with total body irradiation. *British Journal of Haematology, 128,* 496–502. doi:10.1111/j.1365-2141.2004.05330.x

Irwin, M., & Johnson, L.A. (Eds.). (2014). *Putting evidence into practice: A pocket guide to cancer symptom management.* Pittsburgh, PA: Oncology Nursing Society.

Koreth, J., Cutler, C., Djulbegovic, B., Behl, R., Scholossmann, N., & Munshi, N. (2007). High-dose therapy with single autologous transplantation versus chemotherapy for newly diagnosed multiple myeloma: A systematic review and meta-analysis of randomized controlled trials. *Biology of Blood and Marrow Transplantation, 13,* 183–196. doi:10.1016/j.bbmt.2006.09.010

Koreth, J., Stevenson, K.E., Kim, H.T., McDonough, S.M., Bindra, B., Armand, P., ... Alyea, E.P., 3rd. (2012). Bortezomib-based graft-versus-host disease prophylaxis in HLA-mismatched unrelated donor transplantation. *Journal of Clinical Oncology, 30,* 3202–3208. doi:10.1200/JCO.2012.42.0984

Kroger, A., Sumaya, C., Pickering, L., & Atkinson, W. (2011). General recommendations on immunization: Recommendations of the Advisory Committee on Immunization Practices (ACIP). *Morbidity and Mortality Weekly Report, 60,* 1–64.

Kumar, S. (2009). Stem cell transplantation for multiple myeloma. *Current Opinion in Oncology, 21,* 162–170. doi:10.1097/CCO.0b013e328324bc04

Kumar, A., Kharfan-Dabala, M.A., Glasmacher, A., & Djulbegovic, B. (2009). Tandem versus single autologous hematopoietic cell transplantation for the treatment of multiple myeloma: A systematic review and meta-analysis. *Journal of the National Cancer Institute, 101,* 100–106. doi:10.1093/jnci/djn439

Kuruvilla, J., Shepherd, J.D., Sutherland, H.J., Nevill, T.J., Nitta, J., Le, A., ... Song, K.W. (2007). Long-term outcome of myeloablative allogeneic stem cell transplantation for multiple myeloma. *Biology of Blood Marrow Transplantation, 13,* 925–931. doi:10.1016/j.bbmt.2007.04.006

Kyle, R.A., & Rajkumar, S.V. (2008). Multiple myeloma. *Blood, 111,* 2962–2972. doi:10.1182/blood-2007-10-078022

Laffan, A., & Biedrzycki, B. (2006). Immune reconstitution: The foundation for safe living after an allogeneic hematopoietic stem cell transplantation. *Clinical Journal of Oncology Nursing, 10,* 787–794. doi:10.1188/06.CJON.787-794

Lahuerta, J.J., Grande, C., Martinez-Lopez, J., De La Serna, J., Toscano, R., Ortiz, M.C., ... San Miguel, J. (2003). Tandem transplants with different high-dose regimens improve the complete remission rates in multiple myeloma. Results of a Grupo Espanol de Sindromes Linfoproliferativos/Trasplante Autologo de Medula Osea phase II trial. *British Journal of Haematology, 120,* 296–303. doi:10.1046/j.1365-2141.2003.04067.x

Lara, A.R., & Schwarz, M.I. (2010). Diffuse alveolar hemorrhage. *Chest, 137,* 1164–1171. doi:10.1378/chest.08-2084

Lilleby, K., Garcia, P., Gooley, T., McDonnnell, P., Taber, R., Holmberg, L., ... Maloney, D.G. (2006). A prospective, randomized study of cryotherapy during administration of high-dose melphalan to decrease the severity and duration of oral mucositis in patients with multiple myeloma undergoing autologous peripheral blood stem cell transplantation. *Bone Marrow Transplantation, 37,* 1031–1035. doi:10.1038/sj.bmt.1705384

Ljungman, P., Cordonnier, C., Englund, J., Machado, C.M., Storek, J., Small, T., ... Centers for Disease Control and Prevention. (2009). Vaccination of hematopoietic cell transplant recipients. *Bone Marrow Transplantation, 44,* 521–526. doi:10.1038/bmt.2009.263

Lokhorst, H., Einsele, H., Vesole, D., Bruno, B., San Miguel, J., Pérez-Simon, J.A., ... Bensinger, W. (2010). International Myeloma Working Group consensus statement regarding the current status of allogeneic stem-cell transplantation for multiple myeloma. *Journal of Clinical Oncology, 28,* 4521–4530. doi:10.1200/JCO.2010.29.7929

Majhail, N.S., Rizzo, J.D., Lee, S.J., Aljurf, M., Atsuta, Y., Bonfim, C., ... Tichelli, A. (2012). Recommended screening and preventive practices for long-term survivors after hematopoietic cell transplantation. *Bone Marrow Transplantation, 47,* 337–341. doi:10.1038/bmt.2012.5

Martin, P.J., Schoch, G., Fisher, L., Byers, V., Anasetti, C., Appelbaum, F.R., ... Sanders, J.E. (1990). A retrospective analysis of therapy for acute graft-versus-host disease: Initial treatment. *Blood, 76,* 1464–1472.

Mattson, M.R. (2007). Graft-versus-host disease: Review and nursing implications. *Clinical Journal of Oncology Nursing, 11,* 325–328. doi:10.1188/07.CJON.325-328

Mehta, J., & Singhal, S. (1998). Graft versus myeloma. *Bone Marrow Transplantation, 11,* 835–843. doi:10.1038/sj.bmt.1701459

Miceli, T., Lilleby, K., Noonan, K., Kurtin, S., Faiman, B., & Mangan, P.A. (2013). Autologous hematopoietic stem cell transplantation for patients with multiple myeloma: An overview for nurses in community practice. *Clinical Journal of Oncology Nursing, 17*(Suppl. 6), 13–24. doi:10.1188/13.CJON.S2.13-24

Millennium: The Takeda Oncology Company. (2014). *Velcade® (bortezomib)* [Package insert]. Retrieved from http://www.velcade.com/Files/PDFs/VELCADE_PRESCRIBING_INFORMATION.pdf

Moreau, P., Facon, T., Attal, M., Hulin, C., Michallet, M., Maloisel, F., ... Harousseau, J.L. (2002). Comparison of 200 mg/m^2 melphalan and 8 Gy total body irradiation plus 140 mg/m^2 melphalan as conditioning regimens for peripheral blood stem cell transplantation in patients with newly diagnosed multiple myeloma: Final analysis of the Intergroupe Francophone du Myélome 9502 randomized trial. *Blood, 99,* 731–735. doi:10.1182/blood.V99.3.731

Morgan, G.J., Davies, F.E., Gregory, W.M., Bell, S.E., Szubert, A.J., Cook, G., ... Child, J.A. (2013). Long-term follow-up of MRC Myeloma IX trial: Survival outcomes with bisphosphonate and thalidomide treatment. *Clinical Cancer Research, 19,* 6030–6038. doi:10.1158/1078-0432.CCR-12-3211

Nair, B., van Rhee, F., Shaughnessy, J.D., Anaissie, E., Szymonifka, J., Hoering, A., ... Barlogie, B. (2010). Superior results of total therapy 3 (2003-33) in gene expression profiling-defined low-risk multiple myeloma confirmed in subsequent trial 2006-66 with VRD maintenance. *Blood, 115,* 4168–4173. doi:10.1182/blood-2009-11-255620

National Cancer Institute Surveillance, Epidemiology, and End Results Program. (2014). SEER stat facts sheets: Myeloma. Retrieved from http://seer.cancer.gov/statfacts/html/mulmy.html

National Comprehensive Cancer Network. (2015). *NCCN Clinical Practice Guidelines in Oncology (NCCN Guidelines®): Multiple myeloma* [v.3.2015]. Retrieved from http://www.nccn.org/professionals/physician_gls/pdf/myeloma.pdf

Naumann-Winter, F., Greb, A., Borchmann, P., Bohlius, J., Engert, A., & Schnell, R. (2012). First-line tandem high-dose chemotherapy and autologous stem cell transplantation versus single high-dose chemotherapy and autologous stem cell transplantation in multiple myeloma, a systematic review of controlled studies. *Cochrane Database of Systematic Reviews, 2012*(10). doi:10.1002/14651858.CD004626.pub3

Novartis Pharmaceuticals Corporation. (2012a). *Aredia® (pamidronate disodium)* [Package insert]. Retrieved from http://www.pharma.us.novartis.com/product/pi/pdf/aredia.pdf

Novartis Pharmaceuticals Corporation. (2012b). *Zometa® (zoledronic acid)* [Package insert]. Retrieved from http://www.pharma.us.novartis.com/product/pi/pdf/Zometa.pdf

Onyx Pharmaceuticals. (2012). *Kyprolis® (carfilzomib)* [Package insert]. Retrieved from http://kyprolis.com/Content/pdf/PrescribingInformation.pdf

Pallera, A.M., & Schwartzberg, L.S. (2004). Managing the toxicity of hematopoietic stem cell transplant. *Journal of Supportive Oncology, 2,* 223–237.

Palumbo, A., Bringhen, S., Petrucci, M.T., Musto, P., Rossini, F., Nunzi, M., ... Boccadoro, M. (2004). Intermediate-dose melphalan improves survival of myeloma patients aged 50–70: Results of a randomized controlled trial. *Blood, 104,* 3052–3057. doi:10.1182/blood-2004-02-0408

Palumbo, A., & Rajkumar, S.V. (2009). Treatment of newly diagnosed myeloma. *Leukemia, 23*, 449–456. doi:10.1038/leu.2008.325

Pineda-Roman, M., Zangari, M., Haessler, J., Anaissie, E., Tricot, G., van Rhee, F., ... Barlogie, B. (2008). Sustained complete remissions in multiple myeloma linked to bortezomib in total therapy 3: Comparison with total therapy 2. *British Journal of Haematology, 140*, 625–634. doi:10.1111/j.1365-2141.2007.06921.x

Potter, P., Eisenberg, S., Cain, K.C., & Berry, D.L. (2011). Orange interventions for symptoms associated with dimethyl sulfoxide during stem cell reinfusions: A feasibility study. *Cancer Nursing, 34*, 361–368. doi:10.1097/NCC.0b013e31820641a5

Richardson, P.G. (2014). Randomized trial of lenalidomide, bortezomib, dexamethasone vs high-dose treatment with SCT in MM patients up to age 65 (DFCI 10-106). Retrieved from http://clinicaltrials.gov/show/NCT01208662

Rodriguez, A.L. (2010). Treatment of newly diagnosed, transplant-eligible patients. In J.D. Tariman (Ed.), *Multiple myeloma: A textbook for nurses* (pp. 109–124). Pittsburgh, PA: Oncology Nursing Society.

Rosiñol, L., Pérez-Simón, J.A., Sureda, A., de la Rubia, J., de Arriba, F., Lahuerta, J.J., ... Bladé, J. (2008). A prospective PETHEMA study of tandem autologous transplantation versus autograft followed by reduced-intensity conditioning allogeneic transplantation in newly diagnosed multiple myeloma. *Blood, 112*, 3591–3593. doi:10.1182/blood-2008-02-141598

Roxane Laboratories, Inc. (2013). *Cyclophosphamide capsules* [Package insert]. Retrieved from http://bidocs.boehringer-ingelheim.com/BIWebAccess/ViewServlet.ser?docBase=renetnt&folderPath=/Prescribing+Information/PIs/Roxane/Cyclophosphamide+Capsules/10008219+Cyclophosphamide+Capsules.pdf

Russell, N., Douglas, K., Ho, A.D., Mohty, M., Carlson, K., Ossenkoppele, G.J., ... Chabannon, C. (2013). Plerixafor and granulocyte colony-stimulating factor for first-line steady-state autologous peripheral blood stem cell mobilization in lymphoma and multiple myeloma: Results of the prospective PREDICT trial. *Haematologica, 98*, 172–178. doi:10.3324/haematol.2012.071456

Sahebi, F., Frankel, P.H., Farol, L., Krishnan, A.Y., Cai, J.L., Somlo, G., ... Forman, S.J. (2012). Sequential bortezomib, dexamethasone, and thalidomide maintenance therapy after single autologous peripheral stem cell transplantation in patients with multiple myeloma. *Biology of Blood and Marrow Transplantation, 18*, 486–492. doi:10.1016/j.bbmt.2011.12.580

Sahebi, F., Spielberger, R., Kogut, N.M., Fung, H., Falk, P.M., Parker, P., ... Solomo, G. (2006). Maintenance thalidomide following single cycle autologous peripheral blood stem cell transplant in patients with multiple myeloma. *Bone Marrow Transplantation, 37*, 825–829. doi:10.1038/sj.bmt.1705339

Savani, B.N., Griffith, M.L., Jagasia, S., & Lee, S.J. (2011). How I treat late effects in adults after allogeneic stem cell transplantation. *Blood, 117*, 3002–3009. doi:10.1182/blood-2010-10-263095

Singhal, S. (2002). High-dose therapy and autologous transplantation. In J. Mehta & S. Singhal (Eds.), *Myeloma* (pp. 327–347). London, England: Martin Dunitz.

Sonneveld, P., Schmidt-Wolf, I.G., van der Holt, B., El Jarari, L., Bertsch, U., Salwender, H., ... Goldschmidt, S.M. (2012). Bortezomib induction and maintenance treatment in patients with newly diagnosed multiple myeloma: Results of the randomized phase III HOVON-65/GMMG-HD4 trial. *Journal of Clinical Oncology, 30*, 2946–2955. doi:10.1200/JCO.2011.39.6820

Stadtmauer, E.A., Vogl, D.T., Prak, E.L., Boyer, J., Aqui, N.A., Rapoport, A.P., ... Sullivan, K.E. (2011). Transfer of influenza vaccine-primed costimulated autologous T cells after stem cell transplantation for multiple myeloma leads to reconstitution of influenza immunity: Results of a randomized clinical trial. *Blood, 117*, 63–71. doi:10.1182/blood-2010-07-296822

Sung, A.D., & Chao, N.J. (2013). Concise review: Acute graft-versus-host disease: Immunobiology, prevention, and treatment. *Stem Cells Translational Medicine, 2*, 25–32. doi:10.5966/sctm.2012-0115

Tomblyn, M., Chiller, T., Einsele, H., Gress, R., Sepkowitz, K., Storek, J., ... Boeckh, M.J. (2009). Guidelines for preventing infectious complications among hematopoietic cell transplantation recipients: A global perspective. *Biology of Blood and Marrow Transplantation, 15,* 1143–1238. doi:10.1016/j.bbmt.2009.06.019

U.S. Food and Drug Administration. (2012). FDA drug safety communication: Safety review update of cancer drug Revlimid (lenalidomide) and risk of developing new types of malignancies. Retrieved from http://www.fda.gov/Drugs/DrugSafety/ucm302939.htm

Usmani, S.Z., Crowley, J., Hoering, A., Mitchell, A., Waheed, S., Nair, B., ... Barlogie, B. (2013). Improvement in long-term outcomes with successive total therapy trials for multiple myeloma: Are patients now being cured? *Leukemia, 27,* 226–232. doi:10.1038/leu.2012.160

Uy, G.L., Goyal, S.D., Fisher, N.M., Oza, A.Y., Tomasson, M.H., Stockerl-Goldstein, K., ... Vij, R. (2009). Bortezomib administered pre-auto-SCT and as maintenance therapy post- transplant for multiple myeloma: A single institution phase II study. *Bone Marrow Transplantation, 43,* 793–800. doi:10.1038/bmt.2008.384

Zangari, M., van Rhee, F., Anaissie, E., Pineda-Roman, M., Haessler, J., Crowley, J., & Barlogie, B. (2008). Eight-year median survival in multiple myeloma after total therapy 2: Roles of thalidomide and consolidation chemotherapy in the context of Total Therapy 1. *British Journal of Haematology, 141,* 433–444. doi:10.1111/j.1365-2141.2008.06982.x

CHAPTER **6**

Treatment of Newly Diagnosed, Transplant-Ineligible Patients

Beth Faiman, PhD, APRN-BC, AOCN®

Introduction

Multiple myeloma is an incurable plasma cell malignancy that can affect adults at nearly any age. It is estimated that nearly 83,000 individuals are living in the United States with multiple myeloma, and 44.9% will survive at least five years, with the majority of individuals older than age 65 (National Cancer Institute, 2014). The standard treatment for newly diagnosed, transplant-ineligible patients with myeloma was relatively unchanged for 30 years as evidenced in a study from the Myeloma Trialists' Collaborative Group (1998). Data were evaluated on 4,930 patients and an additional 1,703 patients from seven clinical trials to determine whether melphalan and prednisone (MP), the standard treatment for myeloma since the 1960s, was superior to any other available therapy. Although many patients were able to achieve remission from various combination chemotherapy regimens introduced during the decades prior to this analysis, the group noted no difference in overall survival (OS) when comparing MP to other available therapies (Myeloma Trialists' Collaborative Group, 1998). This pivotal analysis demonstrated there was clearly room for improvement in the treatment of patients who are ineligible for stem cell transplantation. In the years since the analysis, numerous drug combinations and strategies have emerged that have led to an OS benefit compared to MP, especially in patients ineligible for stem cell transplantation (Palumbo, Rajkumar, et al., 2014).

A New Era

An era of hope emerged shortly after the Myeloma Trialists' Collaborative Group publication as thalidomide, an older drug with a notorious history, returned. This time, thalidomide shone brightly as the first in a new class of drugs and led the way for novel therapies. Thalidomide renewed optimism and hope for better treatment options among patients with relapsed disease as initial case reports described a new mechanism of action and improved efficacy compared to existing chemotherapy agents (Faiman, 2007; Orlowski et al., 1998; Singhal et al., 1999). This led the way for drug discovery, finding new pathways and newer antimyeloma agents that demonstrated improved response rates and, in many instances, less toxicity than the previously used regimens. The landscape of multiple myeloma management has dramatically changed for the better. Clinicians once had few treatment options and saw little improvement in survival. A cure has not yet been identified, but with the advances of the past decade, the outlook is infinitely more optimistic, as myeloma has transitioned from a short, life-threatening disease course to a chronic disease (Faiman, Miceli, Noonan, & Lilleby, 2013). Multiple factors have played a role in improving outcomes that are seen with multiple myeloma therapy today. Better diagnostic strategies, improved supportive care techniques, and a heightened awareness of multiple myeloma incidence are a few factors that may have contributed to improved survival (Kumar et al., 2008; Kurtin & Faiman, 2013; Ozaki et al., 2014).

Although patients typically are diagnosed at an older age, the approach to treatment is essentially the same for all age groups. Initial therapy for nearly all patients historically consisted of oral MP, which was considered to be the standard of care well into the 1990s. Autologous stem cell transplant (ASCT) became a recognized treatment option in the 1980s, but it was not until the mid-1990s that treatment options were more closely examined based on data from the Intergroupe Francophone du Myélome. A landmark study suggested that tandem ASCTs would successfully improve survival and were superior to single transplant; therefore, all individuals younger than age 65 should be considered for ASCT (Attal et al., 2003). Based on results of this and other trials, attention increased as to whether patients were eligible for ASCT (Barlogie, Kyle, et al., 2006; Palumbo et al., 2004).

Standard Autologous Stem Cell Transplant

Patients diagnosed with multiple myeloma must be evaluated for ASCT eligibility for two main reasons. First, intensive therapy with high-dose chemotherapy not only provides an additional therapeutic option to patients but also has been shown to prolong remissions in a majority of patients

(Attal et al., 1996, 2003; Barlogie, Kyle, et al., 2006; Child et al., 2003). Furthermore, ASCT eligibility must be established prior to therapy that involves preservation of the pluripotent bone marrow stem cell (Miceli et al., 2013). Stem cells of patients who are considered candidates for ASCT must be used or harvested and stored for future use prior to receiving therapies such as alkylating agents. Melphalan is a widely used alkylating agent and can interfere with adequate stem cell mobilization, regardless of whether an early or delayed transplant is contemplated (Kumar et al., 2014). Some data suggest that although adequate stem cell harvest can be achieved with patients who have received lenalidomide, granulocyte–colony-stimulating factor (G-CSF) alone may be inadequate for harvesting of stem cells for reasons that are unclear. Therefore, patients receiving lenalidomide may require cyclophosphamide and G-CSF in order for adequate numbers of stem cells to be harvested (Cook et al., 2008). The CXCR4-binding agent plerixafor can be used in combination with G-CSF to mobilize adequate hematopoietic stem cells (HSCs) (Giralt et al., 2009; Kumar et al., 2014).

A Philosophical Divide

Two principal, but different, philosophical approaches exist to the treatment of patients with newly diagnosed multiple myeloma, and these are centered on transplant eligibility. General criteria exist for determining whether patients are eligible for transplant. Patients are deemed transplant-eligible based on multiple factors, which include physiologic health status, chronologic age, and comorbid medical conditions that would put them at higher risk for transplant-related mortality (Kyle & Rajkumar, 2008; Miceli et al., 2013; Nooka et al., 2014). In addition, patients must be willing to undergo this type of intensive procedure, and not all eligible patients are willing to do so (Miceli et al., 2013). Multiple myeloma traditionally has been viewed as an incurable disease, and although most patients will achieve remission status from ASCT, only a small subset of individuals who undergo aggressive therapies may enjoy the benefits of a prolonged remission until a malignant clone reemerges and disease relapse occurs. For individuals who meet the criteria for diagnosis of symptomatic multiple myeloma and are considered ineligible for transplant, many therapies can be administered to control disease. This was not the case even a few years ago.

Patients with multiple myeloma face the challenge of determining the best treatment for them among the available options. The number of antimyeloma therapies has increased dramatically in the past decade, and selecting the appropriate therapy may be quite overwhelming to patients. Transplant-ineligible patients once had a limited number of treatment options, and most drugs, such as oral MP, had a response rate of only 50% (Alexanian et al., 1969). Furthermore, lower response rates with MP have been noted in modern clinical trials with more stringent response criteria when compared to newer therapies (Palumbo, Bringhen, et al., 2014; San Miguel et al., 2008).

Improved OS is a goal that most clinical trials attempt to achieve as an endpoint, and several have identified treatment options with better OS than the previous standard-of-care regimens (e.g., MP) for patients with multiple myeloma (Facon et al., 2006; Hernandez et al., 2004; San Miguel et al., 2008). ASCT is an effective treatment modality for some, but not all, patients. Although several international groups are continuing to establish the role of transplant in younger patients (Attal et al., 1996; Barlogie, Kyle, et al., 2006; Child et al., 2003; Palumbo et al., 1999), the role of transplant in patients who are ineligible for traditional high-dose therapy or in older adults has yet to be clearly defined. Nurses can take an active role in this era of newer therapies and transplantation to encourage patients and caregivers to participate in shared decision making to better understand treatment options (Tariman, Berry, Cochrane, Doorenbos, & Schepp, 2012).

Reduced-Intensity Autologous Stem Cell Transplant

Reduced-intensity ASCT is a viable treatment option for patients of advanced age. Advanced age has been a poor prognostic factor for patients with multiple myeloma in several conventional chemotherapy trials, characterized by a median survival of less than three years, even after adjusting for major variables such as concurrent illnesses and general health status (Badros et al., 2001; Bringhen et al., 2013). Some researchers hypothesized that by reducing the dose of melphalan chemotherapy, which is the most common chemotherapy regimen used in ASCT, patients who were once deemed ineligible for transplant would now have another treatment option available to them (Gay et al., 2013).

The Italian Myeloma Group investigated the role of reduced-intensity IV melphalan in patients who were not candidates for traditional high-dose chemotherapy. The researchers found it was not well tolerated and patients did not demonstrate improved response or survival rates as compared to conventional therapy (Palumbo et al., 1999). Investigators from the University of Arkansas evaluated 159 patients with multiple myeloma who were older than age 70 from 1992 to 1999. Lower transplant-related doses of IV melphalan were better tolerated than what was received in the higher-dose group, and transplant-related mortality was less in the lower-dose group (Badros et al., 2001). The Italian Study Group also found that response was better with reduced-dose melphalan than the previous standard of care, oral melphalan (Palumbo et al., 1999).

In a study comparing melphalan, prednisone, and thalidomide (MPT) versus MP and ASCT in patients who were not eligible for standard transplant-related doses of melphalan, patients were randomized to MP, MPT, or melphalan 100 mg/m^2 IV as part of ASCT. Patients receiving the MPT regimen had fewer adverse events and improved OS versus the transplant group and showed improved progression-free survival (PFS), suggesting that the MPT regimen is superior to ASCT or MP alone when administered to newly diagnosed, transplant-ineligible patients with multiple myeloma (Facon et al., 2006).

Newer agents that are now widely available tend to be more attractive in transplant-ineligible patients than reduced or standard doses of chemotherapy. Several recent studies have evaluated the role of reduced doses of melphalan chemotherapy in patients not considered eligible for standard doses of melphalan while incorporating newer therapies, but considerable toxicity is associated with even a reduced-dose regimen (Palumbo et al., 2004).

Gay et al. (2013) reported results of a trial that used a sequential approach to treatment with bortezomib induction, then intermediate-dose melphalan consolidation, followed by lenalidomide maintenance. Based on the data, ASCT appears to lead to significant morbidity in individuals older than age 70, and the rate of death related to adverse events was higher in patients older than age 70 compared with younger patients.

Because transplantation in older adults can cause significant toxicity, caution must be exercised when patients select it as a treatment option. Novel therapies may provide patients a better survival advantage than undergoing transplantation even when reduced doses of melphalan are used. Balancing the risks and benefits of the treatment and quality of life is imperative (Tariman et al., 2012). Table 6-1 outlines the alternative treatment options for patients who are not candidates for reduced- or standard-dose-intensity transplant.

Conventional Therapies

Melphalan and Prednisone

The oral MP regimen was the standard-of-care induction regimen for patients with newly diagnosed multiple myeloma since the 1960s (Bergsagel, Sprague, Austin, & Griffith, 1962; Bergsagel & Stewart, 2004). Melphalan is administered via both oral and IV routes and belongs to the alkylating agents group of antineoplastic drugs. Various clinical trials have studied this combination therapy, and as a result, dosing schedules may vary depending on which regimens were used in a particular trial. A common dosing schedule of MP is 12 six-week cycles of melphalan 0.25 mg/kg and prednisone 2 mg/kg given orally for four days (Facon et al., 2006).

Table 6-1. Comparison of Agents Available for Newly Diagnosed, Transplant-Ineligible Patients With Multiple Myeloma

Type of Regimen	Authors	Treatment Schema	Side Effects/Key Conclusions
Bortezomib-based	San Miguel et al., 2008	MP (melphalan, prednisone): Melphalan 9 mg/m^2 plus prednisone 60 mg/m^2 days 1–4 Bortezomib 1.3 mg/m^2 days 1, 4, 8, 11, 22, 25, 29, and 32 for cycles 1–4 and days 1, 8, 22, and 29 during cycles 5–9 (for maintenance) of a 42-day cycle	Myelosuppression, gastrointestinal events, infections, peripheral sensory neuropathy, neuralgias, and dizziness may occur.
	Larocca et al., 2013	VP (bortezomib, prednisone) VCP (bortezomib, cyclophosphamide, prednisone) VMP (bortezomib, melphalan, prednisone) Reduced-intensity subcutaneous bortezomib 1.3 mg/m^2 days 1, 8, 15, and 22 every 28 days N = 152 newly diagnosed patients with multiple myeloma	Similar progression-free survival and overall survival in reduced-intensity subcutaneous bortezomib Patients older than age 75 with no exclusion criteria Patients rated as fit, unfit, or frail based on multiple screening instruments Serious adverse events highest in VMP (30%) compared to VP (22%) and VCP (20%)
Lenalidomide-based	Rajkumar et al., 2010	Lenalidomide 25 mg PO days 1–21 every 28 days Dexamethasone 40 mg PO days 1, 8, 15, and 22 every 28 days	Myelosuppression, rash, change in bowel habits; fatigue, increased risk of venous thromboembolism, hyperglycemia
	Facon et al., 2013	Rd (lenalidomide, low-dose dexamethasone), continuously Rd18: Rd for 18 cycles (72 weeks) MPT (melphalan, prednisone, thalidomide): 12 cycles (72 weeks)	Four-year survival best in Rd group. Safety profile with continuous Rd was manageable. Rd = 59.4% Rd18 = 55.7% MPT = 51.4%

(Continued on next page)

Table 6-1. Comparison of Agents Available for Newly Diagnosed, Transplant-Ineligible Patients With Multiple Myeloma *(Continued)*

Type of Regimen	Authors	Treatment Schema	Side Effects/Key Conclusions
Lenalidomide-based *(cont.)*	Palumbo et al., 2013	Rd MPR (melphalan, lenalidomide, prednisone) or CPR (cyclophosphamide, lenalidomide, prednisone) Dose adjustments made for > 75 years old N = 659 patients (2:1) randomization for triplet and doublet, respectively Newly diagnosed multiple myeloma	The three-drug combination did not lead to different progression-free survival or overall survival benefit over two-drug combination. Grade 3 or higher hematologic adverse events in 51% MPR/CPR vs. 29% Rd ($p < 0.001$) Grade 3 or higher hematologic adverse events in 67% MPR and 31% CPR ($p < 0.001$)
Thalidomide-based	Morgan et al., 2011	CTD (attenuated doses of cyclophosphamide, thalidomide, dexamethasone) in the MRC XI trial	Lower doses of chemotherapy in older patients led to improved progression-free survival benefit. Maintenance therapy was included in the large MRC trial.
	Palumbo et al., 2006	Melphalan 4 mg/m^2 PO days 1–7 Prednisone 40 mg/m^2 PO days 1–7 Thalidomide 100 mg PO each day Given every four weeks for six months	Myelosuppression, constipation, increased infection risk; peripheral neuropathy, rash (rare)
	Facon et al., 2006	Thalidomide maintenance offered until disease progression. Standard doses of MP for 12 courses at 6-week intervals with thalidomide up to 100 mg PO daily (no maintenance)	Myelosuppression and peripheral neuropathy cited as most common side effects

(Continued on next page)

Table 6-1. Comparison of Agents Available for Newly Diagnosed, Transplant-Ineligible Patients With Multiple Myeloma *(Continued)*

Type of Regimen	Authors	Treatment Schema	Side Effects/Key Conclusions
Thalidomide-based *(cont.)*	Palumbo et al., 2012	Melphalan 0.18 mg/kg PO on days 1–4, prednisone 2 mg/kg PO on days 1–4, and lenalidomide 5–10 mg PO on days 1–21 repeated every four to six weeks for nine cycles	Myelosuppression, rash, increased risk of venous thromboembolism
	Gay et al., 2009; Rajkumar et al., 2006	Thalidomide 200 mg PO days 1–28 plus dexamethasone 40 mg PO days 1, 8, 15, and 22 every 28 days	Sedation, somnolence, fatigue, constipation, rash, increased risk of venous thromboembolism
Classical chemotherapy (Not widely used)			
• Dexamethasone	Alexanian et al., 1992	Dexamethasone 40 mg PO days 1–4, 9–12, and 17–21 of a 28-day cycle	Fatigue, asthenia, hyperglycemia, mood swings, increased risk of infection
• Melphalan and prednisone	Palumbo et al., 2006	Six four-week cycles of melphalan 4 mg/m² PO days 1–7 and prednisone 40 mg/m² PO days 1–7	Myelosuppression, fatigue

Alternative dosing of this regimen includes melphalan 9 mg/m²/day on days 1–4 every four weeks with prednisone 60 mg/m² PO daily on days 1–4 (San Miguel et al., 2008). Common side effects of melphalan that occur in at least 15% of patients include leukopenia, thrombocytopenia, and anemia. Gastrointestinal side effects (which include nausea, diarrhea, constipation, and vomiting), infections, and alopecia are rare (Alexanian et al., 1969; San Miguel et al., 2008).

Nursing care and monitoring of patients who are receiving melphalan include evaluation of laboratory parameters prior to each cycle. A complete blood count (CBC) and a renal function panel that includes serum blood urea nitrogen and creatinine are required to assess hematologic status and kidney function, respectively. These laboratory values should be checked before each cycle of MP.

Melphalan is excreted through the kidneys. Therefore, nurses must assess kidney function at baseline in any patient receiving melphalan. Caution must be exercised when administering melphalan to patients with decreased renal function. Dose reduction should be considered to prevent myelosuppression and an increased risk of infection. One study suggested that a 50% reduction in the melphalan dose decreased the incidence of myelosuppression in patients with compromised kidney function (Cornwell, Pajak, McIntyre, Kochwa, & Dosik, 1982).

Corticosteroids

Dexamethasone and prednisone are therapeutic agents that belong to a class of drugs called *corticosteroids*, which are the backbone of antimyeloma therapy. These drugs lead to the inhibition or expression of cytokines such as interleukin-6 (IL-6). IL-6 is a major cytokine growth factor for myeloma cells. Steroids exert their antimyeloma properties by effectively reducing the activity of nuclear factor–kappa-B (NF-κB), which leads to apoptosis, or programmed cell death (Alexanian, Dimopoulos, Delasalle, & Barlogie, 1992; Berenson et al., 2002).

High doses of corticosteroids such as prednisone and dexamethasone have been administered to patients with multiple myeloma for decades and have been shown to induce remissions (Alexanian, Dimopoulos, Delasalle, & Barlogie, 1992; Facon et al., 2006) and prolong remission as maintenance therapy to some degree (Berenson et al., 2002). The mechanism of action for steroids in myeloma includes several pathways. The antitumor effects of steroids have been documented, but recent randomized trials showed high doses of corticosteroids should not be administered to older individuals long-term (Palumbo, Mateos, Bringhen, & San Miguel, 2011; Rajkumar et al., 2010). The toxicity of single-agent dexamethasone has been established and is no longer recommended for frontline management of myeloma. Side effects of therapy must be closely monitored to optimize treatment outcomes (see Table 6-2).

Nurses play a key role in educating patients about the side effects of steroids and providing interventions. Although steroids are effective treatment for myeloma, steroid-related side effects occur in nearly every organ system, as outlined in Table 6-2 (Faiman, Bilotti, Mangan, Rogers, & the IMF Nurse Leadership Board, 2008). Patients may commonly experience side effects such as mood swings and personality changes as a result of steroids. Patients also have reported insomnia and sleeplessness. Weight gain, edema, and shortness of breath, especially in patients with known cardiac disease, should be assessed at each visit. Blurred vision and other vision changes usually are transient and resolve once steroid therapy is completed, but early cataract formation may be a consequence that cannot be avoided. Eye examinations at least every six months are recommended for patients receiving steroid therapy to assess for side effects that may warrant intervention (Faiman et al., 2008).

Table 6-2. Side Effects of Steroids in Patients With Multiple Myeloma

System Affected	Side Effect	Nursing and Patient Intervention
Cardiovascular	Edema	Diuretics; avoidance of excess dietary sodium; compression stockings
Constitutional	Fatigue	Management of activities; timing of medication (dose steroids early in morning or late at night), dose reduction if affecting quality of life
	Insomnia	Good sleep hygiene
	"Let-down" effect after discontinuing steroids	Steroid taper or dose reductions (if severe)
Dermatologic	Acneform rash	Good hygiene with nonirritating soaps; topical or oral antibiotics
	Thinning of skin	Good skin hygiene if skin tears develop
Endocrine	Adrenal insufficiency	Steroid taper if long-term steroids used
	Hyperglycemia	Dietary modifications and avoidance of carbohydrates and sugars; oral hypoglycemic or subcutaneous insulin may be needed in some cases.
	Hypogonadism	Refer to primary care provider or an endocrinologist.
Gastrointestinal	Dyspepsia	H_2 receptor inhibitors and proton pump inhibitors
	Hiccups	Hold breath while drinking water; drink from the other side of the water glass. If severe, may need chlorpromazine or dose reduction of steroids.
	Taste changes	Good oral hygiene; lozenges
Immune	Increased risk of infection	Instruct patient to promptly report signs and symptoms of infection to nurse or healthcare provider.
	Leukocytosis	Surveillance for infection
Musculoskeletal	Avascular necrosis	Prompt reporting of pain symptoms; referral to orthopedist if present

(Continued on next page)

Table 6-2. Side Effects of Steroids in Patients With Multiple Myeloma *(Continued)*

System Affected	Side Effect	Nursing and Patient Intervention
Musculoskeletal (cont.)	Bone thinning or osteoporosis	Monitor bone mineral density; calcium and vitamin D supplements; bisphosphonate therapy for patients with osteoporosis related to steroids or multiple myeloma
	Muscle cramping	L-glutamine, quinine water; rule out restless legs syndrome if occurs only at nighttime.
	Proximal myopathy	Regular exercise; dose reduction of steroids if severe
Ophthalmic	Early cataract formation	Follow with optometry; avoid changing eyeglass prescriptions; may need to be corrected
	Vision changes (blurred)	Routine ophthalmic evaluation
Psychiatric	Mood swings, personality changes	Screen for history of depression or mania before initiating steroids; education regarding this potential side effect; antidepressants or pharmacologic therapy may be warranted.
	Weight gain, "moon face" or cushingoid appearance	Screen for hyperglycemia or insulin resistance with weight gain; screen for depression; provide support and education.
Sexual dysfunction	Decreased libido	Estrogen or testosterone may be indicated, but complete evaluation by primary care provider or urologist is the first step if pharmacologic interventions are warranted.

Note. Based on information from Faiman et al., 2008.

Leukocytosis and an increased risk of infection, such as pneumonia, can occur with short-term and long-term steroid use. Nurses should educate patients regarding the following concepts: increased risk of infection, signs and symptoms that should elicit prompt intervention, and the importance of hand washing. Avascular necrosis of the hip or other joints is a serious side effect of prolonged steroid use. Clinicians should encourage patients to notify their healthcare provider or nurse if symptoms of hip or joint pain present and do not improve within one week (Faiman et al., 2008).

Endocrinopathies are common when steroids are used alone or in combination with other therapies for the treatment of multiple myeloma. Steroid-induced hyperglycemia is one of the greatest concerns, as it places patients at risk for negative short-term and long-term consequences on various organ systems. In some patients, mild postprandial blood glucose levels of less than 200 mg/dl can be managed with a low-carbohydrate and low-sugar diet in combination with exercise. If serum glucose is higher than 300 mg/dl, the short-term effects of electrolyte imbalance and dehydration may occur, as well as potential long-term negative effects of microvascular changes. It is critical that nurses assess for a prior history of elevated blood sugar readings, as patients and family members must be made aware of the risk of developing high blood sugar. Clinicians should discuss the signs and symptoms of hyperglycemia and hypoglycemia and review a baseline assessment of risk (Faiman et al., 2008; Pogach et al., 2004). A primary care practitioner or endocrinologist may be helpful in identifying and managing hyperglycemia if medication intervention and home glucose monitoring are warranted.

Nurses should be aware that adrenal insufficiency, which is characterized by hypotension, hypoglycemia, or altered mental status, may occur from rapid cessation of long-term steroid use. Although tapering steroids over a long period of weeks is not necessary in patients who do not receive steroids on a daily basis, some degree of fatigue may result from steroid withdrawal (Faiman et al., 2008). Patients who are taking steroids on a daily or every-other-day basis for more than a month are at risk for adrenal insufficiency, a potentially life-threatening side effect. Tapering steroids in these patients is suggested (Arlt & Allolio, 2003; Faiman et al., 2008; Wilson & Speiser, 2009).

Steroids are an effective antimyeloma therapy and are used in nearly every regimen. Steroids have been proved to enhance the effects of various novel and chemotherapy agents in nearly every therapeutic clinical trial in which they have been studied. It is critical to communicate to patients the importance of using steroids in combination with other treatments, to reinforce education on side effects, and to implement best management strategies in order to strive for safe and effective delivery of these drugs.

Bortezomib and Dexamethasone

Bortezomib is approved by the U.S. Food and Drug Administration (FDA) for use in combination with MP in patients with newly diagnosed myeloma, but it also can be given with dexamethasone. Aside from use in patients with relapsed or refractory disease, the combination of bortezomib and dexamethasone has been studied in patients with newly diagnosed myeloma and does not impair stem cell harvest in patients who may pursue future transplantation. Therefore, this regimen can be used in all types of patients to include transplant-ineligible patients, older adults, and those who are unsure if they may wish to pursue stem cell transplantation at a later date (Harousseau et al., 2006; Jagannath et al., 2006). Long-term follow-up of patients receiving bortezomib 1.3 mg/m² on days 1, 4, 8, and 11 of a three-week cycle for up to six cycles given with oral dexamethasone 40 mg by mouth on the day of and day after bortezomib showed that while patients responded to single-agent bortezomib, their response was improved by the addition of dexamethasone to the regimen. Dexamethasone generally is administered at a dose of 40 mg by mouth the day of and the day after bortezomib (Harousseau et al., 2006; Jagannath et al., 2005; Richardson et al., 2007) but is generally not well tolerated in older adult patients (Ludwig et al., 2009). Caution must be exercised, and nurses should watch for side effects of high doses of dexamethasone when administered to older adults, as their use is discouraged in this population.

The side effects of bortezomib in combination with dexamethasone were similar to those seen in combination with melphalan, with the exception of myelosuppression. The most common blood count abnormality is the presence of a cyclic and predictable thrombocytopenia that in clinical trials was worse on day 11 of a 21-day cycle. A CBC should be obtained before each dose of bortezomib to evaluate blood counts. Dose reductions for thrombocytopenia rarely are needed with bortezomib and dexamethasone, but reduced dosing is indicated if platelets fall to less than 30,000/mm³. Peripheral sensory neuropathy, increased risk of infection, and gastrointestinal side effects such as diarrhea, nausea, and constipation have all been noted in clinical trials. These adverse effects are milder than what is seen when bortezomib is given in combination with MP and generally are predictable and manageable in most patients (Jagannath et al., 2006).

Thalidomide and Dexamethasone

The history of thalidomide is an interesting one and is not commonly reported. Chemie Grünenthal was a German pharmaceutical company that introduced thalidomide into the market as a sedative in October 1957. By 1960, the drug had been distributed in more than 409 countries and commonly was given to pregnant women to prevent nausea and emesis. The first report of fetal malformations came shortly thereafter and was thought to occur when the drug was taken in the first trimester between days 35 and 49 after the last menstrual period. By the end of 1961, thalidomide was taken off the market in most countries, but almost 10,000 infants already had been affected. The drug was not used in the United States, as FDA had denied approval because of the lack of safety data (Kyle & Rajkumar, 2008). Discussion among the medical community regarding the potential antitumor effects of thalidomide had begun, but given its teratogenic effects, the drug had little use until the mid to late 1990s. At that time, thalidomide was studied in relapsed myeloma and quickly regained favor as a new and effective treatment for patients with relapsed multiple myeloma. Several key clinical studies have subsequently focused on the use of thalidomide alone and in combination with other therapies (Singhal et al., 1999).

Because of the teratogenic effects of thalidomide, FDA has granted approval for its use in patients through a restrictive program designed to monitor the drug's distribution. Celgene Corporation instituted the S.T.E.P.S.® (System for Thalidomide Education and Prescribing Safety) program to educate patients, pharmacists, and providers about the side effects of thalidomide and to restrict its use to the population of patients who can benefit from the drug (Zeldis, Williams, Thomas, & Elsayed, 1999). The program has been modified to encompass safe prescribing of all immunomodulatory drugs and is now called the Thalomid REMS® (Risk Evaluation and Mitigation Strategy) program. Education and awareness of black box warnings, the risk of birth defects, and safe use must be ongoing. Patients must refill thalidomide on a monthly basis and can receive thalidomide only from a registered REMS prescriber. Pharmacists must be specially trained and registered with Celgene to dispense thalidomide in accordance with FDA regulations. Unused drug must be returned to the company. The goal of this program is to eliminate the possibility of fetal exposure to thalidomide while allowing access to individuals who may benefit (Celgene Corporation, 2014).

Thalidomide is a first drug in the class of drugs called *immunomodulatory drugs* approved by FDA for the treatment of newly diagnosed multiple myeloma. In addition, thalidomide is considered an effective treatment regimen in transplant-ineligible patients based on three key studies. In one multicenter, randomized, double-blind, placebo-controlled study, patients were randomized to thalidomide plus dexamethasone (TD) versus dexamethasone alone as initial therapy for newly diagnosed disease. Patients randomized to one arm received thalidomide 50–200 mg PO on days 1–28 and dexamethasone 40 mg on days 1–4, 9–12, and 17–20 of a 28-day cycle. The other group of patients received the same dose of dexamethasone alone. Patients who received TD had a median time to progression of 22.4 months versus 6.5 months in the dexamethasone-only group. OS rates have not been met yet, but many patients in the TD arm remain in remission (Rajkumar et al., 2006).

A third trial conducted by Ludwig et al. (2009) randomized older adult patients to receive oral MP or oral TD for treatment of newly diagnosed myeloma. Patients received thalidomide 50–200 mg PO daily and dexamethasone 40 mg PO on days 1–4, 9–12, and 17–20 of a 28-day regimen. MP was given on a standard dosing schedule. The combination of TD was shown to be superior to MP, with more patients responding to treatment and for a longer duration of time. Despite a higher response to therapy, the results of this trial showed that patients receiving TD had more neuropathy, a higher incidence of deep vein thrombosis (DVT), psychological toxicity, and a higher rate of early treatment discontinuation than patients receiving MP. The data also showed that patients receiving TD had a shorter OS than patients receiving MP therapy even though more hematologic toxicity occurred in patients who had received MP (Ludwig et al., 2009). This suggests that high doses of dexamethasone in combination with other therapies such as thalidomide may not be well tolerated in older adults and should be avoided.

Major side effects of TD include increased risk of venous thromboembolism (VTE), constipation, fatigue or sleepiness, and nervous system disorders such as neuropathy. Myelosuppression occurs in combination with melphalan but is not a side effect of thalidomide. Rash may occur in a small percentage of patients and usually resolves, but in rare cases (less than 1%) Stevens-Johnson syndrome may occur, which produces a widespread rash from head to toe that could be severe (Celgene Corporation, 2014).

Nursing considerations for patients receiving thalidomide in combination with dexamethasone or other agents focus mainly on education regarding drug safety and monitoring for side effects. Patients receiving thalidomide have an increased risk of developing VTE. The nurse's role is to educate patients regarding the increased risk of blood clots, to determine if they are candidates for aspirin or other therapeutic anticoagulation, and to educate patients regarding preventive strategies. Other important nursing interventions and management strategies for constipation, fatigue or sleepiness, and neuropathy also warrant special attention.

Lenalidomide and Dexamethasone

Lenalidomide is an analog of thalidomide and an oral immunomodulatory agent that has demonstrated efficacy in patients with newly diagnosed as well as relapsed disease. Despite its similarity to the first-in-class immunomodulatory agent for myeloma, lenalidomide carries a much different dosing schedule and side effect profile. The mechanism of action has not been well known in lenalidomide (Doss, 2006; Faiman, 2007), but it clearly works in the bone marrow stroma to inhibit proliferation of the plasma cells, prevents angiogenesis, and increases tumoricidal activity (Palumbo, Bringhen, et al., 2014). It is primarily excreted through the kidneys and does not undergo cytochrome P450 metabolism, meaning the risk for drug-drug interactions is low (Celgene Corporation, 2014).

Lenalidomide has been studied extensively in patients with relapsed myeloma and in several newly diagnosed myeloma trials, but the most convincing data for its use in transplant-ineligible patients have resulted from a randomized, controlled, phase III clinical trial sponsored by the Eastern Cooperative Oncology Group. In this trial, patients were randomized to lenalidomide 25 mg PO daily for 21 days with either high-dose dexamethasone (40 mg/day on days 1–4, 9–12, and 17–20 of a 28-day cycle) or low-dose dexamethasone (40 mg/day on days 1, 8, 15, and 22 of a 28-day cycle). The trial was halted early because of the increased one-year survival rate observed in the low-dose dexamethasone arm (96%) compared to the high-dose dexamethasone arm (87%), as the patients receiving high-dose dexamethasone had increased risk of infections and VTE (Rajkumar et al., 2010). Differences in OS favored the low-dose dexamethasone arm in subgroup analysis of patients younger than age 65 and in those age 65 or older, which suggests that all patients with newly diagnosed disease, regardless of age, should receive the lower doses of steroids as opposed to higher doses of steroids, which traditionally was the standard of care (Rajkumar et al., 2010). The three most common grade three or higher toxicities were 26% DVT, 16% infections including pneumonia, and 15% fatigue (Facon et al., 2013).

An important nursing consideration when caring for patients who are receiving lenalidomide is to counsel patients about the risk of birth defects. Preclinical studies suggest that lenalidomide does not appear to cause the same teratogenic effects seen with thalidomide. Despite this finding, no data support its safety in humans, and the potential increased risk for fetal birth defects is not worth taking. The chemical structure closely resembles thalidomide, which warrants caution (Kumar & Rajkumar, 2006). The RevAssist® program of Celgene Corporation is similar to the company's S.T.E.P.S. program and was developed to address the need for safety and education when prescribing lenalidomide. The program has been renamed the Revlimid REMS® program as of 2013. Female patients of childbearing potential must be counseled before the start of lenalidomide therapy and on a monthly basis to avoid becoming pregnant; men receiving the drug must not cause a woman to become pregnant. Two forms of birth control are required at all times, and patients must not donate blood or sperm. Counseling against fetal exposure to lenalidomide should be ongoing and performed at least on a monthly basis prior to prescription refills (Celgene Corporation, 2014).

A second important consideration for patients who are receiving lenalidomide and dexamethasone would be education on the increased risk of VTE. Patients in the Eastern Cooperative Oncology Group trial had an increased risk of VTE in the high-dose dexamethasone group as compared to the low-dose dexamethasone group. Intervention and management of these side effects are the same as with patients receiving thalidomide and should be routinely discussed with patients. Guidelines have been established for the prevention, diagnosis, and management of VTE associated with lenalidomide and thalidomide (Rome, Doss, Miller, Westphal, & the IMF Nurse Leadership Board, 2008).

The proper dosing and schedule of lenalidomide in patients with renal failure and compromised renal function has been described. Little was known about the effects of lenalidomide and renal function until recently, as only patients with serum creatinine levels less than 2.5 mg/dl were allowed to participate in the randomized clinical trials that described its efficacy. As of 2009, FDA has approved changes to the product package insert to reflect renal dosing parameters (Celgene Corporation, 2014). Like many drugs that are excreted through the kidneys, dosing of lenalidomide for patients with myeloma must be done on the basis of creatinine clearance. It is recommended that nurses and healthcare providers calculate serum creatinine clearance so that the correct starting dose of lenalidomide is ordered.

The most common consequence of inappropriate dosing of lenalidomide in patients with renal insufficiency or renal failure is myelosuppression. First reported by Niesvizky et al. (2007), this group observed that patients who received the oral combination of clarithromycin, lenalidomide, and dexamethasone and had concurrent renal dysfunction with a creatinine clearance of less than 40 ml/min experienced more significant myelosuppression than those with normal renal function (Niesvizky et al., 2007). Lenalidomide is safe in patients with renal dysfunction and in patients on dialysis, but it is important to initiate the appropriate dose and implement routine monitoring of serum creatinine clearance. Dose reductions based on decreased renal function should be considered in all patients with myeloma. A CBC and differential should be obtained at least every two weeks at the beginning of therapy; serum creatinine should be monitored at the time of each blood draw (Celgene Corporation, 2014).

Bortezomib, Melphalan, and Prednisone

Many of the newer agents have variable side effect profiles that allow patients to receive combination therapies that produce an improved remission rate with less toxicity. As mentioned, the combination of MP is associated with a median survival of 29–37 months, but for lack of better treatment options, this had been the preferred therapy for treatment of newly diagnosed myeloma for many years (Kyle & Rajkumar, 2004). Preclinical studies suggested that adding bortezomib to MP (VMP) would improve response rates, and a clinical trial was designed to evaluate this combination.

In a phase III clinical trial known as the VISTA (Velcade as Initial Standard Therapy in Multiple Myeloma: Assessment With Melphalan and Prednisone) trial, 682 patients were randomly assigned to receive nine six-week cycles of melphalan (9 mg/m^2 of body surface area) and prednisone (60 mg/m^2) on days 1–4 of a 28-day cycle. MP was given to patients either by itself or in combination with bortezomib (1.3 mg/m^2) on days 1, 4, 8, 11, 22, 25, 29, and 32 of a 42-day cycle. Following the initial treatment phase, the VMP regimen was given to patients during cycles 1–4 and on days 1, 8, 22, and 29 of a 42-day cycle during cycles 5–9, which was considered to be the maintenance phase of therapy. The results of this randomized, controlled trial showed that the combination of VMP was superior to MP alone. Patients randomized to receive VMP experienced an OS benefit, especially if the individual received higher cumulative doses of bortezomib (Mateos et al., 2013; San Miguel et al., 2008).

The route of bortezomib administration should be considered. A randomized, noninferiority trial compared IV bortezomib to subcutaneous (SC) bortezomib in patients with relapsed and refractory multiple myeloma (Moreau et al., 2011). Bortezomib, when given via the SC versus IV route, was shown to be as effective and with statistically significantly lower rates of peripheral neuropathy, which is a dose-limiting toxicity in multiple myeloma.

A trial was designed considering the efficacy of VMP and decreased neurotoxicity observed with SC bortezomib. In the trial, Larocca and colleagues (2013) used reduced doses of SC bortezomib in various schedules and scheduled geriatric assessments as considerations in the treatment selection of elderly patients with newly diagnosed multiple myeloma. Results showed low-dose-intensity, bortezomib-based regimens demonstrated similar PFS and OS estimates as higher doses. Serious adverse events and discontinuations were higher with the three-drug VMP regimen, suggesting that a melphalan-free regimen should be preferred in very elderly or frail patients (Larocca et al., 2013).

Side effects in patients receiving bortezomib-based therapies among the trials were more prevalent than in those who received MP alone, yet no significant increase occurred in treatment-related deaths (Larocca et al., 2013; San Miguel et al., 2008). Key side effects that were noted in most VMP trials include myelosuppression, gastrointestinal events (i.e., nausea, diarrhea, constipation, vomiting), and infections including pneumonia and herpes zoster (Larocca et al., 2013; San Miguel et al., 2008). Nervous system disorders also were common with bortezomib, as peripheral sensory neuropathy, neuralgias, and dizziness occurred.

Nursing implications are focused on patient education and monitoring of treatment-related side effects. Appropriate laboratory monitoring for patients receiving this three-drug regimen is critical. A CBC should be obtained prior to each dose of bortezomib to assess for myelosuppression and hematologic status. Dose reductions according to the package insert should be considered for moderate to severe leukopenia, anemia, or thrombocytopenia, or any other significant side effects that may be related to bortezomib and affect function or quality of life (Millennium Pharmaceuticals, Inc., 2014). Clinicians should evaluate patients' renal function prior to each cycle, as a dose reduction in melphalan may be warranted. It is important to note that patients with renal insufficiency can safely receive the standard dosing schedule of bortezomib (San Miguel et al., 2008). Gastrointestinal side effects of bortezomib are fairly common. Nausea can be prevented by premedication with a 5-HT$_3$ antagonist, such as ondansetron or granisetron, which may decrease the risk of nausea and vomiting associated with bortezomib (Colson, Doss, Swift, Tariman, & Thomas, 2004). Increased dietary fiber intake may help to decrease diarrhea as it reabsorbs water in the colon and acts as a bulking agent. Some patients with predictable diarrhea following meals or bortezomib administration may take loperamide before meals or after each diarrhea stool but not to exceed eight tablets per day. Caution must be exercised when using loperamide and other potent antidiarrheal agents, as watery diarrhea accompanied by abdominal cramping may be a sign of a serious infection. Intermittent laboratory evaluation for *Clostridium difficile* or other serious gastrointestinal infections should be performed by assessing stools for *C. difficile* and cultures (Smith, Bertolotti, Curran, Jenkins, & the IMF Nurse Leadership Board, 2008).

Neuropathy or neurotoxicity is a phenomenon that may occur in patients with cancer as well as noncancer diagnoses, such as peripheral vascular disease and diabetes, but may be present in patients with untreated multiple myeloma as well. Often, nurses and healthcare professionals will identify neuropathy symptoms in multiple myeloma when patients have subjective sensory alteration characterized by burning, numbness, tingling, or a decrease in sensation (Tariman, Love, McCullagh, Sandifer, & the IMF Nurse Leadership Board, 2008). These phenomena can be objectively measured with sensitive neurologic procedures such as electrophysiologic studies, but less expensive techniques may note the presence of neuropathy, such as clinical examination by the practitioner (Mileshkin et al., 2006). Nurses play an ongoing and critical role as educators regarding neuropathy, and this begins by raising patient awareness that peripheral neuropathy may occur. In most instances, the nurse administers the drug and interviews patients just prior to the scheduled treatment and, thus, may have more contact with patients than other providers. Ongoing surveillance, recognition of symptoms, and intervention are critical to alleviating side effects that may impair the delivery of a drug or the patient's ability to stay on the recommended course of treatment (Richardson, Sonneveld, et al., 2009). Changing the route of administration to SC from IV and modifying the dose schedule can alleviate peripheral neuropathy symptoms and contribute to reversibility (Richardson et al., 2012).

Neuropathy in patients receiving bortezomib should be evaluated before each dose and is one of the most serious side effects of bortezomib. Peripheral sensory neuropathy developed in nearly half of patients receiving bortezomib in the VISTA trial, and serious grade 3 toxicity was present in 13% of patients and warranted discontinuation of therapy (Colson et al., 2004; Tariman et al., 2008). Nurses should educate patients about the increased risk, which includes grade 3 dizziness that will occur in approximately 16% of patients. Prompt identification of side effects and dose reduction of bortezomib are critical (Richardson et al., 2012; Tariman et al., 2008).

In a study evaluating the benefits of dose reduction in patients with myeloma who were receiving bortezomib therapy, the dose of bortezomib was held, reduced, or discontinued depending on the severity of peripheral neuropathy as reported by the patient and graded by the nurse or clinician. Overall, 124 of 331 patients (37%) had treatment-emergent peripheral neuropathy, which was lower than in a previous phase II trial that did not include dose reduction guidelines. Efficacy of the bortezomib was not affected by dose reduction in patients who reported painful neuropathy, and the neuropathy was noted in this study to be reversible in the majority of patients (Richardson, Sonneveld, et al., 2009). Based on these findings, close monitoring for neuropathy symptoms and dose reduction of bortezomib in patients with even mildly painful peripheral neuropathy are recommended.

Two types of infections were noted in patients receiving the combination of bortezomib and MP: pneumonia and herpes zoster. Nurses should alert patients to the increased risk of developing respiratory illness and implement intervention strategies such as ambulation, coughing, and deep breathing and prompt report of signs or symptoms of infection (Miceli, Colson, Gavino, Lilleby, & the IMF Nurse Leadership Board, 2008).

The Centers for Disease Control and Prevention (CDC) and the immunizations subcommittee, called the Advisory Committee on Immunization Practices (ACIP), have updated guidelines for pneumococcal vaccination that pertain to patients with multiple myeloma. Currently, two pneumococcal vaccinations exist. ACIP recommends the 13-valent conjugate vaccine be given once and at least 8 weeks prior to the first administration of the standard 23-valent compound (PPSV23) in patients with multiple myeloma who have *not* previously received PPSV23. The Pneumovax® 23 (pneumococcal vaccine polyvalent) is a sterile liquid vaccine for intramuscular or SC injection that includes the 23 most prevalent or invasive pneumococcal types of *Streptococcus pneumoniae* and also includes the 6 serotypes that most frequently cause invasive drug-resistant pneumococcal infections among children and adults in the United States. Pneumococcal vaccination may help to decrease the incidence of pneumococcal infection, a life-threatening condition, for patients with multiple myeloma. Although vaccines against pneumococcus are less effective in older adults than in younger adults, CDC recommends that the vaccine be administered once after age 60 (CDC, 2014). Screening patients to see if they are candidates for the pneumonia vaccine also is important.

Bortezomib has been attributed to an increased risk of herpes zoster or shingles activation in patients with myeloma. The incidence of herpes zoster activation when patients received bortezomib plus MP was 13%, and increased risk was also noted in the APEX (Assessment of Proteasome Inhibition for Extending Remissions) trial (Chanan-Khan et al., 2006; San Miguel et al., 2008). Prophylactic doses of antiviral therapy such as acyclovir or valacyclovir should be given to patients receiving bortezomib, which may prevent the development of shingles or lesions.

Patient education is targeted toward awareness and prompt reporting of symptoms. Signs of a herpetic infection may include a prodrome of a tingling sensation followed by the eruption of a rash that may be described as itchy and painful. An erythematous, vesicular rash typically follows a dermatome, or nerve root, and will become evident. If the virus travels to the nerve root, the resulting pain can be particularly debilitating (Kim et al., 2008). It is especially important to note that although a herpes zoster vaccine called Zostavax® (Merck & Co., Inc., 2014) is available, it is contraindicated in immunosuppressed individuals and those with hematologic malignancies. Zostavax is a live, attenuated vaccine and may reactivate a dormant viral infection in patients who lack an intact immune system (Merck & Co., Inc., 2014).

Melphalan, Prednisone, and Lenalidomide

In prior clinical trials, researchers have added either thalidomide or bortezomib to MP in an attempt to find the best standard of care regimen for older adult or transplant-ineligible patients. Palumbo et al. (2012) studied the combination of MP plus lenalidomide followed by continuous lenalidomide (MPR-R) in newly diagnosed patients older than age 65. A total of 152 patients were randomized to the MPR-R group and received nine four-week cycles of MPR followed by lenalidomide maintenance therapy until a relapse or disease progression occurred. A second group of 153 patients was randomized to receive MPR, and a third group of 154 patients received MP alone. The primary endpoint was PFS. In this trial, the dose of melphalan was 0.18 mg/kg PO on days 1–4, prednisone 2 mg/kg PO on days 1–4, and lenalidomide 5–10 mg PO on days 1–21 repeated every four to six weeks for nine cycles. Patients who received MPR-R experienced a significantly prolonged PFS, and the greatest benefit was observed in patients 65–75 years of age, but not in patients older than 75 years. A 66% reduction in the rate of progression with MPR-R was age-independent, which suggests this is an effective regimen in patients with myeloma (Palumbo et al., 2012).

Palumbo, Bringhen, et al. (2014) reported results of a study designed to compare the efficacy and safety of a non-alkylating agent–containing regimen (Rd) to that of an alkylating agent–containing regimen (MPR/CPR) in transplant-ineligible older adults with newly diagnosed multiple myeloma. Doses of dexamethasone, cyclophosphamide, and melphalan were reduced for individuals age 75 or older. Authors concluded Rd is probably the well-defined treatment for all older adult patients with newly diagnosed multiple myeloma, given that it has the lowest amount of toxicity and similar PFS benefit compared to the three drug regimens (Palumbo, Bringhen, et al., 2014).

The Frontline Investigation of Lenalidomide + Dexamethasone versus Standard Thalidomide (FIRST) trial is a large, randomized, multicenter, open-label, phase III trial comparing the efficacy and safety of Rd versus MPT in transplant-ineligible patients with newly diagnosed multiple myeloma. In the trial, continuous Rd significantly extended PFS, with an OS benefit compared to MPT. Consistent benefit of Rd was sustained across subgroups regardless of age and risk status (Facon et al., 2013).

Side effects of MPR-R are similar to previous trials that used lenalidomide or MP. Neutropenia, thrombocytopenia, and anemia were the most common. Rash and gastrointestinal side effects were noted infrequently. All patients received prophylactic aspirin, and the incidence of VTE in the MPR trial was low and occurred in only three patients, and two patients actually developed DVT after aspirin discontinuation. MPR seems to be fairly well tolerated on the basis of this clinical trial, but clearly more studies are warranted (Palumbo et al., 2012).

Cyclophosphamide, Thalidomide, and Dexamethasone

The Myeloma Research Consortium conducted a large, randomized trial. In the trial, researchers investigated use of attenuated doses of cyclophosphamide, thalidomide, and dexamethasone (CTD) as initial therapy for patients with multiple myeloma who were unsuitable for autologous transplantation (Morgan et al., 2011). One of the treatment arms included 426 patients who received lower doses of cyclophosphamide (500 mg/week), thalidomide 50 mg for four weeks and increased every four weeks in 50-mg increments to a maximum of 200 mg/day, and dexamethasone 20 mg/day on days 1–4 and 15–18 of each 28-day cycle (dexamethasone was reduced from a standard dose of 40 mg). Patients who received the CTD regimen had higher response rates but no increase in survival compared to MP and, in fact, experienced more toxicity. PFS also was similar between groups. Based on findings, the CTD regimen is not an optimal choice for newly diagnosed, transplant-ineligible patients.

Melphalan, Prednisone, and Thalidomide

The FIRST trial randomized patients to receive various doses of lenalidomide and dexamethasone versus MPT. In the trial, the combination of continuous Rd was superior to MPT as a frontline treatment for multiple myeloma (Facon et al., 2013). However, it is important to note the combination of MPT is preferred to MP and has significant activity, and the efficacy of MPT has been reported in three other major randomized trials. Patients in all trials were mainly transplant-ineligible patients and those older than age 65 (Facon et al., 2006; Hulin et al., 2009; Palumbo et al., 2006). One trial randomized patients to receive one of two oral regimens to include MP or MPT. The dose of MP in either arm was the same, and each of the two regimens was administered every month for 12 months. The result of this trial demonstrated that 47% of patients receiving MPT achieved a partial response to therapy versus 7% in the MP group. Researchers also noted a median OS of 51.6 months in the MPT group versus 33.2 months in the MP-alone group, which suggested the MPT regimen was superior to MP alone (Facon et al., 2006). Another trial by Palumbo et al. (2006) randomized patients either to standard-dose

MP for six months or to MPT for six months followed by maintenance therapy with thalidomide. The results of this trial showed a trend toward an improved three-year survival with the combination of MPT followed by maintenance thalidomide. The third trial by the Intergroupe Francophone du Myélome demonstrated the safety and efficacy of MPT in patients older than age 75 and that the combination of MPT was superior to MP with a survival advantage in the MPT group (Hulin et al., 2009).

Despite the higher response rate and improved survival benefit of MPT as compared to MP, side effects with MPT therapy are more frequent than with the two-drug combination therapy, as expected. Incidence of grade 3–4 adverse events occurred in approximately 50% of patients who were treated with MPT compared to 25% of patients receiving MP (Hulin et al., 2009). Common side effects of MPT reported in each of the trials include fatigue, myelosuppression, increased risk of infection, DVT, and nervous system disorders.

Nursing interventions for patients receiving thalidomide include patient and family education about common side effects and strategies to alleviate these effects. Constipation is common in patients who are taking thalidomide for the treatment of multiple myeloma, and higher doses of thalidomide may lead to increased constipation. Patients who are concurrently taking other medicines that have constipation as a side effect, such as pain medications, may have a greater chance of developing constipation. It is important to initiate a bowel regimen and instruct patients to increase fiber in their diet when starting thalidomide therapy. Stool softeners and laxatives may be indicated and are effective as a preventive strategy. Increasing fluid intake will help to decrease the risk of dehydration and constipation (Smith et al., 2008).

Many patients who are taking thalidomide complain of sleepiness and daytime or early-morning fatigue. Nurses must instruct patients that if they are taking thalidomide, they should start slowly with one pill a day taken at bedtime and then titrate the dose in weekly increments to achieve target dosing. To address early-morning fatigue and combat daytime sleepiness and sedation, patients may benefit from taking thalidomide early in the evening. Dose reductions of thalidomide may be warranted if the sleepiness and sedation interfere with daily activities (Faiman, 2007).

Peripheral neuropathy is a side effect of thalidomide that rarely occurs early in the treatment phase but more often develops late in the course of therapy. Thalidomide-induced neurotoxicity may be noted earlier in the treatment phase in patients with other health problems, such as diabetes or long-standing high blood pressure, that lead to microvascular changes and venous insufficiency (Richardson et al., 2012). Although monitoring with electrophysiologic studies provides quantitative data to verify the presence or absence of neuropathy, a clinical neurologic examination also provides important information. In a trial by Mileshkin et al. (2006), clinical examination was as effective as electrophysiologic studies in patients with neuropathy. Patients should be instructed to watch for numbness and tingling in their hands and feet and to promptly report these symptoms to their nurse or healthcare provider. Difficulty with tasks such as buttoning a shirt or opening a jar may be a sign of peripheral neuropathy, but other sensory changes may be present on clinical examination. Dizziness, shakiness, or unsteadiness while walking or standing may be other signs of motor neuropathy that should be reported, and the dose of thalidomide should be decreased (Colson et al., 2004; Faiman, 2007).

Multiple myeloma is intrinsically a hypercoagulable disease, and certain antimyeloma regimens that contain thalidomide and lenalidomide may further increase the risk of VTE. Therefore, patient education about the signs and symptoms of VTE is critical (Rome, Doss, Miller, Westphal, & the IMF Nurse Leadership Board, 2008). For example, when thalidomide was given in combination with MP, the risk of DVT was approximately 20% in the absence of thromboprophylaxis. When patients received enoxaparin, the rate of DVT dropped to approximately 3% (Palumbo et al., 2006). Although VTE can occur with thalidomide and lenalidomide, the risk is low unless given in combination with dexamethasone, doxorubicin, multiagent chemotherapy, or erythropoiesis-stimulating factors, where the risk can be significantly increased up to 75%.

Additional risk factors for VTE exist and must be evaluated before initiation of antimyeloma therapy. Nurses should assess for signs and symptoms of DVT or VTE, including unilateral swelling or cyanosis of the extremity at baseline and at subsequent outpatient or hospital visits. Shortness of breath and anxiety may suggest pulmonary embolism and warrant prompt intervention (Rome et al., 2008; Wiley, 2007). Figure 6-1 lists risk factors and interventions for VTE.

Vincristine, Doxorubicin, and Dexamethasone

The regimen of vincristine, doxorubicin, and dexamethasone (VAD) has been used in transplant-ineligible and transplant-eligible older adult patients with myeloma for many years (Alexanian, Barlogie, & Tucker, 1990; Cavo et al., 2005; Rajkumar, 2005). VAD was one of the few effective chemotherapy regimens available in the past 20 years and became a standard regimen for transplant-eligible patients, as the three-drug therapy does not harm stem cell harvest. In recent years, this regimen has become scarcely used in older adult or transplant-ineligible patients because of the toxicity and relative ineffectiveness compared to newer agents with the potential for fewer side effects and better response rates (Rajkumar, 2005). Vincristine and doxorubicin are administered in this regimen by continuous infusion at the doses of 0.4 mg/day and 9 mg/m^2/day, respectively, on days 1–4 with standard doses of dexamethasone (40 mg PO/IV days 1–4, 9–12, and 17–20

Figure 6-1. Selected Risk Factors and Interventions for Development of Venous Thromboembolism in Multiple Myeloma

Risk Factors
Independent risk factors
- Age
- Obesity (body mass index greater than 30 kg/m^2)
- History of venous thromboembolism
- Central venous catheter

Comorbidities
- Diabetes
- Active infections
- Cardiac disease
- Renal disease
- Surgical procedures (including vertebroplasty and kyphoplasty)
- Inherited thrombophilia or hereditary coagulopathies
- Other concomitant malignancy

Medications: Lenalidomide or thalidomide in combination with
- Erythropoietin
- Estrogens or hormone therapies
- Pegylated liposomal doxorubicin or doxorubicin
- High-dose steroids

Interventions
Education regarding signs and symptoms
- Slight fever
- Tachycardia
- Unilateral swelling
- Shortness of breath
- Cyanosis of extremity
- Pain in extremity
- Dull ache in one extremity
- Venous distention

Prevention
- Avoid dehydration
- Ambulation
- Sequential compression devices
- Prophylactic anticoagulation prior to surgical procedures (enoxaparin, heparin)
- Risk assessment intervention
  - **Low Risk**
    * 0–1 risk factors
    * Aspirin 81–100 mg PO daily
  - **Intermediate Risk**
    * 1–2 risk factors
    * Aspirin 81–325 mg PO daily and watch closely for signs of venous thromboembolism
  - **High Risk**
    * More than 2 risk factors
    * Therapeutic anticoagulation with warfarin, low-molecular-weight heparin, or full-dose heparin for patients with 2 or more risk factors

Note. Based on information from Hussein et al., 2006; Palumbo et al., 2008; Rome et al., 2008; Wiley, 2007.

of a 28-day cycle) and must be given via central venous catheter because doxorubicin is a vesicant (Cavo et al., 2005).

The efficacy of VAD in the era of novel agents has been questioned. Cavo et al. (2005) compared the infusional VAD regimen to the oral TD regimen in 200 patients. Participants who received TD had a significantly higher response rate (76%) than those receiving IV VAD (52%). VAD also was found to have inferior outcome when compared to bortezomib and dexamethasone (Harousseau et al., 2008). With the neurotoxicity seen with vincristine, the steroid side effect profile of high-dose dexamethasone, cost, inconvenience, and infection risk associated with implanted central venous catheter placement, most institutions do not use VAD in patients with newly diagnosed disease any longer, and it is not considered standard of care (Rajkumar, 2005).

Nurses should be aware that although VAD has been used for many years, it is no longer the best frontline option for transplant-eligible or transplant-ineligible patients, given the plethora of newer, more effective therapies. Major side effects of VAD include myelosuppression and constipation, which may be attributed to doxorubicin, and neurotoxicity secondary to vincristine, which may provide little if any contribution to the regimen. Nausea and vomiting may occur but generally is mild and can be prevented with the administration of antiemetic agents. Oral mucositis can develop, and good oral hygiene is encouraged. Cardiotoxicity may occur; nurses should be aware of the cumulative dose of doxorubicin prior to each infusion, as patients should not receive a cumulative dose of greater than 550 mg/m^2. Baseline left ventricular ejection fraction should be obtained to assess for stable cardiac function. As discussed in previous sections, transplant-ineligible patients often are older, and high doses of dexamethasone used in the VAD regimen may lead to increased toxicity (Facon et al., 2006; Ludwig et al., 2009). As with any treatment decision that is to be made, the risks, benefits, and alternatives should be weighed carefully before proceeding with VAD therapy, especially in older adults.

Maintenance Therapy

The role of maintenance therapy in newly diagnosed patients with multiple myeloma who have not received high-dose therapy remains controversial. Maintaining a result following induction therapy is an important goal in multiple myeloma, yet no clear consensus as to the length of therapy exists (Ludwig et al., 2012). Clinical trials are ongoing to answer this question, which primarily focuses on individual patients' response to therapy. Maintenance has been incorporated into cancer treatment for years in an effort to prevent the reemergence of a malignant clone and maintain control of the disease. Interferon, corticosteroids, immunomodulatory agents, and proteasome inhibitors have all been studied to varying degrees. Continuous doses of thalidomide, lenalidomide, and bortezomib have been the most widely studied maintenance agents in randomized, controlled trials with non–transplant-eligible patients (Ludwig et al., 2012).

Lenalidomide

Lenalidomide has shown effectiveness when used as a single agent in relapsed disease and prolongs OS following stem cell transplantation even in high-risk patients with multiple myeloma (McCarthy, Einsele, Attal, & Giralt, 2014; Nooka et al., 2014; Palumbo, Mina, Cerrato, & Cavallo, 2013; Richardson, Jagannath, et al., 2009). In older adult patients ineligible for transplantation, continuous lenalidomide prolongs remission and response rate, as seen in the MPR and MPR-R trials regimens that resulted in significantly higher response rates with approximately three times as many complete responses in the maintenance arm compared with MP only (Palumbo et al., 2012). Analysis of results of the 459 patients in the MM-015 trial showed induction with lenalidomide, melphalan, and prednisone followed by lenalidomide maintenance improved health-related quality of life compared with those who did not receive maintenance therapy (Dimopoulos et al., 2013). Another study demonstrated the efficacy of lenalidomide and prednisone (RP) induction, followed by lenalidomide, melphalan, and prednisone consolidation and finally RP maintenance in elderly patients (Falco et al., 2013).

A third study conducted in Canada reported preliminary safety information among older adult patients who were not transplantation candidates (White et al., 2013). Higher doses of MP and lenalidomide were administered. The authors cautioned readers about the dose-limiting hematologic toxicity of melphalan in combination with lenalidomide. Therefore, careful attention to blood counts must be exercised.

Bortezomib

Bortezomib has demonstrated efficacy when used to treat patients with newly diagnosed and relapsed disease. The use of bortezomib as a maintenance drug has been incorporated into several published clinical trials in relapsed myeloma and up-front use in the transplant-ineligible population (Goyal, Uy, DiPersio, & Vij, 2007; Richardson et al., 2007; San Miguel et al., 2008). Recent studies have demonstrated efficacy of bortezomib in older adults after induction in combination with thalidomide (Gay et al., 2013; Palumbo, Bringhen, et al., 2014).

In the VISTA trial, patients ineligible for stem cell transplantation received VMP versus MP. In a landmark survival analysis, patients who received doses of bortezomib greater than 39 mg/m² experienced an improved OS benefit compared to MP (Mateos et al., 2013).

Another study compared VMP plus thalidomide (VMPT) induction followed by two years of bortezomib-thalidomide maintenance (VMPT-VT) with nine five-week cycles of VMP in newly diagnosed patients with multiple myeloma ineligible for transplantation (Palumbo, Bringhen, et al., 2014). At 54 months follow-up, a median PFS advantage with VMPT-VT (35.3 months) compared with VMP (24.8 months; hazard ratio [HR] = 0.58; $p < 0.001$) was observed. The time to next therapy was 46.6 months in the VMPT-VT group and 27.8 months in the VMP group (HR = 0.52; $p < 0.001$). The five-year OS was also greater with VMPT-VT (61%) than with VMP (51%; HR = 0.70; $p = 0.01$) (Palumbo, Bringhen, et al., 2014).

Side effects of VT maintenance primarily include myelosuppression. Short-term side effects, directed toward thalidomide such as increased risk for thrombosis, constipation, sedation, and dizziness, and long-term side effects, such as neurotoxicity, provide a questionable risk-benefit ratio that should be balanced before maintenance with thalidomide is initiated (Ludwig et al., 2012).

Each practitioner is strongly encouraged to consider current data to make an informed recommendation based on each patient's individual situation. When possible, participation in a clinical trial to evaluate the role of maintenance therapy is recommended (National Comprehensive Cancer Network®, 2014).

Thalidomide

Thalidomide is an active antimyeloma therapy and is safe for use in patients who are not candidates for a transplant. Numerous trials have examined the use of thalidomide as maintenance therapy in patients following stem cell transplantation (Attal et al., 2006; Barlogie, Tricot, et al., 2006; Brinker et al., 2006). Three mature trials have investigated thalidomide as a maintenance strategy in older adults with multiple myeloma (Ludwig et al., 2010; Morgan et al., 2012; Palumbo, Rajkumar, et al., 2014). The Morgan et al. (2012) study compared attenuated doses of CTD to MP. Results showed a late PFS benefit in the CTD group versus MP (Morgan et al., 2012).

In another study of 289 patients older than 65 years of age, patients were randomized to receive thalidomide and interferon maintenance therapy compared to interferon alone. The combination of thalidomide and interferon led to a significantly longer PFS compared to interferon (27.7 versus 13.2 months, P = 0.0068), but no difference in OS was seen between groups (52.6 versus 51.4 months, p = 0.81) or between patients age 75 or older and younger patients (p = 0.39). Patients also experienced more toxicity from the two-drug maintenance combination compared to interferon alone. Based on the lack of survival benefit, thalidomide and interferon maintenance is not recommended (Ludwig et al., 2010).

Results of continuous lenalidomide (FIRST) and bortezomib (VISTA) studies demonstrate better tolerability than with thalidomide. Thalidomide can be used in certain individuals but must be used with caution in older adults with newly diagnosed multiple myeloma.

Glucocorticoids

For patients who have received standard combination therapy as the induction regimen for the treatment of myeloma, steroids may play a role in maintaining an initial response. In a Southwest Oncology Group trial, patients received VAD chemotherapy and were randomized to different alternate-day schedules of oral prednisone. Two different doses of prednisone were used, either 10 mg PO every other day or 50 mg PO every other day for remission maintenance. Patients who received prednisone 50 mg PO every other day had improved PFS (14 months versus 5 months) and improved OS (37 months versus 26 months) compared to patients who received 10 mg PO every other day. This suggests that using oral prednisone 50 mg every other day following induction chemotherapy may prolong PFS intervals (Berenson et al., 2002) and is independent of whether the patient underwent transplantation.

Interferon

Interferon has been studied in patients with multiple myeloma, but it seldom is used in the maintenance phase because of its poor tolerability, conflicting efficacy data, high cost, and relatively low benefit associated with therapy (Sirohi, Treleaven, & Powles, 2002). Interferon is a less attractive option than other available novel agents and is rarely used in current practice.

Conclusion

Patients undoubtedly have benefited from the advances in multiple myeloma clinical research in the past decades. Patients who are ineligible for transplant or who decide not to pursue transplant have many different options that were not available in the past. An enormous amount of dedication is needed on behalf of investigators, patients, nurses, study coordinators, and support staff to complete a clinical trial. Each trial, no matter how big or small, provides valuable information for the next group of patients and researchers. Numerous clinical trials are ongoing, and each strives to find a more effective and better tolerated antimyeloma therapy with the hope of ultimately achieving a cure. Nurses will continue to play a critical role as they guide patients through the maze of treatment and side effect management. Nurses are improving patients' clinical outcomes and quality of life with their knowledge, education, and expertise.

References

Alexanian, R., Barlogie, B., & Tucker, S. (1990). VAD-based regimens as primary treatment for multiple myeloma. *American Journal of Hematology, 33,* 86–89. doi:10.1002/ajh.2830330203

Alexanian, R., Dimopoulos, M.A., Delasalle, K., & Barlogie, B. (1992). Primary dexamethasone treatment of multiple myeloma. *Blood, 80,* 887–890.

Alexanian, R., Haut, A., Khan, A.U., Lane, M., McKelvey, E.M., Migliore, P.J., ... Wilson, H.E. (1969). Treatment for multiple myeloma: Combination chemotherapy with different melphalan dose regimens. *JAMA, 208,* 1680–1685. doi:10.1001/jama.208.9.1680

Arlt, W., & Allolio, B. (2003). Adrenal insufficiency. *Lancet, 361,* 1881–1893. doi:10.1016/S0140-6736(03)13492-7

Attal, M., Harousseau, J.-L., Facon, T., Guilhot, F., Doyen, C., Fuzibet, J.G., ... Bataille, R. (2003). Single versus double autologous stem-cell transplantation for multiple myeloma. *New England Journal of Medicine, 349,* 2495–2502. doi:10.1056/NEJMoa032290

Attal, M., Harousseau, J.-L., Leyvraz, S., Doyen, C., Hulin, C., Benboubkher, L., ... Facon, T. (2006). Maintenance therapy with thalidomide improves survival in patients with multiple myeloma. *Blood, 108,* 3289–3294. doi:10.1182/blood-2006-05-022962

Attal, M., Harousseau, J.-L., Stoppa, A.M., Sotto, J.J., Fuzibet, J.G., Rossi, J.F., ... Bataille, R. (1996). A prospective, randomized trial of autologous bone marrow transplantation and chemotherapy in multiple myeloma: Intergroupe Français du Myélome. *New England Journal of Medicine, 335,* 91–97. doi:10.1056/NEJM199607113350204

Badros, A., Barlogie, B., Siegel, E., Morris, C., Desikan, R., Zangari, M., ... Tricot, G. (2001). Autologous stem cell transplantation in elderly multiple myeloma patients over the age of 70 years. *British Journal of Haematology, 114,* 600–607. doi:10.1046/j.1365-2141.2001.02976.x

Barlogie, B., Kyle, R.A., Anderson, K.C., Greipp, P.R., Lazarus, H.M., Hurd, D.D., ... Crowley, J.C. (2006). Standard chemotherapy compared with high-dose chemoradiotherapy for multiple myeloma: Final results of phase III US Intergroup Trial S9321. *Journal of Clinical Oncology, 24,* 929–936. doi:10.1200/JCO.2005.04.5807

Barlogie, B., Tricot, G., Anaissie, E., Shaughnessy, J., Rasmussen, E., van Rhee, F., ... Crowley, J. (2006). Thalidomide and hematopoietic-cell transplantation for multiple myeloma. *New England Journal of Medicine, 354,* 1021–1030. doi:10.1056/NEJMoa053583

Berenson, J.R., Crowley, J.J., Grogan, T.M., Zangmeister, J., Briggs, A.D., Mills, G.M., ... Salmon, S.E. (2002). Maintenance therapy with alternate-day prednisone improves survival in multiple myeloma patients. *Blood, 99,* 3163–3168. doi:10.1182/blood.V99.9.3163

Bergsagel, D.E., Sprague, C.C., Austin, C., & Griffith, K.M. (1962). Evaluation of new chemotherapeutic agents in the treatment of multiple myeloma. IV. L-Phenylalanine mustard (NSC-8806). *Cancer Chemotherapy Reports, 21,* 87–99.

Bergsagel, D.E., & Stewart, A.K. (2004). Conventional-dose chemotherapy of myeloma. In J.S. Malpas, D.E. Bergsagel, R. Kyle, & K. Anderson (Eds.), *Myeloma: Biology and management* (3rd ed., pp. 203–217). Philadelphia, PA: Saunders.

Bringhen, S., Mateos, M.V., Zweegman, S., Larocca, A., Falcone, A.P., Oriol, A., ... Palumbo, A. (2013). Age and organ damage correlate with poor survival in myeloma patients: Meta-analysis of 1435 individual patient data from 4 randomized trials. *Haematologica, 98,* 980–987. doi:10.3324/haematol.2012.075051

Brinker, B.T., Waller, E.K., Leong, T., Heffner, L.T., Jr., Redei, I., Langston, A.A., & Lonial, S. (2006). Maintenance therapy with thalidomide improves overall survival after autologous hematopoietic progenitor cell transplant with multiple myeloma. *Cancer, 106,* 2171–2180. doi:10.1002/cncr.21852

Cavo, M., Zamagni, E., Tosi, P., Tacchetti, P., Cellini, C., Cangini, D., ... Baccarani, M. (2005). Superiority of thalidomide and dexamethasone over vincristine-doxorubicin-dexamethasone (VAD) as primary therapy in preparation for autologous transplantation for multiple myeloma. *Blood, 106,* 35–39. doi:10.1182/blood-2005-02-0522

Celgene Corporation. (2014). *Revlimid® (lenalidomide)* [Package insert]. Summit, NJ: Author.

Centers for Disease Control and Prevention. (2014). PCV13 (Pneumococcal conjugate) vaccine: Recommendations, scenarios and Q&As for healthcare professionals about PCV13 for adults. Retrieved from http://www.cdc.gov/vaccines/vpd-vac/pneumo/vac-PCV13-adults.htm

Chanan-Khan, A.A., Sonneveld, P., Schuster, M., Irwin, D., Stadtmauer, E.A., Facon, T., ... Richardson, P.G. (2006). Analysis of varicella zoster virus reactivation among bortezomib-treated patients in the APEX study [Abstract No. 3535]. Retrieved from http://abstracts.hematologylibrary.org/cgi/content/abstract/108/11/3535

Child, J.A., Morgan, G.J., Davies, F.E., Owen, R.G., Bell, S.E., Hawkins, K., ... Selby, P.J. (2003). High-dose chemotherapy with hematopoietic stem-cell rescue for multiple myeloma. *New England Journal of Medicine, 348,* 1875–1883. doi:10.1056/NEJMoa022340

Colson, K., Doss, D.S., Swift, R., Tariman, J., & Thomas, T.E. (2004). Bortezomib, a newly approved proteasome inhibitor for the treatment of multiple myeloma: Nursing implications. *Clinical Journal of Oncology Nursing, 8,* 473–480. doi:10.1188/04.CJON.473-480

Cook, R.J., Vogl, D., Mangan, P.A., Cunningham, K., Luger, S., Porter, D.L., ... Stadtmauer, E.A. (2008). Lenalidomide and stem cell collection in patients with multiple myeloma [Abstract No. 8547]. Retrieved from http://meeting.ascopubs.org/cgi/content/abstract/26/15_suppl/8547

Cornwell, G.G., 3rd, Pajak, T.F., McIntyre, O.R., Kochwa, S., & Dosik, H. (1982). Influence of renal failure on myelosuppressive effects of melphalan: Cancer and Leukemia Group B experience. *Cancer Treatment Reports, 66,* 475–481.

Dimopoulos, M.A., Delforge, M., Hajek, R., Kropff, M., Petrucci, M.T., Lewis, P., ... Palumbo, A. (2013). Lenalidomide, melphalan, and prednisone, followed by lenalidomide maintenance, improves health-related quality of life in newly diagnosed multiple myeloma patients aged 65 years or older: Results of a randomized phase III trial. *Haematologica, 98,* 784–788. doi:10.3324/haematol.2012.074534

Doss, D.S. (2006). Advances in oral therapy in the treatment of multiple myeloma. *Clinical Journal of Oncology Nursing, 10,* 514–520. doi:10.1188/06.CJON.514-520

Facon, T., Dimopoulos, M.A., Dispenzieri, A., Catalano, J.V., Belch, A.R., Hulin, C., ... Benboubker, L. (2013). Initial phase 3 results of the FIRST (Frontline Investigation of Lenalidomide + Dexamethasone Versus Standard Thalidomide) Trial (MM-020/IFM 07 01) in newly diagnosed multiple myeloma (NDMM) patients (Pts) ineligible for stem cell transplantation (SCT) [Abstract No. 2]. *Blood, 122.* Retrieved from http://bloodjournal.hematologylibrary.org/content/122/21/2

Facon, T., Mary, J.-Y., Pegourie, B., Attal, M., Renaud, M., Sadoun, A., ... Bataille, R. (2006). Dexamethasone-based regimens versus melphalan-prednisone for elderly multiple myeloma patients ineligible for high-dose therapy. *Blood, 107,* 1292–1298. doi:10.1182/blood-2005-04-1588

Faiman, B. (2007). Clinical updates and nursing considerations for patients with multiple myeloma. *Clinical Journal of Oncology Nursing, 11,* 831–840. doi:10.1188/07.CJON.831-840

Faiman, B., Bilotti, E., Mangan, P.A., Rogers, K., & the IMF Nurse Leadership Board. (2008). Steroid-associated side effects in patients with multiple myeloma: Consensus statement of the IMF Nurse Leadership Board. *Clinical Journal of Oncology Nursing, 12*(Suppl. 3), 53–63. doi:10.1188/08.CJON.S1.53-62

Faiman, B., Miceli, T., Noonan, K., & Lilleby, K. (2013). Clinical updates in blood and marrow transplantation in multiple myeloma. *Clinical Journal of Oncology Nursing, 17*(Suppl. 6), 33–41. doi:10.1188/13.CJON.S2.33-41

Falco, P., Cavallo, F., Larocca, A., Rossi, D., Guglielmelli, T., Rocci, A., ... Palumbo, A. (2013). Lenalidomide-prednisone induction followed by lenalidomide-melphalan-prednisone consolidation and lenalidomide-prednisone maintenance in newly diagnosed elderly unfit myeloma patients. *Leukemia, 27,* 695–701. doi:10.1038/leu.2012.271

Gay, F., Hayman, S., Lacy, M.Q., Buadi, F., Gertz, M.A., Kumar, S., ... Rajkumar, S.V. (2009). Superiority of lenalidomide-dexamethasone versus thalidomide-dexamethasone as initial therapy for newly diagnosed multiple myeloma [Abstract No. 3884]. Retrieved from http://ash.confex.com/ash/2009/webprogram/Paper20613.html

Gay, F., Magarotto, V., Crippa, C., Pescosta, N., Guglielmelli, T., Cavallo, F., ... Palumbo, A. (2013). Bortezomib induction, reduced-intensity transplantation, and lenalidomide consolidation-maintenance for myeloma: Updated results. *Blood, 122,* 1376–1383. doi:10.1182/blood-2013-02-483073

Giralt, S., Stadtmauer, E.A., Harousseau, J.L., Palumbo, A., Bensinger, W., Comenzo, R.L., ... Durie, B.G. (2009). International Myeloma Working Group (IMWG) consensus statement and guidelines regarding the current status of stem cell collection and high-dose therapy for multiple myeloma and the role of plerixafor (AMD 3100). *Leukemia, 23,* 1904–1912. doi:10.1038/leu.2009.127

Goyal, S.D., Uy, G., DiPersio, J.R., & Vij, R. (2007). Bortezomib (BTZ) prior to and as maintenance therapy after autologous stem cell transplant (ASCT) in multiple myeloma (MM): Long-term follow-up of a phase II study [Abstract No. 8044]. *Journal of Clinical Oncology, 25*(Suppl. 19). Retrieved from http://meeting.ascopubs.org/cgi/content/abstract/25/18_suppl/8044

Harousseau, J.-L., Attal, M., Leleu, X., Troncy, J., Pegourie, B., Stoppa, A.M., ... Avet-Loiseau, H. (2006). Bortezomib plus dexamethasone as induction treatment prior to autologous stem cell transplantation in patients with newly diagnosed multiple myeloma: Results of an IFM phase II study. *Haematologica, 91,* 1498–1505.

Harousseau, J.-L., Mathiot, C., Attal, M., Marit, G., Caillot, D., Hullin, C., ... Moreau, P. (2008). Bortezomib/dexamethasone versus VAD as induction prior to autologous stem cell transplantation (ASCT) in previously untreated multiple myeloma (MM): Updated data from IFM 2005/01 trial [Abstract No. 8505]. *Journal of Clinical Oncology, 31,* 3279–3287. doi:10.1200/JCO.2009.27.9158

Hernández, J.M., García-Sanz, R., Golvano, E., Bladé, J., Fernandez-Calvo, J., Trujillo, J., ... San Miguel, J.F. (2004). Randomized comparison of dexamethasone combined with melphalan versus melphalan with prednisone in the treatment of elderly patients with multiple myeloma. *British Journal of Haematology, 127,* 159–164. doi:10.1111/j.1365-2141.2004.05186.x

Hulin, C., Facon, T., Rodon, P., Pegourie, B., Benboubker, L., Doyen, C., ... Moreau, P. (2009). Efficacy of melphalan and prednisone plus thalidomide in patients older than 75 years with newly diagnosed multiple myeloma: IFM 01/01 trial. *Journal of Clinical Oncology, 27,* 3664–3670. doi:10.1200/JCO.2008.21.0948

Hussein, M.A., Baz, R., Srkalovic, G., Agrawal, N., Suppiah, R., Hsi, E., ... Walker, E. (2006). Phase 2 study of pegylated liposomal doxorubicin, vincristine, decreased-frequency dexamethasone and thalidomide in newly diagnosed and relapsed-refractory multiple myeloma. *Mayo Clinic Proceedings, 81,* 889–895. doi:10.4065/81.7.889

Jagannath, S., Barlogie, B., Berenson, J.R., Singhal, S., Alexanian, R., Srkalovic, G., ... Anderson, K.C. (2005). Bortezomib in recurrent and/or refractory multiple myeloma: Initial clinical experience in patients with impaired renal function. *Cancer, 103,* 1195–1200. doi:10.1002/cncr.20888

Jagannath, S., Durie, B.G.M., Wolf, J.L., Camacho, E.S., Irwin, D., Lutzky, J., ... Vescio, R. (2006). Long-term follow-up of patients treated with bortezomib alone and in combination with dexamethasone as frontline therapy for multiple myeloma [Abstract No. 796]. *Blood, 108.* Retrieved from http://abstracts.hematologylibrary.org/cgi/content/abstract/108/11/796

Kim, S.J., Kim, K., Kim, B.S., Lee, H.J., Kim, H., Lee, N.R., ... Shin, H.J. (2008). Bortezomib and the increased incidence of herpes zoster in patients with multiple myeloma. *Clinical Lymphoma and Myeloma, 8,* 237–240. doi:10.3816/CLM.2008.n.031

Kumar, S.K., Mikhael, J., Laplant, B., Lacy, M.Q., Buadi, F.K., Dingli, D., ... Winters, J.L. (2014). Phase 2 trial of intravenously administered plerixafor for stem cell mobilization in patients with multiple myeloma following lenalidomide-based initial therapy. *Bone Marrow Transplantation, 49,* 201–205. doi:10.1038/bmt.2013.175

Kumar, S., & Rajkumar, S.V. (2006). Thalidomide and lenalidomide in the treatment of multiple myeloma. *European Journal of Cancer, 42,* 1612–1622. doi:10.1016/j.ejca.2006.04.004

Kumar, S.K., Rajkumar, S.V., Dispenzieri, A., Lacy, M.Q., Hayman, S.R., Buadi, F.K., ... Gertz, M.A. (2008). Improved survival in multiple myeloma and the impact of novel therapies. *Blood, 111,* 2516–2520. doi:10.1182/blood-2007-10-116129

Kurtin, S., & Faiman, B. (2013). The changing landscape of multiple myeloma: Implications for oncology nurses. *Clinical Journal of Oncology Nursing, 17*(Suppl. 6), 7–11. doi:10.1188/13 .CJON.S2.7-11

Kyle, R.A., & Rajkumar, S.V. (2004). Multiple myeloma. *New England Journal of Medicine, 351,* 1860–1873. doi:10.1056/NEJMra041875

Kyle, R.A., & Rajkumar, S.V. (2008). Multiple myeloma. *Blood, 111,* 2962–2972. doi:10.1182/ blood-2007-10-078022

Larocca, A., Cavallo, F., Magarotto, V., Offidani, M., Federico, V., Innao, V., ... Palumbo, A. (2013). Reduced dose-intensity subcutaneous bortezomib plus prednisone (VP) or plus cyclophosfamide (VCP) or plus melphalan (VMP) for newly diagnosed multiple myeloma patients older than 75 years of age [Abstract No. 539]. *Blood, 122.* Retrieved from http:// bloodjournal.hematologylibrary.org/content/122/21/539

Ludwig, H., Adam, Z., Tóthová, E., Hajek, R., Labar, B., Egyed, M., ... Zojer, N. (2010). Thalidomide maintenance treatment increases progression-free but not overall survival in elderly patients with myeloma. *Haematologica, 95,* 1548–1554. doi:10.3324/haematol.2009 .020586

Ludwig, H., Durie, B.G., McCarthy, P., Palumbo, A., San Miguel, J., Barlogie, B., ... Attal, M. (2012). IMWG consensus on maintenance therapy in multiple myeloma. *Blood, 119,* 3003–3015. doi:10.1182/blood-2011-11-374249

Ludwig, H., Hajek, R., Tothova, E., Drach, J., Adam, Z., Labar, B., ... Hinke, A. (2009). Thalidomide-dexamethasone compared with melphalan-prednisolone in elderly patients with multiple myeloma. *Blood, 113,* 3435–3442. doi:10.1182/blood-2008-07-169565

Mateos, M.V., Richardson, P.G., Shi, H., Niculescu, L., Elliott, J., Dow, E., ... San Miguel, J.F. (2013). Higher cumulative bortezomib dose results in better overall survival (OS) in patients with previously untreated multiple myeloma (MM) receiving bortezomib-melphalan-prednisone (VMP) in the phase 3 VISTA study [Abstract No. 1968]. *Blood, 122.* Retrieved from http://bloodjournal.hematologylibrary.org/content/122/21/1968

McCarthy, P.L., Einsele, H., Attal, M., & Giralt, S. (2014). The emerging role of consolidation and maintenance therapy for transplant-eligible multiple myeloma patients. *Expert Review of Hematology, 7,* 55–66. doi:10.1586/17474086.2014.878645

Merck & Co., Inc. (2014). *Zostavax® (zoster vaccine live)* [Package insert]. Retrieved from http:// www.merck.com/product/usa/pi_circulars/z/zostavax/zostavax_pi.pdf

Miceli, T., Colson, K., Gavino, M., Lilleby, K., & the IMF Nurse Leadership Board. (2008). Myelosuppression associated with novel therapies in patients with multiple myeloma: Consensus statement of the IMF Nurse Leadership Board. *Clinical Journal of Oncology Nursing, 12*(Suppl. 3), 13–19. doi:10.1188/08.CJON.S1.13-19

Miceli, T., Lilleby, K., Noonan, K., Kurtin, S., Faiman, B., & Mangan, P.A. (2013). Autologous hematopoietic stem cell transplantation for patients with multiple myeloma: An overview for nurses in community practice. *Clinical Journal of Oncology Nursing, 17*(Suppl. 6), 13–24. doi:10.1188/13.CJON.S2.13-24

Mileshkin, L., Stark, R., Day, B., Seymour, J.F., Zeldis, J.B., & Prince, H.M. (2006). Development of neuropathy in patients with myeloma treated with thalidomide: Patterns of occurrence and the role of electrophysiologic monitoring. *Journal of Clinical Oncology, 24*, 4507–4514. doi:10.1200/JCO.2006.05.6689

Millennium Pharmaceuticals, Inc. (2014). *Velcade® (bortezomib)* [Package insert]. Retrieved from http://www.velcade.com/files/PDFs/VELCADE_PRESCRIBING_INFORMATION.pdf

Moreau, P., Pylypenko, H., Grosicki, S., Karamanesht, I., Leleu, X., Grishunina, M., ... Harousseau, J.-L. (2011). Subcutaneous versus intravenous administration of bortezomib in patients with relapsed multiple myeloma: A randomised, phase 3, non-inferiority study. *Lancet Oncology, 12*, 431–440. doi:10.1016/S1470-2045(11)70081-X

Morgan, G.J., Davies, F.E., Gregory, W.M., Russell, N.H., Bell, S.E., Szubert, A.J., ... Child, J.A. (2011). Cyclophosphamide, thalidomide, and dexamethasone (CTD) as initial therapy for patients with multiple myeloma unsuitable for autologous transplantation. *Blood, 118*, 1231–1238. doi:10.1182/blood-2011-02-338665

Morgan, G.J., Gregory, W.M., Davies, F.E., Bell, S.E., Szubert, A.J., Brown, J.M., ... Child, J.A. (2012). The role of maintenance thalidomide therapy in multiple myeloma: MRC Myeloma IX results and meta-analysis. *Blood, 119*, 7–15. doi:10.1182/blood-2011-06-357038

Myeloma Trialists' Collaborative Group. (1998). Combination chemotherapy versus melphalan plus prednisone as treatment for multiple myeloma: An overview of 6,633 patients from 27 randomized trials. *Journal of Clinical Oncology, 16*, 3832–3842.

National Cancer Institute. (2014). SEER cancer statistics review, 1975–2011. Retrieved from http://seer.cancer.gov/csr/1975_2011

National Comprehensive Cancer Network. (2014). *NCCN Clinical Practice Guidelines in Oncology (NCCN Guidelines®): Multiple myeloma* [v.2.2014]. Retrieved from http://www.nccn.org/professionals/physician_gls/pdf/myeloma.pdf

Niesvizky, R., Jayabalan, D., Zafar, F., Christos, P., Pearse, R., Jalbrzikowski, J.B., ... Coleman, M. (2007). BiRD (Biaxin®/Revlimid®/dexamethasone) in myeloma (MM) [Abstract No. PO-714]. *Haematologica, 92*(Suppl. 2), 178.

Nooka, A.K., Kaufman, J.L., Muppidi, S., Langston, A., Heffner, L.T., Gleason, C., ... Lonial, S. (2014). Consolidation and maintenance therapy with lenalidomide, bortezomib and dexamethasone (RVD) in high-risk myeloma patients. *Leukemia, 28*, 690–693. doi:10.1038/leu.2013.335

Orlowski, R.Z., Eswara, J.R., Lafond-Walker, A., Grever, M.R., Orlowski, M., & Dang, C.V. (1998). Tumor growth inhibition induced in a murine model of human Burkitt's lymphoma by a proteasome inhibitor. *Cancer Research, 58*, 4342–4348.

Ozaki, S., Harada, T., Saitoh, T., Shimazaki, C., Itagaki, M., Asaoku, H., ... Shimizu, K. (2014). Survival of multiple myeloma patients aged 65–70 years in the era of novel agents and autologous stem cell transplantation: A multicenter retrospective collaborative study of the Japanese Society of Myeloma and the European Myeloma Network. *Acta Haematologica, 132*, 211–219. doi:10.1159/000357394

Palumbo, A., Bringhen, S., Caravita, T., Merla, E., Capparella, V., Callea, V., ... Galli, M. (2006). Oral melphalan and prednisone chemotherapy plus thalidomide compared with melphalan and prednisone alone in elderly patients with multiple myeloma: Randomised controlled trial. *Lancet, 367*, 825–831. doi:10.1016/S0140-6736(06)68338-4

Palumbo, A., Bringhen, S., Larocca, A., Rossi, D., Di Raimondo, F., Magarotto, V., ... Cavo, M. (2014). Bortezomib-melphalan-prednisone-thalidomide followed by maintenance with bortezomib-thalidomide compared with bortezomib-melphalan-prednisone for initial treatment of multiple myeloma: Updated follow-up and improved survival. *Journal of Clinical Oncology, 32*, 634–640. doi:10.1200/JCO.2013.52.0023

Palumbo, A., Bringhen, S., Petrucci, M.T., Musto, P., Rossini, F., Nunzi, M., ... Boccadoro, M. (2004). Intermediate-dose melphalan improves survival of myeloma patients aged 50 to 70:

Results of a randomized controlled trial. *Blood, 104,* 3052–3057. doi:10.1182/blood-2004-02-0408

Palumbo, A., Hajek, R., Delforge, M., Kropff, M., Petrucci, M.T., Catalano, J., ... Dimopoulos, M.A. (2012). Continuous lenalidomide treatment for newly diagnosed multiple myeloma. *New England Journal of Medicine, 366,* 1759–1769. doi:10.1056/NEJMoa1112704

Palumbo, A., Mateos, M.-V., Bringhen, S., & San Miguel, J.-F. (2011). Practical management of adverse events in multiple myeloma: Can therapy be attenuated in older patients? *Blood, 25,* 181–191. doi:10.1016/j.blre.2011.03.005

Palumbo, A., Mina, R., Cerrato, C., & Cavallo, F. (2013). Role of consolidation/maintenance therapy in multiple myeloma. *Clinical Lymphoma, Myeloma and Leukemia, 13*(Suppl. 2), S349–S354. doi:10.1016/j.clml.2013.05.009

Palumbo, A., Rajkumar, S.V., Dimopoulos, M.A., Richardson, P.G., San Miguel, J., Barlogie, B., ... Hussein, M.A. (2008). Prevention of thalidomide- and lenalidomide-associated thrombosis in myeloma. *Leukemia, 22,* 414–423. doi:10.1038/sj.leu.2405062

Palumbo, A., Rajkumar, S.V., San Miguel, J.-F., Larocca, A., Niesvizky, R., Morgan, G., ... Orlowski, R.Z. (2014). International Myeloma Working Group consensus statement for the management, treatment, and supportive care of patients with myeloma not eligible for standard autologous stem cell transplantation. *Journal of Clinical Oncology, 32,* 587–600. doi:10.1200/JCO.2013.48.7934

Palumbo, A., Triolo, T., Argentino, C., Bringhen, S., Dominietto, A., Rus, C., ... Boccadoro, M. (1999). Dose-intensive melphalan with stem cell support (MEL100) is superior to standard treatment in elderly myeloma patients. *Blood, 94,* 1248–1253.

Pogach, L.M., Brietzke, S.A., Cowan, C.L., Conlin, P., Walder, D.J., & Sawin, C.T. (2004). Development of evidence-based clinical practice guidelines for diabetes: The Department of Veterans Affairs/Department of Defense guidelines initiative. *Diabetes Care, 27*(Suppl. 2), B82–B89. doi:10.2337/diacare.27.suppl_2.B82

Rajkumar, S.V. (2005). Multiple myeloma: The death of VAD as initial therapy. *Blood, 106,* 2–3. doi:10.1182/blood-2005-04-1451

Rajkumar, S.V., Blood, E., Vesole, D., Fonseca, R., & Greipp, P.R. (2006). Phase III clinical trial of thalidomide plus dexamethasone compared with dexamethasone alone in newly diagnosed multiple myeloma: A clinical trial coordinated by the Eastern Cooperative Oncology Group. *Journal of Clinical Oncology, 24,* 431–436. doi:10.1200/JCO.2005.03.0221

Rajkumar, S.V., Jacobus, S., Callander, N.S., Fonseca, R., Vesole, D.H., Williams, M.E., ... Greipp, P.R. (2010). Lenalidomide plus high-dose dexamethasone versus lenalidomide plus low-dose dexamethasone as initial therapy for newly diagnosed multiple myeloma: An open-label randomised controlled trial. *Lancet Oncology, 11,* 29–37. doi:10.1016/S1470-2045(09)70284-0

Richardson, P.G., Delforge, M., Beksac, M., Wen, P., Jongen, J.L., Sezer, O., ... Sonneveld, P. (2012). Management of treatment-emergent peripheral neuropathy in multiple myeloma. *Leukemia, 26,* 595–608. doi:10.1038/leu.2011.346

Richardson, P., Jagannath, S., Hussein, M., Berenson, J., Singhal, S., Irwin, D., ... Anderson, K.C. (2009). Safety and efficacy of single-agent lenalidomide in patients with relapsed and refractory multiple myeloma. *Blood, 114,* 772–778. doi:10.1182/blood-2008-12-196238

Richardson, P.G., Sonneveld, P., Schuster, M.W., Irwin, D., Stadtmauer, E.A., Facon, T., ... Anderson, K.C. (2007). Safety and efficacy of bortezomib in high-risk and elderly patients with relapsed multiple myeloma. *British Journal of Haematology, 137,* 429–435. doi:10.1111/j.1365-2141.2007.06585.x

Richardson, P.G., Sonneveld, P., Schuster, M.W., Stadtmauer, E.A., Facon, T., Harousseau, J.-L., ... San Miguel, J. (2009). Reversibility of symptomatic peripheral neuropathy with bortezomib in the phase III APEX trial in relapsed multiple myeloma: Impact of dose-modification guidelines. *British Journal of Haematology, 144,* 895–903. doi:10.1111/j.1365-2141.2008.07573.x

Rome, S., Doss, D.S., Miller, K.C., Westphal, J., & the IMF Nurse Leadership Board. (2008). Thromboembolic events associated with novel therapies in patients with multiple myeloma: Consensus statement of the IMF Nurse Leadership Board. *Clinical Journal of Oncology Nursing, 12*(Suppl. 3), 21–28. doi:10.1188/08.CJON.S1.21-27

San Miguel, J.F., Schlag, R., Khuageva, N.K., Dimopoulos, M.A., Shpilberg, O., Kropff, M., ... Richardson, P.G. (2008). Bortezomib plus melphalan and prednisone for initial treatment of multiple myeloma. *New England Journal of Medicine, 359*, 906–917. doi:10.1056/NEJMoa0801479

Singhal, S., Mehta, J., Desikan, R., Ayers, D., Roberson, P., Eddlemon, P., ... Barlogie, B. (1999). Antitumor activity of thalidomide in refractory multiple myeloma. *New England Journal of Medicine, 341*, 1565–1571. doi:10.1056/NEJM199911183412102

Sirohi, B., Treleaven, J., & Powles, R. (2002). Role of interferon. In J. Mehta & S. Singhal (Eds.), *Myeloma* (pp. 383–396). London, England: Martin Dunitz.

Smith, L.C., Bertolotti, P., Curran, K., Jenkins, B., & the IMF Nurse Leadership Board. (2008). Gastrointestinal side effects associated with novel therapies in patients with multiple myeloma: Consensus statement of the IMF Nurse Leadership Board. *Clinical Journal of Oncology Nursing, 12*(Suppl. 3), 37–52. doi:10.1188/08.CJON.S1.37-51

Tariman, J.D., Berry, D.L., Cochrane, B., Doorenbos, A., & Schepp, K.G. (2012). Physician, patient, and contextual factors affecting treatment decisions in older adults with cancer and models of decision making: A literature review [Online exclusive]. *Oncology Nursing Forum, 39*, E70–E83. doi:10.1188/12.ONF.E70-E83

Tariman, J., Love, G., McCullagh, E., Sandifer, S., & the IMF Nurse Leadership Board. (2008). Peripheral neuropathy associated with novel therapies in patients with multiple myeloma: Consensus statement of the IMF Nurse Leadership Board. *Clinical Journal of Oncology Nursing, 12*(Suppl. 3), 29–36. doi:10.1188/08.CJON.S1.29-35

White, D.J., Bahlis, N.J., Marcellus, D.C., Belch, A., Stewart, A.K., Chen, C., ... Couban, S. (2013). Lenalidomide plus melphalan without prednisone for previously untreated older patients with multiple myeloma: A phase II trial. *Clinical Lymphoma, Myeloma and Leukemia, 13*, 19–24. doi:10.1016/j.clml.2012.08.009

Wiley, K.E. (2007). Multiple myeloma and treatment-related thromboembolism: Oncology nurses' role in prevention, assessment, and diagnosis. *Clinical Journal of Oncology Nursing, 11*, 847–851. doi:10.1188/07.CJON.847-851

Wilson, T.A., & Speiser, P. (2009). Adrenal insufficiency. Retrieved from http://emedicine.medscape.com/article/919077-overview

Zeldis, J.B., Williams, B.A., Thomas, S.D., & Elsayed, M.E. (1999). S.T.E.P.S.: A comprehensive program for controlling and monitoring access to thalidomide. *Clinical Therapeutics, 21*, 319–330. doi:10.1016/S0149-2918(00)88289-2

CHAPTER 7

Treatment of Relapsed and Refractory Multiple Myeloma

Kevin Brigle, PhD, ANP

Introduction

For the decade of the 1990s, the mainstay of treatment for multiple myeloma included chemotherapy in combination with steroids followed by an autologous stem cell transplant (ASCT) (Kyle & Rajkumar, 2004). In this setting, five-year overall survival (OS) hovered around 30%. In the past decade, however, the discovery and use of new agents has dramatically improved patient outcomes, resulting in a doubling of OS, and long-term remissions of 8–10 years are not uncommon (Kumar et al., 2008, 2014). For the majority of patients, this success has been mainly attributed to the introduction of novel agents that include bortezomib, a proteasome inhibitor, and the two immunomodulatory agents, thalidomide and lenalidomide. The safety and efficacy of both bortezomib and lenalidomide in the up-front and relapsed settings, either alone or in combination with other agents, has been well documented over the past 10 years. In spite of these successes, the majority of patients will experience multiple relapses of their disease and eventually become "double refractory" to both of these agents. For these relapsed and refractory patients who are resistant or intolerant to both lenalidomide/thalidomide and bortezomib, the picture is particularly grim. Until recently, treatment options have been few, and median OS is only about nine months (Kumar et al., 2012). Within the past two years, however, two new novel agents were approved by the U.S. Food and Drug Association (FDA) to meet the unmet needs of this patient population. Carfilzomib, a second-generation proteasome inhibitor, was approved in July 2012 (Onyx Pharmaceuticals, Inc., 2012) and pomalidomide, a novel third-in-class immunomodulatory agent, was approved in February 2013 (Celgene Corporation, 2013a). Both gained approval for use in patients who have received at least two prior therapies, including lenalidomide and bortezomib, and who have demonstrated disease progression on or within 60 days of completion of their last therapy. These agents have modest and relatively equal activity in this heavily pretreated patient population, and their optimal sequencing has not been established. Side effects of each agent are quite manageable, and the choice of which one to use in this patient population is based on previous therapy as well as disease- and patient-specific factors. For those patients who eventually exhaust all of these novel agents and their various combinations, there remain several older but fairly effective chemotherapy-based salvage regimens that show reasonable activity in the relapsed setting.

Clinical and Biochemical Relapse

The International Myeloma Workshop Consensus Panel has established definitions used to describe relapsed myeloma. *Relapsed and refractory* myeloma is defined as disease that is nonresponsive while on salvage therapy or as disease that progresses within 60 days of discontinuing the last treatment. The more general term of *relapsed myeloma* is defined as previously treated myeloma that now shows evidence of progression but does not fit the previously mentioned definition of *relapsed and refractory* myeloma. At initial diagnosis of multiple myeloma, the start of treatment often is delayed until there is evidence of end-organ damage as reflected by the CRAB criteria of hyperCalcemia, Renal impairment, Anemia, and Bone lesions (Durie et al., 2006, 2007). Likewise, in the case of relapsed disease, not all patients will require immediate therapy.

More broadly, relapsed disease can be defined as being *biochemical* or *clinical*. As suggested by its name, clinical relapse is characterized by the presence of worsening end-organ damage per the CRAB criteria. Biochemical relapse is characterized by an increase in the monoclonal protein that meets the definitions set forth by the International Myeloma Working Group (IMWG) criteria (Durie et al., 2006, 2007) but without evidence of end-organ damage. While patients in clinical relapse obviously require intervention, the decision to treat a patient in biochemical relapse is not always so clear. Some patients may have a slow biochemical relapse that does not merit the risks of committing them to start what would likely become indefinite therapy. Conversely, other patients will show evidence of a more rapidly progressing biochemical relapse that merits intervention even in the absence of the clinical signs and symptoms of the CRAB criteria. To help clinicians with this decision, the International Myeloma Workshop Consensus Panel put forth a set of guidelines for beginning treatment in patients with biochemical relapse for whom evidence of end-organ damage is not yet apparent (Rajkumar et al., 2011). These criteria focus on both the absolute level and the rate of increase of the abnormal monoclonal protein that is present in the blood or urine.

Despite advances in first-line and salvage therapy, multiple myeloma is still considered an incurable disease. In the absence of a definitive cure, the goal of myeloma therapy has been to improve a patient's long-term progression-free survival (PFS) and, in turn, OS. An important factor associated with these goals is a patient's quality of response to treatment and, in particular, the attainment of a complete response (CR) at any treatment point in the disease trajectory. A CR is defined as the elimination of detectable disease by currently available laboratory means. At present, this means the disappearance of the abnormal myeloma protein as determined by a negative immunofixation of the serum and/or urine. Ongoing research is seeking to develop even more sensitive tests aimed at making the definition of a CR more stringent. These tests are looking to identify the presence of very low levels of disease, known as *minimal residual disease* or MRD, with the ultimate goal of eradicating all traces of residual myeloma (Compagno, Mantoan, Astolfi, Boccadoro, & Ladetto, 2005; Owen & Rawstron, 2005). Numerous studies have shown that a CR in the frontline setting is associated with both prolonged PFS and OS (Rawstron et al., 2013; van de Velde et al., 2007). With the development of the novel agents, similar evidence is now available as to the benefit of attaining a CR in the setting of relapsed disease as well (Chanan-Khan & Giralt, 2010; Niesvizky et al., 2008). As such, an increasing number of patients are living longer as a result of the high response rates (including CRs) seen by using these novel agents in the up-front, relapsed, and double refractory setting.

IMWG has established response criteria in order to standardize and uniformly analyze outcomes in the treatment of multiple myeloma. It has defined six categories of response: CR, stringent complete response (sCR), very good partial response (VGPR), partial response (PR), stable disease (SD), and progressive disease (PD). Of these, the three main categories most often described in clinical practice roughly include CR as defined above; VGPR, whereby patients achieve a 90% or greater reduction from baseline abnormal protein values in the serum plus a urine protein level of less than 100 mg/24 hours; and PR, which is defined as a 50%–90% reduction in the abnormal protein in serum or urine (Durie et al., 2006).

Imaging Patients With Relapsed Multiple Myeloma

The development of specific bone lesions, osteopenia, or plasmacytomas occurs commonly in patients with multiple myeloma. Up to 90% of patients will develop bone lesions at some time in the course of their disease, and the pain associated with these lesions may be the first indication of relapse. While some patients may have asymptomatic bony lesions, the vast majority will experience pain at the site of bone damage (Raje & Roodman, 2011). In addition to the painful areas of bone involvement, it is critical to identify asymptomatic areas of bone loss that may be at risk for pathologic fracture. The sites most commonly affected are those with active hematopoiesis, including the vertebrae (65%), ribs (45%) skull (40%), shoulders (40%), pelvis (30%), and long bones (25%) (Dimopoulos, Terpos, et al., 2009). Imaging of the skeletal system is an essential component for evaluating and identifying areas of bone disease that may require localized treatment. Conventionally, plain film radiography, or x-rays, has been used to diagnose bone disease. The metastatic skeletal survey with plain radiographs is recommended as the imaging technique choice, and it includes a series of x-rays of the skull, pelvis, long bones, and extremities to identify areas of myeloma-related bone damage. Unfortunately, this is not an exquisitely sensitive technique, and it may reveal lytic disease only when 30% or more of the trabecular bone has been lost (Roodman, 2008). Because of this limitation, magnetic resonance imaging (MRI), computed tomography (CT), and positron-emission tomography (PET) are gaining wider use (Dimopoulos et al., 2011). These imaging techniques are more sensitive and are useful to visualize soft tissue, spinal cord, and nerve root involvement and to discriminate between malignant and benign vertebral compression fractures (VCFs). These painful fractures involve the collapse of a vertebra as a result of myeloma bone destruction, and they appear as a wedge deformity on conventional x-rays. The collapse results in a vertebral loss of height that is greater anteriorly than posteriorly, causing the spinal column above it to bend forward (Hussein et al., 2008).

While radiation therapy is effective in palliating pain of VCFs or decreasing the tumor size, other procedures such as percutaneous vertebroplasty (injection of a bone cement) or balloon kyphoplasty (use of an inflatable balloon to restore vertebral height followed by installation of a bone cement) may be used to correct the vertebral body deformity associated with the VCF (Terpos et al., 2013). These procedures often provide rapid pain relief, help to stabilize the deformity, and provide improvement in functional status and quality of life (Berenson et al., 2011; Hussein et al., 2008; McDonald et al., 2008). It is important to note that although a VCF may occur in a patient with multiple myeloma and often is related to the tumor, a VCF also may be the result of osteoporosis and unrelated to the cancer. In this instance, balloon kyphoplasty or vertebroplasty may be warranted, but radiation would be of no benefit (Terpos et al., 2013).

Bisphosphonates in Relapsed Multiple Myeloma

Bone disease in multiple myeloma may lead to hypercalcemia of malignancy, pain, or an increase in skeletal-related events (SREs) such as pathologic fractures, spinal cord compression, and the requirement for surgery or palliative radiotherapy. The IV bisphosphonates (BPs) pamidronate and zoledronate play a fundamental role in minimizing and managing skeletal-related complications in multiple myeloma (Palumbo et al., 2014; Terpos et al., 2013). These agents have a strong affinity for hydroxyapatite (the major constituent of bone) and achieve high concentrations at sites of active osteoclast-mediated bone destruction (Drake, Clarke, & Khosla, 2008). Clinical trials have shown that these two agents are equally effective at limiting both SREs and pain in patients with multiple myeloma, with zoledronate having the practical advantage of a shorter infusion time (Palumbo et al., 2014; Rosen et al., 2003). Zoledronate has been associated with improved survival in patients with myeloma who have bone disease, but only when compared to the oral BP clodronate (Morgan et al., 2010). For pamidronate, no survival data are available, but doses of 30 mg versus 90 mg were similarly efficacious, and patients had better physical functioning at 12 months with the lower dose (Gimsing et al., 2010).

IMWG recently released guidelines concerning the management of multiple myeloma–related bone disease (Terpos et al., 2013). An expert panel recommended that all patients with multiple myeloma receive IV BP therapy regardless of the presence of bone disease at diagnosis. Starting at diagnosis, these agents are to be administered every three to four weeks and should be given continuously in patients with active disease for up to two years. They may be discontinued in patients achieving a CR or VGPR but should be resumed upon relapse of disease (Terpos et al., 2013). While the BPs generally are well tolerated, potential adverse events include hypocalcemia, acute-phase reactions, renal impairment, osteonecrosis of the jaw (ONJ), and atypical fractures (Chang et al., 2012; Kennel & Drake, 2009; Miceli et al., 2011). Nursing management of patients receiving BPs includes side effect education and assessment for complications (Miceli et al., 2011).

Hypocalcemia generally is mild, but all patients receiving BPs should receive oral calcium (600 mg/day) in combination with 400 IU/day of vitamin D_3 (Peter, Mishra, & Fraser, 2004). Acute-phase reactions, manifested as flulike symptoms, are rare but often occur following the first BP infusion. Symptoms generally respond to acetaminophen 650 mg PO taken every four to six hours following the infusion (Miceli et al., 2011).

Some degree of renal impairment is present in about 20% of patients with multiple myeloma and is not an uncommon finding in the relapsed patient. The BPs are associated with both dose-dependent and rate-dependent adverse effects on renal function (Perazella & Markowitz, 2008). Thus, a reduced dose or longer infusion time is indicated in the setting of mild to moderate renal impairment (estimated creatinine clearance of 30–60 ml/min). Zoledronic acid is administered as a 4 mg IV infusion over 15 minutes in patients with normal renal function, but dose adjustments are recommended for patients with even mild renal impairment (Terpos, Berenson, Raje, & Roodman, 2014). Pamidronate is administered as a 30–90 mg IV infusion, and no dose adjustment is recommended for renal impairment when given monthly. Previously, it has been given over four to six hours, but recent studies have demonstrated safety with infusion times of only 60 minutes in patients with normal renal function (Chantzichristos, Andreasson, & Johansson, 2008; Gimsing et al., 2010). For patients at risk for worsening renal function, increasing the interval between BP infusions and slowing the infusion rate may help to reduce the potential for cumulative chronic renal toxicity. Maintenance of good hydration is important for patients receiving IV BPs, as is monitoring of the serum creatinine before each dose to assess for renal dysfunction (Miceli et al., 2011).

The development of ONJ is a rare but more serious complication of prolonged BP therapy (Palumbo et al., 2014; Van den Wyngaert et al., 2013). It typically manifests as a painful, exposed, necrotic area of the maxilla or mandible that does not heal within six to eight weeks of therapy. ONJ more commonly is seen with zoledronate than with pamidronate; other factors that increase the risk of ONJ include poor oral hygiene, invasive dental procedures, and concomitant treatment with corticosteroids. To limit the risk of ONJ, good oral hygiene should be encouraged, and patients should have a careful dental exam prior to starting BP therapy to identify active or anticipated dental issues. Dental exams should continue throughout BP therapy, and invasive dental procedures such as tooth extractions and dental implants should be avoided (Cafro et al., 2008; Miceli et al., 2011). The IMWG guidelines recommend suspending BP therapy 90 days prior to and for 90 days following such procedures, although routine cleaning, root canals, and fillings may proceed without BP interruption (Terpos et al., 2013). A recent retrospective study by Montefusco et al. (2008) suggests that antibiotic prophylaxis prior to invasive dental procedures, may be helpful in limiting the incidence of ONJ in patients with multiple myeloma receiving BP therapy, but further studies are needed to validate this practice (Montefusco et al., 2008).

Radiation Therapy in Relapsed Multiple Myeloma

Plasma cells generally are quite sensitive to the effects of radiation, and nearly 40% of patients with multiple myeloma will require radiation therapy at some point during the course of their disease. It has long been considered an effective treatment modality for local control of myeloma-related skeletal and soft tissue lesions (Featherstone, Delaney, Jacob, & Barton, 2005; Terpos et al., 2013). Radiation may be curative in a small percentage of patients who present with a solitary plasmacytoma, but this is a rare presentation and only occurs in approximately 5% of patients (Anderson et al., 2011). Soft tissue and extramedullary plasmacytomas may deposit in the skin or other organs and generally confer a particularly poor prognosis (Liu, Bakst, Phelps, Jagannath, & Blacksburg, 2013).

Radiation most often is administered with palliative intent to provide pain relief, although other indications include relief of symptoms associated with a tumor mass (e.g., cranial nerve, organ, or joint dysfunction), treatment of an impending pathologic fracture, or reduction of a tumor on the spine that is causing a spinal cord compression with neurologic compromise. Radiation may be administered in patients who are not candidates for systemic treatment or as an adjunct to systemic therapy at any stage of the disease (Palumbo et al., 2014).

The most commonly used approach to treat myeloma-related bone disease is conventional external beam radiation. The dose delivered and the number of fractions given is 4,000–5,000 centigray and is given in a single fraction or over a period of days to weeks depending on the anatomic location being irradiated (Bosch & Frias, 1988; Wernicke et al., 2012).

For most patients with relapsed disease, the intent of radiation is simply palliation. However, some patients in relapse may be under consideration for ASCT, and as such, there is a need to preserve as much bone marrow as possible when planning a course of radiation. Likewise, preserving hematopoietic function is important because it may affect the ability to administer additional effective but potentially myelosuppressive systemic therapy in the future (Miceli et al., 2011).

Nursing care of patients receiving involved-field radiation includes alleviating the side effects related to the irradiated field. Patients receiving head and neck radiation may have difficulty chewing or swallowing and are prone to mouth sores. Patients receiving mediastinal radiation often develop nausea, loss of appetite, and painful swallowing associated with irritation of the esophagus. In both instances, good oral hygiene needs to be encouraged, and pain medications may be warranted (Harris, Eilers, Harriman, Cashavelly, & Maxwell, 2008). Pain medications also can help patients to tolerate uncomfortable positions that may be required during the radiation session, and they are quite effective to treat the pain of radiation burns. Fatigue is a common side effect of cumulative radiation therapy, and patients need to be educated about self-care strategies such as balancing activity with rest and managing their activities to conserve energy (Erickson, Spurlock, Kramer, & Davis, 2013).

Choice of Therapy for Relapsed Multiple Myeloma

For patients with multiple myeloma, increased survival and quality of life have been aided by improvements in supportive care, including the institution of prophylactic strategies, and by better management of the complications of both therapy and the disease itself (Kurtin & Faiman, 2013; Ludwig et al., 2013; Palumbo et al., 2014). Even with these successes, remissions generally are temporary, and the majority of patients will undergo multiple successive therapies punctuated with increasingly shorter remissions.

Despite better supportive care in these relapsed patients, the combination of preexisting medical problems and the comorbidities associated with both progressive disease and therapy-related side effects make continued treatment a clinical challenge (Jakubowiak, 2012; Mohty et al., 2012; Stephens, McKenzie, & Jordens, 2014). With a median age of 69 at diagnosis, many patients have preexisting medical conditions, including hypertension, cardiac disease, peripheral vascular disease, chronic kidney disease, and diabetes along with its associated comorbidities. Therapy-related toxicities most prominently include cytopenias and neuropathies but also may be associated with cardiac, renal, pulmonary, and venous thrombotic events (VTEs) (Faiman, Mangan, Spong, Tariman, & the IMF Nurse Leadership Board, 2011; Niesvizky & Badros, 2010). Finally, the disease itself commonly manifests with cytopenias, marked immunosuppression, and signs of end-organ damage including renal insufficiency, bone disease, and hypercalcemia (Kyle et al., 2003). Thus, selection of therapy for the treatment of relapsed disease requires careful consideration of these factors plus the type, efficacy, and tolerance of the previous treatment including the time interval from the last therapy (Mohty et al., 2012). The chance that a patient will respond to a previously used agent increases with the duration of the treatment-free interval of remission. According to the National Comprehensive Cancer Network® (NCCN®), retreatment with the same agent should be considered if the patient had a good response to the therapy, tolerated it well, and demonstrated an unmaintained PFS of greater than six months (NCCN, 2015b). IMWG has recommended more durable response criteria that include a remission of 20–24 months after induction at diagnosis and more than 9–12 months following therapy for relapsed disease (Palumbo et al., 2014). On the other hand, changing the treatment regimen and the drug class is recommended for those patients who had a poor response to therapy, did not tolerate the therapy, or had rapid relapse of their disease (see Figure 7-1).

For younger patients who achieve good remission, a second ASCT may be considered if they responded well to the initial transplant and had a disease-free interval of at least one year (NCCN, 2015b). Likewise, an ASCT may be recommended for appropriate patients who did not pursue a transplant in the up-front setting. Ultimately, patients who are refractory to all novel agents may be offered a clinical trial or palliative treatment using older regimens such as cyclophosphamide, dexamethasone, etoposide, and cisplatin (DCEP), dexamethasone, thalidomide, cisplatin, doxorubicin, cyclophosphamide, and etoposide (DT-PACE), or bendamustine-containing regimens as per the NCCN guidelines (see Figure 7-2).

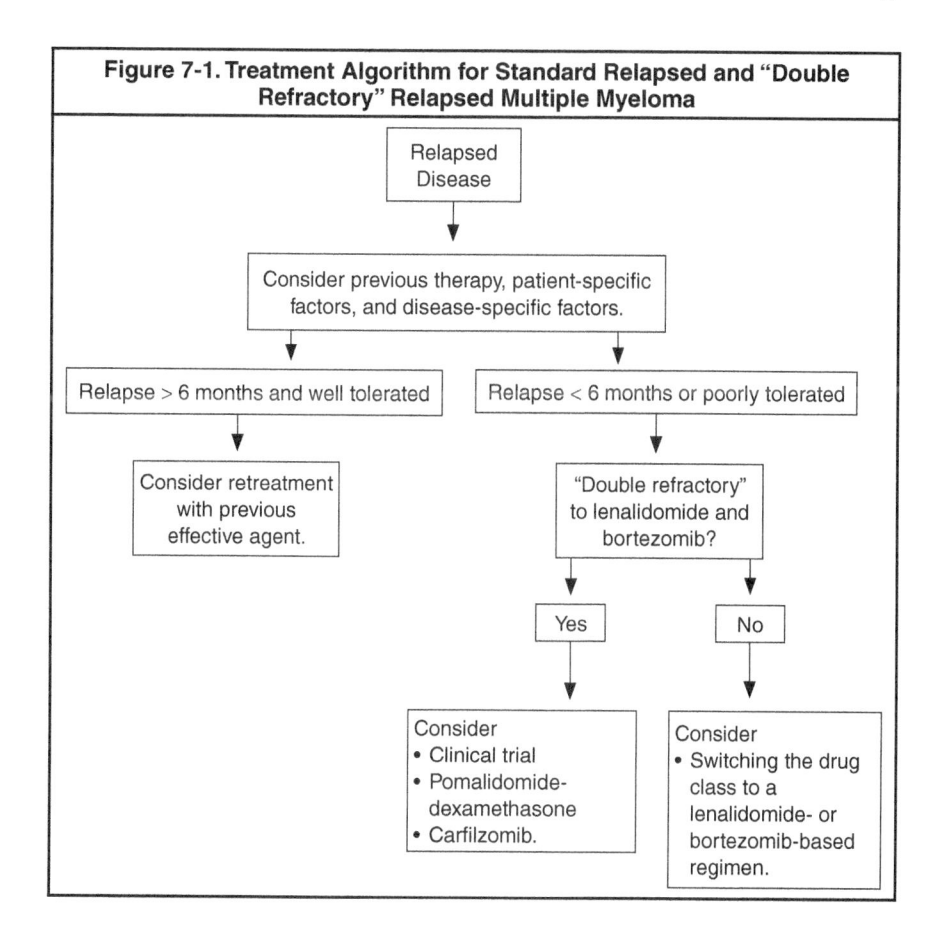

Figure 7-1. Treatment Algorithm for Standard Relapsed and "Double Refractory" Relapsed Multiple Myeloma

```
Relapsed Disease
      │
      ▼
Consider previous therapy, patient-specific
factors, and disease-specific factors.
      │
      ├──────────────────────────┬──────────────────────────┐
      ▼                                                     ▼
Relapse > 6 months and well tolerated      Relapse < 6 months or poorly tolerated
      │                                                     │
      ▼                                                     ▼
Consider retreatment                         "Double refractory"
with previous                                to lenalidomide and
effective agent.                             bortezomib?
                                                     │
                                            ┌────────┴────────┐
                                            ▼                 ▼
                                           Yes                No
                                            │                 │
                                            ▼                 ▼
                                     Consider          Consider
                                     • Clinical trial  • Switching the drug
                                     • Pomalidomide-     class to a
                                       dexamethasone     lenalidomide- or
                                     • Carfilzomib.      bortezomib-based
                                                         regimen.
```

The vast majority of patients with myeloma will experience multiple relapses and receive many different treatment regimens to fight their disease. Therefore, nurses need to be well aware of the different regimens, the agents used in each of them, the side effect profiles of the various agents, and nursing interventions to help patients deal with those side effects (see Table 7-1).

Bortezomib

Bortezomib is a first-in-class, reversible proteasome inhibitor with a novel mechanism of action. As compared to traditional chemotherapeutic agents, bortezomib has many different actions, including the inhibition of nuclear factor–kappa-B (NF-κB), a protein complex that functions as a cellular transcription factor (Richardson et al., 2003). The efficacy of bortezomib in newly diagnosed multiple myeloma has been established (San Miguel et al.,

> **Figure 7-2. Preferred Regimens for Treatment of Patients With Relapsed and Refractory Multiple Myeloma per National Comprehensive Cancer Network Guidelines**
>
> **Category 1**
> - Bortezomib
> - Bortezomib + liposomal doxorubicin
> - Lenalidomide + dexamethasone
> - Panobinostat + bortezomib + dexamethasone
>
> **Category 2A**
> - Bortezomib + dexamethasone
> - Bortezomib + lenalidomide + dexamethasone
> - Bortezomib + thalidomide + dexamethasone
> - Carfilzomib*
> - Cyclophosphamide + bortezomib + dexamethasone
> - Cyclophosphamide + lenalidomide + dexamethasone
> - Dexamethasone + cyclophosphamide + etoposide + cisplatin (DCEP)
> - Dexamethasone + thalidomide + cisplatin + doxorubicin + cyclophosphamide + etoposide (DT-PACE) ± bortezomib
> - High-dose cyclophosphamide
> - Pomalidomide* + dexamethasone
> - Thalidomide + dexamethasone
>
> **Not on Preferred List**
> - Bendamustine-containing regimens
> - Bortezomib + vorinostat
>
> **Notes**
> - Repeat previous therapy if relapse occurs at > 6 months.
> - Clinical trial should always be considered.
>
> *Indicated for patients who have received at least two prior therapies including bortezomib and an immunomodulatory agent and have demonstrated disease progression on or within 60 days of completion of last therapy.
>
> *Note.* Based on information from National Comprehensive Cancer Network®, 2015b.

2008), and it has been successfully used in patients with relapsed disease as well. Richardson et al. (2003) was the first to report on the efficacy of bortezomib in patients with relapsed disease; that same year, it received FDA approval for treatment of this patient population.

Based on the positive efficacy data from the original trials, Richardson et al. (2005) initiated APEX (Assessment of Proteasome Inhibition for Extending Remissions), a phase III multicenter study comparing bortezomib versus dexamethasone in patients with relapsed multiple myeloma. Bortezomib was dosed at 1.3 mg/m² IV on days 1, 4, 8, and 11 every 21 days, and if a suboptimal response was seen after four cycles of bortezomib, patients were given 20 mg PO dexamethasone the day of and the day following each bortezomib infusion. For patients receiving bortezomib, the one-year survival

Table 7-1. Summary of Available Agents and Nursing Considerations in the Treatment of Patients With Relapsed and Refractory Multiple Myeloma

Regimen	Major Side Effects and Nursing Considerations
Bortezomib plus dexamethasone	Myelosuppression, GI toxicities, peripheral neuropathy Risk of HSV reactivation is increased (acyclovir or valacyclovir recommended). Obtain CBC with differential before each cycle. Regimen is safe in patients with renal failure. Watch for steroid side effects with high-dose dexamethasone. Premedicate with 5-HT$_3$ receptor antagonist to prevent nausea. (Richardson et al., 2005, 2007)
Bortezomib plus PLD	Myelosuppression, GI toxicities, peripheral neuropathy, PPE, mucositis Risk of HSV reactivation is increased (acyclovir or valacyclovir recommended). Obtain CBC with differential before each cycle. Regimen is safe in patients with renal failure. Educate patient to prevent PPE due to PLD. Educate patient to prevent mucositis due to PLD. Premedicate with 5-HT$_3$ receptor antagonist to prevent nausea. (Orlowski et al., 2007)
Lenalidomide plus dexamethasone	Neutropenia, thrombocytopenia, anemia, pneumonia, VTE Risk stratify patient for thromboprophylaxis. Obtain CBC with differential every 2 weeks for the first 12 weeks of treatment, then monthly thereafter. Check serum Cr frequently, and adjust lenalidomide dose for renal insufficiency. Modify doses for grade 3 toxicities (myelosuppression, GI toxicities). Lenalidomide is distributed only through Celgene's REMS program. (Dimopoulos et al., 2009; Weber et al., 2007)
Lenalidomide plus bortezomib and dexamethasone	Myelosuppression, fatigue, mild GI toxicities (no nausea, vomiting), VTE Risk stratify patient for thromboprophylaxis. Risk of HSV reactivation is increased (acyclovir or valacyclovir recommended). Obtain CBC with differential prior to each dose of bortezomib. Check serum Cr frequently and adjust lenalidomide dose for renal insufficiency. Assess for nausea; vomiting was rare in clinical trials. Lenalidomide is distributed only through Celgene's REMS program. (Dimopoulos et al., 2010; Richardson et al., 2014)
Carfilzomib	Fatigue, anemia, thrombocytopenia, mild GI toxicities, dyspnea, mild transient serum Cr elevations Carefully monitor patients with cardiac history. Hydrate prior to administration in cycle 1 only. Premedicate with low-dose dexamethasone to infusion reactions. Dose is capped for patients with BSA greater than 2.2 m^2.

(Continued on next page)

Table 7-1. Summary of Available Agents and Nursing Considerations in the Treatment of Patients With Relapsed and Refractory Multiple Myeloma *(Continued)*

Regimen	Major Side Effects and Nursing Considerations
Carfilzomib *(cont.)*	First cycle is dosed at 20 mg/m² and increased to 27 mg/m² with subsequent cycles. Risk of HSV reactivation is increased (acyclovir or valacyclovir recommended). (Badros et al., 2013; Siegel et al., 2012, 2013)
Panobinostat	Diarrhea, fatigue, anorexia, fever, vomiting, weakness, prolongation of QTc interval Consider monitoring blood counts. All patients should receive acyclovir prophylaxis to prevent shingles (with bortezomib). Loperamide can be recommended after each loose bowel movement, not to exceed 16 mg/day.
Pomalidomide plus dexamethasone	Neutropenia, anemia, thrombocytopenia, pneumonia, fatigue, increased risk for VTE Risk stratify patient for thromboprophylaxis. Obtain CBC with differential weekly for the first 8 weeks of treatment and then monthly thereafter. Modify doses for grade 3 hematologic toxicities. Regimen has not been studied in patients with Cr greater than 3 mg/dl. Pomalidomide is distributed only through Celgene's REMS program. (Richardson et al., 2014)
DCEP: Dexamethasone, cyclophosphamide, etoposide, cisplatin	Neutropenia, thrombocytopenia, anemia, pneumonia, GI toxicities Administer G-CSF or pegylated G-CSF. Obtain CBC with differential weekly. Premedicate with 5-HT$_3$ receptor antagonist to prevent nausea. (Dadacaridou et al., 2007)
DT-PACE: Dexamethasone, thalidomide, cisplatin, doxorubicin, cyclophosphamide, etoposide	Neutropenia, thrombocytopenia, anemia, pneumonia, GI toxicities, VTE Risk stratify patient for thromboprophylaxis (increased risk with thalidomide and doxorubicin). Obtain CBC with differential weekly. Administer G-CSF or pegylated G-CSF. Use central line for doxorubicin infusion. Premedicate with 5-HT$_3$ receptor antagonist to prevent nausea. (Lee et al., 2003)

BSA—body surface area; CBC—complete blood count; Cr—creatinine; 5-HT$_3$—5-hydroxytryptamine-3; G-CSF—granulocyte–colony-stimulating factor; GI—gastrointestinal; HSV—herpes simplex virus; PLD—pegylated liposomal doxorubicin; PPE—palmar-plantar erythrodysesthesia; REMS—Risk Evaluation and Mitigation Strategy; VTE—venous thromboembolism rate was 80%, compared to 66% in patients receiving dexamethasone alone. As a result, the study was terminated early, and all patients who initially were randomized to dexamethasone were offered bortezomib regardless of their disease status (Richardson et al., 2005). At 22 months median follow-up, an updated analysis showed a median survival of 30 months for the bortezomib arm versus 24 months in the dexamethasone-alone arm (Richardson et al., 2007).

Both the hematologic and nonhematologic side effects of bortezomib are quite manageable. A complete blood count should be obtained prior to each dose of bortezomib to assess for leukopenia, anemia, and thrombocytopenia. Dose reductions as per the package insert should be considered for moderate to severe leukopenia or thrombocytopenia or for any significant nonhematologic side effects that affect function or quality of life (Millennium Pharmaceuticals, Inc., 2014). Patients receiving bortezomib in clinical trials experienced an increased risk of herpes zoster virus reactivation of up to 13%. As such, all patients who are under treatment with this agent should also be receiving prophylactic doses of acyclovir or valacyclovir (Kim et al., 2008).

Bortezomib is oxidatively metabolized via cytochrome P450 enzymes. Therefore, it is safe for use in patients with renal insufficiency or concurrent renal failure and requires no dose modifications for renal dysfunction. For patients undergoing hemodialysis, the agent is given following the dialysis session (San Miguel et al., 2008).

Gastrointestinal side effects are common but preventable. The emetogenic potential of bortezomib is low compared to other forms of chemotherapy, and nausea and vomiting can be prevented with prophylactic antiemetics and dietary modifications (Colson, Doss, Swift, Tariman, & Thomas, 2004). Patients may experience either diarrhea or constipation when receiving bortezomib. Many over-the-counter options are available to help to prevent and alleviate constipation. Increased dietary fiber and loperamide may help to decrease the number of stools in patients experiencing diarrhea. For patients with recurrent refractory diarrhea, it is important to assess stools for *Clostridium difficile*, especially if the diarrhea is accompanied by nausea, fever, or abdominal cramping (Smith, Bertolotti, Curran, Jenkins, & the IMF Nurse Leadership Board, 2008).

Patients with relapsed and refractory multiple myeloma often experience peripheral neuropathy (PN) as a result of their disease or toxicity from prior treatments (Richardson, 2010; Richardson, Laubach, Schlossman, Mitsiades, & Anderson, 2010). Treatment-related PN typically presents in a distal-to-proximal stocking-and-glove pattern. Symptoms can include numbness, tingling, burning, pain, and in severe cases, motor weakness (Colson et al., 2004; Tariman, Love, McCullagh, Sandifer, & the IMF Nurse Leadership Board, 2008). In the case of bortezomib, PN is the dose-limiting toxicity, and it is the most common reason for both dose reduction and discontinuation of therapy.

Fortunately, measures can be taken to reduce both the frequency and severity of PN when administering bortezomib by changing the dose and the schedule of administration. When given in the standard, twice-weekly IV schedule, bortezomib-related PN occurs in 35%–65% of patients, including 10%–15% of these patients in whom it is severe (grade 3 or higher). In the previously discussed APEX trial, a dose modification schedule was adopted, which resulted in a reduction in the overall frequency and severity of the problem (Richardson et al., 2007). To improve tolerability in patients with treatment-emergent PN, bortezomib has been given on a weekly schedule rather than twice weekly. This reduced schedule of bortezomib has similar efficacy to twice-weekly dosing but with a lower incidence of all grades of PN (Richardson et al., 2012).

Finally, based on the results of a randomized clinical trial, subcutaneous (SC) administration is recommended to reduce the onset and severity of treatment-emergent PN. A noninferiority trial of IV versus SC bortezomib in relapsed and refractory patients demonstrated a reduced incidence and severity of all grades of PN without sacrificing efficacy (Moreau et al., 2011). As such, in January 2012, FDA approved SC administration of the drug in all indications. It also should be noted that bortezomib-induced PN is reversible, and in the APEX study, 64% of patients experienced improvement or resolution of PN to baseline in three to four months by following the dose modification schedule (Richardson et al., 2007). Nurses play a critical role in assessing patients for PN at baseline and then prior to the administration of each subsequent dose of bortezomib. In relapsed patients, the proper combination of dose, frequency, and route of administration allows them to remain on effective therapy for a longer period of time (Tariman et al., 2008).

Bortezomib and Liposomal Doxorubicin

Based on efficacy data from a phase II study, FDA approved the combination of bortezomib and pegylated liposomal doxorubicin (PLD) for use in relapsed myeloma (Orlowski et al., 2007). In this study, all patients received IV bortezomib on days 1, 4, 8, and 11 of a 21-day cycle, but half of the patients also received PLD at a dose of 30 mg/m^2 on day 4 of therapy. Results showed that the bortezomib-PLD combination significantly increased time to progression (9.3 months) compared with single-agent bortezomib (6.5 months). Patients tolerated this regimen well and the most common side effects of therapy were myelosuppression (thrombocytopenia and neutropenia), nausea, diarrhea, constipation, and fatigue (Orlowski et al., 2007).

Side effects unique to the bortezomib-PLD combination included stomatitis and hand-foot syndrome or palmar-plantar erythrodysesthesia (PPE). These side effects occurred in fewer than 15% of patients and only 5% had serious grade 3 or grade 4 complications. Ongoing nursing assessment, patient education, and adjustments to either the dose or dosing schedule can reduce the severity and frequency of these occurrences (Orlowski et al., 2007).

Management of stomatitis includes good oral hygiene. Mouth rinses with a saline–baking soda solution may help to prevent the development of mouth sores, and patients should avoid over-the-counter rinses that contain alcohol. If mouth sores develop, a swish-and-swallow preparation of topical viscous lidocaine with or without other agents (e.g., nystatin, tetracycline, diphenhydramine, Maalox®) can relieve pain. While all patients receiving bortezomib should be taking a prophylactic dose of acyclovir or valacyclovir, a higher treatment dose may be indicated if a viral infection, such as with the herpes zoster virus, is suspected. If patients continue to experience persistent stomatitis symptoms, a change in the dose and/or the schedule of PLD should be considered (Harris et al., 2008).

Symptoms of PPE often are equated to a burn-like rash on the hands and feet that may result in a painful sloughing of skin that varies from a slight peel to a severe burn. The mechanism responsible for PPE is not clear but may be caused by localized extravasation of liposomes through capillaries in the skin that results in a vesicant-type burn. Patients should be discouraged from immersing their hands or feet in warm water for extended periods of time within 24–48 hours of PLD administration, and they should avoid repetitive activities and exercise. They need to minimize sun exposure and avoid applying direct heat to any one area, such as wearing heavy socks or restrictive clothing (Lorusso et al., 2007; von Moos et al., 2008). Cold compresses, cushioning of the affected area, and over-the-counter analgesics such as acetaminophen may help to decrease pain. Patients with multiple myeloma who are experiencing painful PPE should avoid nonsteroidal anti-inflammatory drugs (NSAIDs) such as naproxen and ibuprofen, as agents have been implicated in contributing to acute renal failure in patients with multiple myeloma (Faiman et al., 2011). If acetaminophen does not provide effective pain relief, prescription narcotic or non-narcotic analgesics should be considered.

Lenalidomide and Dexamethasone

Based on the results of a large international phase III study, FDA approved the use of lenalidomide in combination with high-dose dexamethasone (LD) in patients with relapsed or refractory multiple myeloma (Dimopoulos et al., 2009). In this trial, patients in relapse who had received at least one prior therapy were randomly assigned to receive either 25 mg PO lenalidomide or placebo on days 1–21 of a 28-day cycle. For both groups, dexamethasone was given PO at a dose of 40 mg/day on days 1–4, 9–12, and 17–20 in each of the first four cycles, followed by 40 mg/day PO on days 1–4 of each subsequent 28-day cycle. In the LD arm, the time to progression was 11.1

months and median OS was 29.6 months, compared with 4.7 months and 20.2 months, respectively, in patients who received dexamethasone in combination with placebo (Weber et al., 2007).

Common side effects of the LD combination include myelosuppression, gastrointestinal toxicities (constipation or diarrhea), and an increased risk of VTE. Patients receiving lenalidomide also require counseling on birth control, as it has the potential to cause embryo-fetal harm, having a chemical structure that closely resembles the known teratogen thalidomide (Celgene Corporation, 2013b). To address the concern of birth defects and safeguard against the risk of fetal exposure in women of childbearing potential, Celgene Corporation administers the Revlimid REMS® (formerly RevAssist®) program. This is a restricted-access program developed to address the need for patient safety and education when prescribing lenalidomide. Prior to starting lenalidomide and throughout treatment, patients must be counseled about the black box warnings, which include hematologic toxicity, an increased risk of VTE, and the potential embryo-fetal toxicity of the drug. Females of childbearing potential must avoid becoming pregnant while taking the drug and for four weeks after discontinuation. Males who are taking the drug are required to use two forms of birth control to prevent a female partner from becoming pregnant. Males are not allowed to donate sperm and neither gender may donate blood while taking lenalidomide. Counseling against fetal exposure to lenalidomide is an ongoing process and must occur at least once monthly prior to each prescription refill (Celgene Corporation, 2013b).

Myelosuppression is a common side effect of LD, but appropriate dose modifications lessen the likelihood of blood counts becoming critically low. Lenalidomide undergoes limited metabolism, and the vast majority of the dose is eliminated as unchanged drug in the urine. As such, lenalidomide needs to be dosed based on patients' renal function. Inappropriate dosing of lenalidomide in patients with renal insufficiency or renal failure may lead to significant myelosuppression. Lenalidomide can be safely given to patients on hemodialysis when properly dosed, and it should be administered after the dialysis session is complete. A complete blood count (CBC) with differential should be obtained at least every two weeks at the beginning of therapy, and serum creatinine should be checked at each blood draw. Nurses should monitor serum creatinine levels in patients with compromised renal function to assess for worsening renal failure that may warrant further dose reductions (Celgene Corporation, 2013b).

The gastrointestinal side effects of lenalidomide generally are mild and mainly include constipation and diarrhea. Nausea and vomiting, although reported in the original registration trial, are extremely rare. Most of the adverse gastrointestinal effects of lenalidomide can be managed with education and dietary modification combined with over-the-counter preparations that target the complaint. Before any intervention is recommended, however, a thorough patient history and examination should be performed. The history should establish a time course for when the symptoms began, their frequency and severity, and should include a review of other medications that may be contributing to the problem. Examination of the abdomen for the presence and character of bowel sounds, accompanied by palpation of the abdomen to evaluate the presence of abdominal pain, may be indicated for prolonged periods of constipation (Smith et al., 2008). Constipation can be managed by increasing dietary fiber and adding senna-containing laxatives. More potent over-the-counter medications for constipation may be indicated but are rarely needed in patients receiving lenalidomide. Diarrhea may be managed with the use of bulking agents such as a psyllium dietary fiber supplement combined with mild antidiarrheal agents such as loperamide (Smith et al., 2008). Patients who continue to have troublesome gastrointestinal difficulties should be encouraged to keep a food diary, which may help to identify certain foods that are triggering the problem. All patients experiencing diarrhea or constipation should be instructed to increase their fluid intake and avoid becoming dehydrated. Avoiding excessive alcohol and caffeine intake also should be encouraged for patients experiencing mild to moderate gastrointestinal symptoms. It is important to note that the physical effects related to oral therapies can lead to decreased medication adherence. Further, severe uncontrolled gastrointestinal difficulties also may have negative psychological effects, including anxiety and depression, both of which adversely affect patients' overall well-being (Smith et al., 2008).

The incidence of VTE in patients with cancer is higher than in unaffected cohorts. Among hematologic malignancies, patients with multiple myeloma have the highest risk of thrombosis (Larocca et al., 2012). The exact mechanisms behind VTE in multiple myeloma are unknown, but the type of drug therapy used to treat the disease appears to be the dominant factor in determining risk. As a single agent, lenalidomide does not appear to significantly increase risk of VTE in relapsed patients, but when combined with dexamethasone or other agents, the incidence of VTE rises considerably (Palumbo et al., 2008; Zonder et al., 2006). Patients need to be counseled about the risk of VTE while taking lenalidomide, and they should be educated about the signs and symptoms of both deep vein thrombosis and the potentially lethal complication of pulmonary embolism (Rome, Doss, Miller, Westphal, & the IMF Nurse Leadership Board, 2008). A number of studies have shown the benefit of VTE prophylaxis in relapsed and refractory patients receiving immunomodulatory drugs (Larocca et al., 2012; Niesvizky & Badros, 2010).

The choice of thromboprophylaxis agent should be tailored to the baseline risk of VTE associated with a particular regimen along with the presence of additional factors that may increase that baseline risk. In several reported studies, aspirin has been shown to be an effective prophylaxis in patients who receive lenalidomide in combination with low-dose dexamethasone (once-weekly dosing) and a number of other agents such as PLD. The use of high-dose dexamethasone as given in the original LD regimen is an additional risk factor and may mandate a more aggressive thromboprophylaxis regimen. IMWG has published guidelines for the prevention, diagnosis, and management of VTE associated with both lenalidomide and thalidomide (Palumbo et al., 2008; Rome et al., 2008).

Panobinostat, Bortezomib, and Dexamethasone

Panobinostat is the newest drug to be approved for multiple myeloma. Panobinostat received FDA approval February 23, 2015, to be given in combination with bortezomib and dexamethasone to patients who failed at least two prior therapies. Panobinostat is the first histone deacetylase inhibitor approved for use in myeloma. The safety and efficacy of the drug was tested in 193 patients and in combination with bortezomib and dexamethasone. Patients were randomized to receive panobinostat, bortezomib, and dexamethasone or bortezomib and dexamethasone alone. Results showed that patients who received the three-drug regimen had a longer PFS of 10.6 months versus 5.8 months, respectively. The recommended starting dose is 20 mg PO taken once every other day, three times a week, for weeks 1 and 2 of a 28-day cycle (Novartis Pharmaceuticals Corporation, 2015).

Bortezomib, Lenalidomide, and Dexamethasone

Bortezomib and lenalidomide are two of the most effective antimyeloma therapies currently available. Richardson, Xie, et al. (2014) evaluated a combination of these two agents with dexamethasone (RVD) in patients with relapsed and refractory disease having had one to three prior regimens. In this phase II study, 64 patients received up to eight 21-day cycles of lenalidomide 15 mg PO (days 1–14), bortezomib 1 mg/m^2 IV (days 1, 4, 8, and 11), and dexamethasone the day of and the day following bortezomib administration (40 mg PO cycles 1–4 and 20 mg PO all subsequent cycles). A maintenance phase was included for patients who had stable disease or who were still responding to the therapy. In maintenance, lenalidomide was given PO days 1–14, and bortezomib was administered IV days 1 and 8 at doses tolerated at the completion of cycle 8. Dexamethasone was given 10 mg PO days 1, 2, 8, and 9, and therapy continued until disease progression or toxicity. In this heavily pretreated group of patients, the overall response rate (ORR) was 64% with median PFS and median OS of 9.5 months and 30 months, respectively. The most common side effects of the RVD regimen included fatigue (50%), neutropenia (42%), and as expected, sensory neuropathy in 53% of patients (Richardson et al., 2014).

A randomized phase III study by Dimopoulos et al. (2010) compared the impact of adding bortezomib to RD on outcomes in relapsed and refractory patients having adverse cytogenetics. In this study, ORR, median PFS, and median OS were similar between the RD and RVD arms. Patients with poor-risk cytogenetics, excluding del(17p), had higher response rates using the RVD regimen compared to RD, but this did not translate to increased PFS or OS. Interestingly, study results also noted that the addition of bortezomib to bortezomib and dexamethasone was unable to overcome the major detrimental effect of having demonstrated previous resistance to thalidomide (Dimopoulos et al., 2010).

Carfilzomib

Carfilzomib is a second-generation epoxyketone proteasome inhibitor. Unlike the first-generation inhibitor bortezomib, it binds irreversibly to its catalytic target site in the proteasome resulting in sustained inhibition of cellular protein degradation (Siegel et al., 2012; Stewart, 2009). It is metabolized via extra-renal pathways, and neither its efficacy nor its side effect profile is influenced by renal function (Badros et al., 2013). Carfilzomib is administered twice weekly at a daily dose of 20 mg/m^2 IV in cycle 1 and then, if well tolerated, at a dose of 27 mg/m^2 in subsequent cycles until evidence of disease progression or unacceptable toxicity.

The efficacy of the drug was demonstrated in a phase II clinical trial in a heavily pretreated population of relapsed and refractory patients, most of whom had progressive disease at the time of entry into the study (Siegel et al., 2012). Of these patients, 73% had disease refractory to bortezomib, and 80% were either double refractory or intolerant to both bortezomib and lenalidomide. The ORR with single-agent carfilzomib was 23.7% with a median OS of 15.6 months. In the subpopulation of patients who were double refractory to both bortezomib and lenalidomide, ORR was 15.4% and median OS was 11.9 months. Both of these survival rates are an improvement over the approximately nine months typically seen for these heavily pretreated patients.

With respect to carfilzomib's safety profile, combined data from four phase II clinical trials representing 526 patients show it to be well tolerated (Siegel et al., 2013). The most common adverse events of any grade were fatigue (55.5%), anemia (46.8%), nausea (44.9%), thrombocytopenia (36.3%), and dyspnea (34.6%). Nonhematologic side effects including gastrointestinal events, constitutional symptoms, and dyspnea were generally mild and easily managed.

The incidence of treatment-emergent PN was uncommon (13.9%) with grade 3 events occurring in only 1.3% of patients. Only one patient discontinued treatment due to neuropathic pain, and only four patients required a dose reduction. This is an important finding considering the majority of the patients (71.9%) in these combined carfilzomib studies had active grade

1 or grade 2 PN at the time of study entry, most of which was attributable to previous therapy. The majority of new-onset PN that did occur appeared early in treatment (within the first six cycles), suggesting a lack of cumulative toxicity that supports the extended use of carfilzomib in these relapsed and refractory patients.

In the combined analysis, respiratory adverse events were reported in 69% of patients. Dyspnea was the most commonly reported respiratory adverse event and generally occurred early in the course of treatment on the day of or the day following treatment. It was most often transient and resolved spontaneously without dose reduction or discontinuation. The cause of this dyspnea was not clear, but fluid retention, especially with hydration in the first cycle of therapy, may be a contributing factor.

Cardiac adverse events occurred in 22.1% of patients, with grade 1 and grade 2 hypertension (14.3%) and arrhythmias (11%) most commonly reported. Cardiac failure events including congestive heart failure, decreased ejection fraction, and pulmonary edema occurred in 7.2% of patients. Seventy percent of patients enrolled in these four studies had baseline cardiac risk factors, and thus, the extent to which the reported cardiac adverse events were due to carfilzomib toxicity as opposed to comorbidities or prior treatment is unclear. Patients with significant cardiac risk factors should be cleared by a cardiologist prior to the start of therapy, and in the clinic, nurses should carefully monitor blood pressure and assess for signs of fluid overload. Some patients may require a reduction in hydration or the addition of a diuretic if they have symptoms of fluid overload.

Pomalidomide

Pomalidomide, the newest of the immunomodulatory agents, is a potent structural analog of thalidomide and lenalidomide. Like these other two agents, pomalidomide manifests multiple cellular effects, and it works synergistically with dexamethasone. Besides having direct antimyeloma activity, it inhibits stromal support cells and has a host of immunomodulatory properties (Zhu, Kortuem, & Stewart, 2013). Pomalidomide is an oral medication that is metabolized primarily by the cytochrome P450 pathway, and less than 2% is excreted unchanged in the urine (Zhu et al., 2013). As such, renal function should have no impact on dosing of the drug, but this has not been formally studied and caution should be exercised in patients with severe renal impairment. The recommended starting dose of pomalidomide is 4 mg PO on days 1–21 of a 28-day cycle in combination with once-weekly low-dose dexamethasone (40 mg PO). In older or less-fit patients, the dexamethasone dose may be reduced to 20 mg PO weekly to increase tolerability of the regimen. Treatment should be continued until evidence of disease progression or unacceptable toxicity (Celgene Corporation, 2013a; Dimopoulos et al., 2014).

The efficacy of the drug was demonstrated in a phase II randomized trial population of relapsed and refractory patients comparing pomalidomide 4 mg daily plus low-dose dexamethasone versus pomalidomide alone (Richardson, Siegel, et al., 2014). In the combination arm, ORR was 33% compared to 18% with single-agent pomalidomide, confirming the synergistic effect with dexamethasone. Median OS was 16.5 months, which is a big improvement compared to the 9-month survival rate typically seen for these patients. There appeared to be no cross-resistance between pomalidomide and lenalidomide, as there was no change in the efficacy of the regimen in patients who had received a lenalidomide-based treatment as their last therapy. Finally, among the 50 patients in this study who had previously received carfilzomib, ORR in the pomalidomide-dexamethasone arm was 37%, and median OS was 17.7 months, numbers that are essentially identical to the study group as a whole. Thus, double refractory patients who have exhausted lenalidomide and both proteasome inhibitors (bortezomib and carfilzomib) still demonstrated a relatively robust response to the pomalidomide-dexamethasone regimen.

With respect to its safety profile, the primary grade 3 or 4 adverse events were hematologic, with fairly significant rates of neutropenia (41%), anemia (22%), and thrombocytopenia (19%). Despite the high rate of neutropenia, the incidence of febrile neutropenic events was low (3%), although approximately 50% of patients were treated with granulocyte–colony-stimulating factor. From a nursing perspective, patients need to be educated about the risk of neutropenia and the practices necessary to prevent infection. They should practice strict handwashing techniques and avoid individuals with signs of overt illness. Nurses need to reinforce the prompt reporting of febrile episodes and instruct patients when to call the clinic or go directly to the emergency department. Neutropenic fever can pose a life-threatening event, and early intervention is critical for good outcomes (Miceli, Colson, Gavino, Lilleby, & the IMF Nurse Leadership Board, 2008).

The most common grade 3 or 4 nonhematologic adverse events were pneumonia (22%), fatigue (14%), and dyspnea (13%), all of which likely bear some relation to the hematologic side effects. The incidence of VTE was only 2%, and thromboprophylaxis consisted of aspirin 81–100 mg daily. Approximately one-third of patients required a dose reduction or dose interruption because of a serious adverse event, but discontinuation was fairly uncommon and occurred in only 3% of patients.

Like thalidomide and lenalidomide, pomalidomide also may have the potential for fetal-embryo toxicity, and patients receiving this drug require the same counseling on birth control as for the other two agents. Registration and counseling is done through a restricted access program administered through Celgene Corporation known as Pomalyst REMS™. Restrictions concerning birth control with pomalidomide are identical to those set forth for thalidomide and lenalidomide, and counseling must occur prior to starting the agent and at least once monthly prior to each prescription refill (Celgene Corporation, 2013a).

Dexamethasone, Cyclophosphamide, Etoposide, and Cisplatin

For patients who have exhausted the novel agents and their various combinations, there remain several chemotherapy-based regimens that show reasonable activity in the relapsed setting. The combination of cyclophosphamide, high-dose dexamethasone, etoposide, and cisplatin (DCEP) was evaluated in the mid-1990s as a salvage regimen for patients with multiple myeloma who relapsed following ASCT (Munshi et al., 1996). The DCEP regimen generally requires hospitalization and includes 40 mg PO dexamethasone days 1–4 along with continuous infusion on days 1–4 of cyclophosphamide (400 mg/m^2 daily), etoposide (40 mg/m^2 daily), and cisplatin (15 mg/m^2 daily). Filgrastim or pegfilgrastim is administered following completion of treatment, and the course is repeated every 28 days. In this study, the DCEP regimen produced a partial response in 41% of patients, and 10% of patients achieved a CR. It was during this time that the effectiveness of thalidomide for the treatment of multiple myeloma was beginning to emerge (Singhal et al., 1999), and investigators at the University of Arkansas evaluated the benefit of adding this novel agent to the DCEP regimen. After a median follow-up of 17 months, the ORR after three cycles of DCEP-thalidomide was 36% compared to just 18% in the DCEP arm (Barlogie et al., 2001).

The DCEP regimen was evaluated more recently by Dadacaridou et al. (2007) in a small study of 11 patients with refractory multiple myeloma. In this study, the ORR was 58.3% with a median duration of response of only nine months. While this is a relatively low response rate in the era of novel agents, this regimen still represents a reasonable, well-tolerated therapeutic option for patients with relapsed and refractory disease who have exhausted other options (Dadacaridou et al., 2007).

In 2005, Corso et al. published the results of a study comparing the inpatient infusional-DCEP regimen with a shortened, outpatient version (DCEP-short) as a pretransplant mobilization regimen. In this study, patients with newly diagnosed multiple myeloma were treated with two cycles of DCEP or DCEP-short. The response rate and safety profile were similar between the two regimens. Based on these results, a less-intensive DCEP dosing schedule that allows for outpatient administration may be a consideration for patients with relapsed multiple myeloma (Corso et al., 2005).

The most common toxicity of the DCEP regimen is moderate to severe myelosuppression. Depending on the baseline blood cell counts, patients should have a CBC with differential at least weekly if not more regularly following the DCEP regimen. Filgrastim or pegfilgrastim should be implemented to facilitate white blood cell count recovery, and patients should expect their white blood cell count to nadir between days 10 and 14 of each cycle.

Severe anemia and thrombocytopenia can be managed by red blood cell or platelet transfusions in symptomatic patients or if bone marrow recovery is not imminent. Patients need to be educated regarding the increased risk of bleeding and given thrombocytopenic precautions. Severe anemia may lead to dizziness, hypotension, and cardiac dysfunction, especially in patients with a history of renal insufficiency or cardiac conduction abnormalities. Fatigue associated with anemia is quite common, and patients should be given recommendations for managing their activities to conserve energy while still staying active during chemotherapy (Erickson et al., 2013; Miceli et al., 2008).

Erythropoiesis-stimulating agents (ESAs) can be used in the management of anemia to maintain the blood hemoglobin at the lowest level to avoid transfusion. According to the NCCN (2015a) guidelines for the treatment of cancer- and chemotherapy-induced anemia, darbepoetin can be initiated at a weekly dose of 2.25 mcg/kg SC or 500 mcg SC every three weeks. Alternatively, epoetin alfa can be given at a weekly dose of 40,000 units SC or 150 units/kg SC three times weekly. For patients with cancer, the revised FDA black box warnings for these products state that ESAs only should be given for chemotherapy-induced anemia and should be discontinued once the course is complete. To promote safety and ensure that patients have a full understanding of the black box warnings, ESAs only may be administered with informed consent under the REMS program for patients with cancer known as ESA APPRISE (Assisting Providers and Cancer Patients with Risk Information for the Safe Use of ESAs). It is important to note that ESAs have been implicated in increasing the risk of VTEs in patients with multiple myeloma. Therefore, clinicians must carefully balance the risks and benefits of ESA therapy versus the risks of blood transfusion or observation (Zonder et al., 2006). Finally, functional iron deficiency may develop in patients who are receiving long-term ESA therapy, and in fact, most patients receiving ESAs eventually will require iron supplementation. As such, serum iron, ferritin, and serum total iron-binding capacity tests are recommended prior to initiating treatment with ESAs.

Dexamethasone, Thalidomide, Cisplatin, Doxorubicin, Cyclophosphamide, and Etoposide

Prior to the development of the DCEP-thalidomide regimen, the Arkansas group had successfully treated patients with refractory multiple myeloma using a regimen (VAD) that contained high-dose dexamethasone (40 mg PO dexamethasone days 1–4) along with continuous infusion on days 1–4 of doxorubicin (9 mg/m^2 daily) and vincristine (0.4 mg/m^2 daily) (Barlogie, Smith, & Alexanian, 1984). In 2003, Lee et al. reported on the development of another salvage regimen, DT-PACE, that combined the successes of this older VAD regimen with the newer DCEP-thalidomide regimen discussed earlier. The dose and schedule of the agents in DT-PACE are similar to those in the individual regimens except that thalidomide was given at 400 mg PO daily, and there were minor changes in the dosing of cisplatin (reduced from 15 mg/m^2 daily to 10 mg/m^2 daily) and doxorubicin (increased from 9 mg/m^2 daily to 10 mg/m^2 daily). This regimen was given on an inpatient basis, and cycles were repeated every four to six weeks depending upon recovery of the patient's neutrophil and platelet counts. Following two cycles of therapy, 32% of patients in the study experienced a PR, and an impressive 16% attained a CR (Lee et al., 2003).

Patients receiving DT-PACE experienced a wide range of mild to moderate and relatively infrequent hematologic and nonhematologic side effects. Sensory neuropathy was fairly common and was thought to be related to these patients' previous vincristine exposure combined with the known neuropathic toxicity of thalidomide in the DT-PACE regimen. Doses of thalidomide were reduced or withheld to manage neuropathic toxicity. Regimens containing the combination of thalidomide and doxorubicin pose an increased risk of VTE, and this regimen was no exception (Zangari et al., 2002). Following a 15% incidence of DVTs early in the study, all patients were given low-molecular-weight heparin as thromboprophylaxis. As with the DCEP regimen, DT-PACE remains a consideration for relapsed refractory patients who have exhausted all nonchemotherapeutic options.

Conclusion

The incurable nature of multiple myeloma makes it necessary to develop new drugs and investigate unique combinations of existing agents in an effort to transform it into a chronic disease. Patients with relapsed and refractory disease have more options now than just a few years ago. With the addition of the five novel agents (three immunomodulatory agents and two proteasome inhibitors) in the past 12 years, patients with multiple myeloma are living longer and experiencing better-quality lives. And while both the number and efficacy of therapeutic options have increased, improved supportive care and patient management also has contributed to this success. With ongoing research, promising new agents are poised to become available in the next several years, and the number of unique therapeutic combinations will continue to grow. Ultimately, researchers are in search of a cure for multiple myeloma, but even when that time arrives, oncology nurses will remain integral to care of these patients and their improved outcomes.

References

Anderson, K.C., Alsina, M., Bensinger, W., Biermann, J.S., Chanan-Khan, A., Cohen, A.D., ... National Comprehensive Cancer Network. (2011). Multiple myeloma. *Journal of the National Comprehensive Cancer Network, 9,* 1146–1183.

Badros, A.Z., Vij, R., Martin, T., Zonder, J.A., Kunkel, L., Wang, Z., ... Niesvizky, R. (2013). Carfilzomib in multiple myeloma patients with renal impairment: Pharmacokinetics and safety. *Leukemia, 27,* 1707–1714. doi:10.1038/leu.2013.29

Barlogie, B., Smith, L., & Alexanian, R. (1984). Effective treatment of advanced multiple myeloma refractory to alkylating agents. *New England Journal of Medicine, 310,* 1353–1356. doi:10.1056/NEJM198405243102104

Barlogie, B., Zangari, M., Spencer, T., Fassas, A., Anaissie, E., Badros, A., ... Tricot, G. (2001). Thalidomide in the management of multiple myeloma. *Seminars in Hematology, 38,* 250–259. doi:10.1016/S0037-1963(01)90017-4

Berenson, J., Pflugmacher, R., Jarzem, P., Zonder, J., Schechtman, K., Tillman, J.B., ... Vrlonis, F. (2011). Balloon kyphoplasty versus non-surgical fracture management for treatment of painful vertebral body compression fractures in patients with cancer: A multicentre, randomised controlled trial. *Lancet Oncology, 12,* 225–235. doi:10.1016/S1470-2045(11)70008-0

Bosch, A., & Frias, Z. (1988). Radiotherapy in the treatment of multiple myeloma. *International Journal of Radiation Oncology, Biology, Physics, 15,* 1363–1369. doi:10.1016/0360-3016(88)90232-5

Cafro, A.M., Barbarano, L., Nosari, A.M., D'Avanzo, G., Nichelatti, M., Bibas, M., ... Andriani, A. (2008). Osteonecrosis of the jaw in patients with multiple myeloma treated with bisphosphonates: Definition and management of the risk related to zoledronic acid. *Clinical Lymphoma and Myeloma, 8,* 111–116. doi:10.3816/CLM.2008.n.013

Celgene Corporation. (2013a). *Pomalyst® (pomalidomide)* [Package insert]. Retrieved from https://www.celgene.com/content/uploads/2014/03/POMMG.002_03_2014.pdf

Celgene Corporation. (2013b). *Revlimid® (lenalidomide)* [Package insert]. Retrieved from http://www.revlimid.com/wp-content/uploads/2013/11/PI.pdf

Chanan-Khan, A.A., & Giralt, S. (2010). Importance of achieving a complete response in multiple myeloma, and the impact of novel agents. *Journal of Clinical Oncology, 28,* 2612–2624. doi:10.1200/JCO.2009.25.4250

Chang, S.T., Tenforde, A.S., Grimsrud, C.D., O'Ryan, F.S., Gonzalez, J.R., Baer, D.M., ... Lo, J.C. (2012). Atypical femur fractures among breast cancer and multiple myeloma patients receiving intravenous bisphosphonate therapy. *Bone, 51,* 524–527. doi:10.1016/j.bone.2012.05.010

Chantzichristos, D., Andreasson, B., & Johansson, P. (2008). Safe and tolerable one-hour pamidronate infusion for multiple myeloma patients. *Therapeutics and Clinical Risk Management, 4,* 1371–1374.

Colson, K., Doss, D.S., Swift, R., Tariman, J., & Thomas, T.E. (2004). Bortezomib, a newly approved proteasome inhibitor for the treatment of multiple myeloma: Nursing implications. *Clinical Journal of Oncology Nursing, 8,* 473–480. doi:10.1188/04.CJON.473-480

Compagno, M., Mantoan, B., Astolfi, M., Boccadoro, M., & Ladetto, M. (2005). Real-time polymerase chain reaction of immunoglobulin rearrangements for quantitative evaluation of minimal residual disease in myeloma. *Methods in Molecular Medicine, 113,* 145–163.

Corso, A., Mangiacavalli, S., Nosari, A., Castagnola, C., Zappasodi, P., Cafro, A.M., ... Lazzarino, M. (2005). Efficacy, toxicity and feasibility of a shorter schedule of DCEP regimen for stem cell mobilization in multiple myeloma. *Bone Marrow Transplantation, 36,* 951–954. doi:10.1038/sj.bmt.1705166

Dadacaridou, M., Papanicolaou, X., Maltesas, D., Megalakaki, C., Patos, P., Panteli, K., ... Mitsouli-Mentzikof, C. (2007). Dexamethasone, cyclophosphamide, etoposide and cisplatin

(DCEP) for relapsed or refractory multiple myeloma patients. *Journal of the Balkan Union of Oncology, 12,* 41–44.

Dimopoulos, M., Kyle, R., Fermand, J.P., Rajkumar, S.V., San Miguel, J., Chanan-Khan, A., ... Jagannath, S. (2011). Consensus recommendations for standard investigative workup: Report of the International Myeloma Workshop Consensus Panel 3. *Blood, 117,* 4701–4705. doi:10.1182/blood-2010-10-299529

Dimopoulos, M., Terpos, E., Comenzo, R.L., Tosi, P., Beksac, M., Sezer, O., ... Durie, B.G.M. (2009). International Myeloma Working Group consensus statement and guidelines regarding the current role of imaging techniques in the diagnosis and monitoring of multiple myeloma. *Leukemia, 23,* 1545–1556. doi:10.1038/leu.2009.89

Dimopoulos, M.A., Chen, C., Spencer, A., Niesvizky, R., Attal, M., Stadtmauer, E.A., ... Weber, D.M. (2009). Long-term follow-up on overall survival from the MM-009 and MM-010 phase III trials of lenalidomide plus dexamethasone in patients with relapsed or refractory multiple myeloma. *Leukemia, 23,* 2147–2152. doi:10.1038/leu.2009.147

Dimopoulos, M.A., Kastritis, E., Christoulas, D., Migkou, M., Gavriatopoulou, M., Gkotzamanidou, M., ... Terpos, E. (2010). Treatment of patients with relapsed/refractory multiple myeloma with lenalidomide and dexamethasone with or without bortezomib: Prospective evaluation of the impact of cytogenetic abnormalities and of previous therapies. *Leukemia, 24,* 1769–1778. doi:10.1038/leu.2010.175

Dimopoulos, M.A., Leleu, X., Palumbo, A., Moreau, P., Delforge, M., Cavo, M., ... Miguel, J.F. (2014). Expert panel consensus statement on the optimal use of pomalidomide in relapsed and refractory multiple myeloma. *Leukemia, 28,* 1573–1585. doi:10.1038/leu.2014.60

Drake, M.T., Clarke, B.L., & Khosla, S. (2008). Bisphosphonates: Mechanism of action and role in clinical practice. *Mayo Clinic Proceedings, 83,* 1032–1045. doi:10.4065/83.9.1032

Durie, B.G.M., Harousseau, J., Miguel, J.S., Bladé, J., Barlogie, B., Anderson, K., ... Kyle, R. (2006). International uniform response criteria for multiple myeloma. *Leukemia, 20,* 1467–1473. doi:10.1038/sj.leu.2404284

Durie, B.G.M., Harousseau, J., Miguel, J.S., Bladé, J., Barlogie, B., Anderson, K., ... Kyle, R. (2007). International uniform response criteria for multiple myeloma. Corrigendum. *Leukemia, 21,* 1134–1134. doi:10.1038/sj.leu.2404582

Erickson, J.M., Spurlock, L.K., Kramer, J.C., & Davis, M.A. (2013). Self-care strategies to relieve fatigue in patients receiving radiation therapy. *Clinical Journal of Oncology Nursing, 17,* 319–324. doi:10.1188/13.CJON.319-324

Faiman, B.M., Mangan, P., Spong, J., Tariman, J.D., & the IMF Nurse Leadership Board. (2011). Renal complications in multiple myeloma and related disorders: Survivorship care plan of the International Myeloma Foundation Nurse Leadership Board. *Clinical Journal of Oncology Nursing, 15*(Suppl. 4), 66–76. doi:10.1188/11.CJON.S1.66-76

Featherstone, C., Delaney, G., Jacob, S., & Barton, M. (2005). Estimating the optimal utilization rates of radiotherapy for hematologic malignancies from a review of the evidence: Part II—Leukemia and myeloma. *Cancer, 103,* 393–401. doi:10.1002/cncr.20755

Gimsing, P., Carlson, K., Turesson, I., Fayers, P., Waage, A., Vangsted, A., ... Wisloff, F. (2010). Effect of pamidronate 30 mg versus 90 mg on physical function in patients with newly diagnosed multiple myeloma (Nordic Myeloma Study Group): A double-blind, randomised controlled trial. *Lancet Oncology, 11,* 973–982. doi:10.1016/S1470-2045(10)70198-4

Harris, D.J., Eilers, J., Harriman, A., Cashavelly, B.J., & Maxwell, C. (2008). Putting Evidence Into Practice®: Evidence-based interventions for the management of oral mucositis. *Clinical Journal of Oncology Nursing, 12,* 141–152. doi:10.1188/08.CJON.141-152

Hussein, M.A., Vrionis, F.D., Allison, R., Berenson, J., Berven, S., Erdem, E., ... Durie, G.M. (2008). The role of vertebral augmentation in multiple myeloma: International Myeloma Working Group consensus statement. *Leukemia, 22,* 1479–1484. doi:10.1038/leu.2008.127

Jakubowiak, A. (2012). Management strategies for relapsed/refractory multiple myeloma: Current clinical perspectives. *Seminars in Hematology, 49*(Suppl. 1), S16–S32. doi:10.1053/j.seminhematol.2012.05.003;

Kennel, K.A., & Drake, M.T. (2009). Adverse effects of bisphosphonates: Implications for osteoporosis management. *Mayo Clinic Proceedings, 84,* 632–638. doi:10.1016/S0025-6196(11)60752-0

Kim, S.J., Kim, K., Kim, B.S., Lee, H.J., Kim, H., Lee, N.R., ... Korean Multiple Myeloma Working Party. (2008). Bortezomib and the increased incidence of herpes zoster in patients with multiple myeloma. *Clinical Lymphoma and Myeloma, 8,* 237–240. doi:10.3816/CLM.2008.n.031

Kumar, S.K., Dispenzieri, A., Lacy, M.Q., Gertz, M.A., Buadi, F.K., Pandey, S., ... Rajkumar, S.V. (2014). Continued improvement in survival in multiple myeloma: Changes in early mortality and outcomes in older patients. *Leukemia, 28,* 1122–1128. doi:10.1038/leu.2013.313

Kumar, S.K., Lee, J.H., Lahuerta, J.J., Morgan, G., Richardson, P.G., Crowley, J., ... Orlowski, R. (2012). Risk of progression and survival in multiple myeloma relapsing after therapy with IMiDs and bortezomib: A multicenter International Myeloma Working Group study. *Leukemia, 26,* 149–157. doi:10.1038/leu.2011.196

Kumar, S.K., Rajkumar, S.V., Dispenzieri, A., Lacy, M.Q., Hayman, S.R., Buadi, F.K., ... Gertz, M.A. (2008). Improved survival in multiple myeloma and the impact of novel therapies. *Blood, 111,* 2516–2520. doi:10.1182/blood-2007-10-116129

Kurtin, S., & Faiman, B. (2013). The changing landscape of multiple myeloma: Implications for oncology nurses. *Clinical Journal of Oncology Nursing, 17*(Suppl. 6), 7–11. doi:10.1188/13.CJON.S2.7-11

Kyle, R.A., Gertz, M.A., Witzig, T.E., Lust, J.A., Lacy, M.Q., Dispenzieri, A., ... Greipp, P.R. (2003). Review of 1027 patients with newly diagnosed multiple myeloma. *Mayo Clinic Proceedings, 78,* 21–33. doi:10.4065/78.1.21

Kyle, R.A., & Rajkumar, S.V. (2004). Multiple myeloma. *New England Journal of Medicine, 351,* 1860–1873. doi:10.1056/NEJMra041875

Larocca, A., Cavallo, F., Bringhen, S., Di Raimondo, F., Falanga, A., Evangelista, A., ... Palumbo, A. (2012). Aspirin or enoxaparin thromboprophylaxis for patients with newly diagnosed multiple myeloma treated with lenalidomide. *Blood, 119,* 933–939. doi:10.1182/blood-2011-03-344333

Lee, C.K., Barlogie, B., Munshi, N., Zangari, M., Fassas, A., Jacobson, J., ... Tricot, G. (2003). DTPACE: An effective, novel combination chemotherapy with thalidomide for previously treated patients with myeloma. *Journal of Clinical Oncology, 21,* 2732–2739. doi:10.1200/JCO.2003.01.055

Liu, J., Bakst, R., Phelps, R., Jagannath, S., & Blacksburg, S. (2013). Radiation therapy for secondary cutaneous plasmacytomas. *Case Reports in Hematology, 2013,* Article ID 739230. doi:10.1155/2013/739230

Lorusso, D., Di Stefano, A., Carone, V., Fagotti, A., Pisconti, S., & Scambia, G. (2007). Pegylated liposomal doxorubicin-related palmar-plantar erythrodysesthesia ('hand-foot' syndrome). *Annals of Oncology, 18,* 1159–1164. doi:10.1093/annonc/mdl477

Ludwig, H., Miguel, J.S., Dimopoulos, M.A., Palumbo, A., Sanz, R.G., Powles, R., ... Durie, B. (2013). International Myeloma Working Group recommendations for global myeloma care. *Leukemia, 28,* 981–992. doi:10.1038/leu.2013.293

McDonald, R.J., Trout, A.T., Gray, L.A., Dispenzieri, A., Thielen, K.R., & Kallmes, D.F. (2008). Vertebroplasty in multiple myeloma: Outcomes in a large patient series. *American Journal of Neuroradiology, 29,* 642–648. doi:10.3174/ajnr.A0918

Miceli, T.S., Colson, K., Faiman, B.M., Miller, K., Tariman, J.D., & the IMF Nurse Leadership Board. (2011). Maintaining bone health in patients with multiple myeloma: Survivorship care plan of the International Myeloma Foundation Nurse Leadership Board. *Clinical Journal of Oncology Nursing, 15*(Suppl. 4), 9–23. doi:10.1188/11.S1.CJON.9-23

Miceli, T., Colson, K., Gavino, M., Lilleby, K., & the IMF Nurse Leadership Board. (2008). Myelosuppression associated with novel therapies in patients with multiple myeloma: Consensus statement of the IMF Nurse Leadership Board. *Clinical Journal of Oncology Nursing, 12*(Suppl. 3), 13–20. doi:10.1188/08.CJON.S1.13-19

Millennium Pharmaceuticals, Inc. (2014). *Velcade® (bortezomib)* [Package insert]. Retrieved from http://www.velcade.com/files/pdfs/velcade_prescribing_information.pdf

Mohty, B., El-Cheikh, J., Yakoub-Agha, I., Avet-Loiseau, H., Moreau, P., & Mohty, M. (2012). Treatment strategies in relapsed and refractory multiple myeloma: A focus on drug sequencing and 'retreatment' approaches in the era of novel agents. *Leukemia, 26,* 73–85. doi:10.1038/leu.2011.310

Montefusco, V., Gay, F., Spina, F., Miceli, R., Maniezzo, M., Teresa Ambrosini, M., ... Corradini, P. (2008). Antibiotic prophylaxis before dental procedures may reduce the incidence of osteonecrosis of the jaw in patients with multiple myeloma treated with bisphosphonates. *Leukemia and Lymphoma, 49,* 2156–2162. doi:10.1080/10428190802483778

Moreau, P., Pylypenko, H., Grosicki, S., Karamanesht, I., Leleu, X., Grishunina, M., ... Harousseau, J.L. (2011). Subcutaneous versus intravenous administration of bortezomib in patients with relapsed multiple myeloma: A randomised, phase 3, non-inferiority study. *Lancet Oncology, 12,* 431–440. doi:10.1016/S1470-2045(11)70081-X

Morgan, G.J., Davies, F.E., Gregory, W.M., Cocks, K., Bell, S.E., Szubert, A.J., ... Child, J.A.. (2010). First-line treatment with zoledronic acid as compared with clodronic acid in multiple myeloma (MRC Myeloma IX): A randomised controlled trial. *Lancet, 376,* 1989–1999. doi:10.1016/S0140-6736(10)62051-X

Munshi, N., Desikan, K., Jagannath, S., Bracy, D., Tricot, G., & Barlogie, B. (1996). Dexamethasone, cyclophosphamide, etoposide and cis-platinum (DCEP), an effective regimen for relapse after high-dose chemotherapy and autologous transplantation. *Blood, 88*(Suppl.1), 586a.

National Comprehensive Cancer Network. (2015a). *NCCN Clinical Practice Guidelines in Oncology (NCCN Guidelines®): Cancer- and chemotherapy-induced anemia* [v.2.2015]. Retrieved from http://www.nccn.org/professionals/physician_gls/pdf/anemia.pdf

National Comprehensive Cancer Network. (2015b). *NCCN Clinical Practice Guidelines in Oncology (NCCN Guidelines®): Multiple myeloma* [v.2.2015]. Retrieved from http://www.nccn.org/professionals/physician_gls/pdf/myeloma.pdf

Niesvizky, R., & Badros, A.Z. (2010). Complications of multiple myeloma therapy, part 2: Risk reduction and management of venous thromboembolism, osteonecrosis of the jaw, renal complications, and anemia. *Journal of the National Comprehensive Cancer Network, 8*(Suppl. 1), S13–S20.

Niesvizky, R., Richardson, P.G., Rajkumar, S.V., Coleman, M., Rosiñol, L., Sonneveld, P., ... Bladé, J. (2008). The relationship between quality of response and clinical benefit for patients treated on the bortezomib arm of the international, randomized, phase 3 APEX trial in relapsed multiple myeloma. *British Journal of Haematology, 143,* 46–53. doi:10.1111/j.1365-2141.2008.07303.x

Novartis Pharmaceuticals Corporation. (2015). *Farydak® (panobinostat)* [Package insert]. Retrieved from http://www.pharma.us.novartis.com/product/pi/pdf/farydak.pdf

Onyx Pharmaceuticals, Inc. (2012). *Kyprolis® (carfilzomib)* [Package insert]. Retrieved from http://www.onyx.com/file.cfm/611/docs/PrescribingInformation.pdf

Orlowski, R.Z., Nagler, A., Sonneveld, P., Bladé, J., Hajek, R., Spencer, A., ... Harousseau, J.L. (2007). Randomized phase III study of pegylated liposomal doxorubicin plus bortezomib compared with bortezomib alone in relapsed or refractory multiple myeloma: Combination therapy improves time to progression. *Journal of Clinical Oncology, 25,* 3892–3901. doi:10.1200/JCO.2006.10.5460

Owen, R.G., & Rawstron, A.C. (2005). Minimal residual disease monitoring in multiple myeloma: Flow cytometry is the method of choice. *British Journal of Haematology, 128,* 732–733. doi:10.1111/j.1365-2141.2005.05376.x

Palumbo, A., Rajkumar, S.V., Dimopoulos, M.A., Richardson, P.G., San Miguel, J., Barlogie, B., … Hussein, M.A. (2008). Prevention of thalidomide- and lenalidomide-associated thrombosis in myeloma. *Leukemia, 22,* 414–423. doi:10.1038/sj.leu.2405062

Palumbo, A., Rajkumar, S.V., San Miguel, J.F., Larocca, A., Niesvizky, R., Morgan, G., … Orlowski, R.Z. (2014). International Myeloma Working Group consensus statement for the management, treatment, and supportive care of patients with myeloma not eligible for standard autologous stem-cell transplantation. *Journal of Clinical Oncology, 32,* 587–600. doi:10.1200/JCO.2013.48.7934

Perazella, M.A., & Markowitz, G.S. (2008). Bisphosphonate nephrotoxicity. *Kidney International, 74,* 1385–1393. doi:10.1038/ki.2008.356

Peter, R., Mishra, V., & Fraser, W.D. (2004). Severe hypocalcaemia after being given intravenous bisphosphonate. *BMJ, 328,* 335–336. doi:10.1136/bmj.328.7435.335

Raje, N., & Roodman, G.D. (2011). Advances in the biology and treatment of bone disease in multiple myeloma. *Clinical Cancer Research, 17,* 1278–1286. doi:10.1158/1078-0432.CCR-10-1804

Rajkumar, S.V., Harousseau, J.L., Durie, B., Anderson, K.C., Dimopoulos, M., Kyle, R., … San Miguel, J. (2011). Consensus recommendations for the uniform reporting of clinical trials: Report of the International Myeloma Workshop Consensus Panel 1. *Blood, 117,* 4691–4695. doi:10.1182/blood-2010-10-299487

Rawstron, A.C., Child, J.A., de Tute, R.M., Davies, F.E., Gregory, W.M., Bell, S.E., … Owen, R.G. (2013). Minimal residual disease assessed by multiparameter flow cytometry in multiple myeloma: Impact on outcome in the Medical Research Council Myeloma IX study. *Journal of Clinical Oncology, 31,* 2540–2547. doi:10.1200/JCO.2012.46.2119

Richardson, P.G. (2010). Towards a better understanding of treatment-related peripheral neuropathy in multiple myeloma. *Lancet Oncology, 11,* 1014–1016. doi:10.1016/S1470-2045(10)70248-5

Richardson, P.G., Barlogie, B., Berenson, J., Singhal, S., Jagannath, S., Irwin, D., … Anderson, K.C. (2003). A phase 2 study of bortezomib in relapsed, refractory myeloma. *New England Journal of Medicine, 348,* 2609–2617. doi:10.1056/NEJMoa030288

Richardson, P.G., Delforge, M., Beksac, M., Wen, P., Jongen, J.L., Sezer, O., … Sonneveld, P. (2012). Management of treatment-emergent peripheral neuropathy in multiple myeloma. *Leukemia, 26,* 595–608. doi:10.1038/leu.2011.346

Richardson, P.G., Laubach, J.P., Schlossman, R.L., Mitsiades, C., & Anderson, K. (2010). Complications of multiple myeloma therapy, part 1: Risk reduction and management of peripheral neuropathy and asthenia. *Journal of the National Comprehensive Cancer Network, 8*(Suppl. 1), S4–S12.

Richardson, P.G., Siegel, D.S., Vij, R., Hofmeister, C.C., Baz, R., Jagannath, S., … Anderson, K.C. (2014). Pomalidomide alone or in combination with low-dose dexamethasone in relapsed and refractory multiple myeloma: A randomized phase 2 study. *Blood, 123,* 1826–1832. doi:10.1182/blood-2013-11-538835

Richardson, P.G., Sonneveld, P., Schuster, M.W., Irwin, D., Stadtmauer, E.A., Facon, T., … Anderson, K.C. (2005). Bortezomib or high-dose dexamethasone for relapsed multiple myeloma. *New England Journal of Medicine, 352,* 2487–2498. doi:10.1056/NEJMoa043445

Richardson, P.G., Sonneveld, P., Schuster, M., Irwin, D., Stadtmauer, E., Facon, T., … Anderson, K.C. (2007). Extended follow-up of a phase 3 trial in relapsed multiple myeloma: Final time-to-event results of the APEX trial. *Blood, 110,* 3557–3560. doi:10.1182/blood-2006-08-036947

Richardson, P.G., Xie, W., Jagannath, S., Jakubowiak, A., Lonial, S., Raje, N.S., … Anderson, K.C. (2014). A phase 2 trial of lenalidomide, bortezomib, and dexamethasone in patients with relapsed and relapsed/refractory myeloma. *Blood, 123,* 1461–1469. doi:10.1182/blood-2013-07-517276

Rome, S., Doss, D., Miller, K., Westphal, J., & IMF Nurse Leadership Board. (2008). Thromboembolic events associated with novel therapies in patients with multiple myeloma: Consensus statement of the IMF Nurse Leadership Board. *Clinical Journal of Oncology Nursing, 12*(Suppl. 3), 21–28. doi:10.1188/08.CJON.S1.21-27

Roodman, G.D. (2008). Skeletal imaging and management of bone disease. *ASH Education Book, 2008,* 313–319. doi:10.1182/asheducation-2008.1.313

Rosen, L.S., Gordon, D., Kaminski, M., Howell, A., Belch, A., Mackey, J., ... Seaman, J.J. (2003). Long-term efficacy and safety of zoledronic acid compared with pamidronate disodium in the treatment of skeletal complications in patients with advanced multiple myeloma or breast carcinoma: A randomized, double-blind, multicenter, comparative trial. *Cancer, 98,* 1735–1744. doi:10.1002/cncr.11701

San Miguel, J.F., Schlag, R., Khuageva, N.K., Dimopoulos, M.A., Shpilberg, O., Kropff, M., ... Richardson, P.G. (2008). Bortezomib plus melphalan and prednisone for initial treatment of multiple myeloma. *New England Journal of Medicine, 359,* 906–917. doi:10.1056/NEJMoa0801479

Siegel, D., Martin, T., Nooka, A., Harvey, R.D., Vij, R., Niesvizky, R., ... Lonial, S. (2013). Integrated safety profile of single-agent carfilzomib: Experience from 526 patients enrolled in 4 phase II clinical studies. *Haematologica, 98,* 1753–1761. doi:10.3324/haematol.2013.089334

Siegel, D.S., Martin, T., Wang, M., Vij, R., Jakubowiak, A.J., Lonial, S., ... Jagannath, S. (2012). A phase 2 study of single-agent carfilzomib (PX-171-003-A1) in patients with relapsed and refractory multiple myeloma. *Blood, 120,* 2817–2825. doi:10.1182/blood-2012-05-425934

Singhal, S., Mehta, J., Desikan, R., Ayers, D., Roberson, P., Eddlemon, P., ... Barlogie, B. (1999). Antitumor activity of thalidomide in refractory multiple myeloma. *New England Journal of Medicine, 341,* 1565–1571. doi:10.1056/NEJM199911183412102

Smith, L.C., Bertolotti, P., Curran, K., Jenkins, B., & the IMF Nurse Leadership Board. (2008). Gastrointestinal side effects associated with novel therapies in patients with multiple myeloma: Consensus statement of the IMF Nurse Leadership Board. *Clinical Journal of Oncology Nursing, 12*(Suppl. 3), 37–52. doi:10.1188/08.CJON.S1.37-51

Stephens, M., McKenzie, H., & Jordens, C.F. (2014). The work of living with a rare cancer: Multiple myeloma. *Journal of Advanced Nursing, 70,* 2800–2809. doi:10.1111/jan.12430

Stewart, A.K. (2009). Novel therapies for relapsed myeloma. *ASH Education Book, 2009,* 578–586. doi:10.1182/asheducation-2009.1.578

Tariman, J.D., Love, G., McCullagh, E., Sandifer, S., & the IMF Nurse Leadership Board. (2008). Peripheral neuropathy associated with novel therapies in patients with multiple myeloma: Consensus statement of the IMF Nurse Leadership Board. *Clinical Journal of Oncology Nursing, 12*(Suppl. 3), 29–36. doi:10.1188/08.CJON.S1.29-35

Terpos, E., Berenson, J., Raje, N., & Roodman, G.D. (2014). Management of bone disease in multiple myeloma. *Expert Review of Hematology, 7,* 113–125. doi:10.1586/17474086.2013.874943

Terpos, E., Morgan, G., Dimopoulos, M.A., Drake, M.T., Lentzsch, S., Raje, N., ... Roodman, G.D. (2013). International Myeloma Working Group recommendations for the treatment of multiple myeloma-related bone disease. *Journal of Clinical Oncology, 31,* 2347–2357. doi:10.1200/JCO.2012.47.7901

Van den Wyngaert, T., Delforge, M., Doyen, C., Duck, L., Wouters, K., Delabaye, I., ... Wildiers, H. (2013). Prospective observational study of treatment pattern, effectiveness and safety of zoledronic acid therapy beyond 24 months in patients with multiple myeloma or bone metastases from solid tumors. *Supportive Care in Cancer, 21,* 3483–3490. doi:10.1007/s00520-013-1934-0

van de Velde, H.J., Liu, X., Chen, G., Cakana, A., Deraedt, W., & Bayssas, M. (2007). Complete response correlates with long-term survival and progression-free survival in high-dose therapy in multiple myeloma. *Haematologica, 92,* 1399–1406. doi:10.3324/haematol.11534

von Moos, R., Thuerlimann, B.J., Aapro, M., Rayson, D., Harrold, K., Sehouli, J., ... Hauschild, A. (2008). Pegylated liposomal doxorubicin-associated hand-foot syndrome: Recommendations of an international panel of experts. *European Journal of Cancer, 44,* 781–790. doi:10.1016/j.ejca.2008.01.028

CHAPTER 7. TREATMENT OF RELAPSED AND REFRACTORY MULTIPLE MYELOMA

Weber, D.M., Chen, C., Niesvizky, R., Wang, M., Belch, A., Stadtmauer, E.A., ... Knight, R.D. (2007). Lenalidomide plus dexamethasone for relapsed multiple myeloma in North America. *New England Journal of Medicine, 357,* 2133–2142. doi:10.1056/NEJMoa070596

Wernicke, A.G., Sabbas, A., Kulidzhanov, F., Shamis, M., Golster, Y., Niesvizky, R., & Lane, J. (2012). A single-dose conformal delivery of radiotherapy following osteoplasty: A novel approach to treatment of osteolytic metastasis in the setting of multiple myeloma. *HSS Journal, 8,* 169–174. doi:10.1007/s11420-011-9213-4

Zangari, M., Siegel, E., Barlogie, B., Anaissie, E., Saghafifar, F., Fassas, A., ... Tricot, G. (2002). Thrombogenic activity of doxorubicin in myeloma patients receiving thalidomide: Implications for therapy. *Blood, 100,* 1168–1171. doi:10.1182/blood-2002-01-0335

Zhu, Y.X., Kortuem, K.M., & Stewart, A.K. (2013). Molecular mechanism of action of immunemodulatory drugs thalidomide, lenalidomide and pomalidomide in multiple myeloma. *Leukemia and Lymphoma, 54,* 683–687. doi:10.3109/10428194.2012.728597

Zonder, J.A., Barlogie, B., Durie, B.G., McCoy, J., Crowley, J., & Hussein, M.A. (2006). Thrombotic complications in patients with newly diagnosed multiple myeloma treated with lenalidomide and dexamethasone: Benefit of aspirin prophylaxis. *Blood, 108,* 403–404. doi:10.1182/blood-2006-01-0154

CHAPTER 8

Living With Multiple Myeloma

Sandra Kurtin, RN, MS, AOCN®, ANP

Introduction

The concept of survivorship care in oncology emerged following the release of the groundbreaking report from the Institute of Medicine (IOM) in 2005 titled *From Cancer Patient to Cancer Survivor: Lost in Transition* (Hewitt, Greenfield, & Stovall, 2006). This report was generated based on a belief that, upon completion of their cancer treatment, the growing number of cancer survivors may not transition back to prevention- and health promotion–focused models of care with effective integration of continued cancer surveillance (Hewitt et al., 2006). For the patient with multiple myeloma, which often involves multiple periods of remission and recurrence, treatment is likely to continue from the time of diagnosis until death and include episodes of improvement and deterioration; thus, "care" is never really completed.

This chapter will focus on adaptation of key survivorship initiatives for patients with multiple myeloma, with consideration of episodes of care, shared decision making and self-management, surveillance for both multiple myeloma recurrence and development of other cancers, strategies for staying well, and management of common disease- or treatment-emergent adverse events. Every cancer survivor, regardless of disease type or prognosis, wants to experience a good quality of life. Elements of health-related quality of life (HRQOL) will be interwoven throughout this chapter.

Who Are Multiple Myeloma Survivors?

Multiple myeloma represents 1.4% of all cancer diagnoses and 13% of hematologic malignancies. In 2015, 26,850 new cases of multiple myeloma and 11,240 deaths from multiple myeloma are projected (Siegel, Miller, & Jemal, 2015). The five-year relative survival has almost doubled since 1975, increasing from 26.3% that year to an estimated 44.9% in 2014 (see Figure 8-1). The improvement in survival has been attributed primarily to the development of novel agents and better supportive care strategies (Kumar et al., 2013). Despite these advances, multiple myeloma remains an incurable disease fraught with relapses, each with unique clinical characteristics, patient attributes, and treatment options (Kurtin & Faiman, 2013; Palumbo & Anderson, 2011; Siegel & Bilotti, 2009).

The median age at diagnosis for multiple myeloma is 69 years; 62% of patients are over the age of 65, and 34% of patients are over the age of 75. Both the incidence and prevalence of multiple myeloma in older patients are expected to increase in the future because of expected increases in life expectancy of the general population and the improved survival times achieved with the introduction of novel agents (Palumbo et al., 2014). Roughly 38%

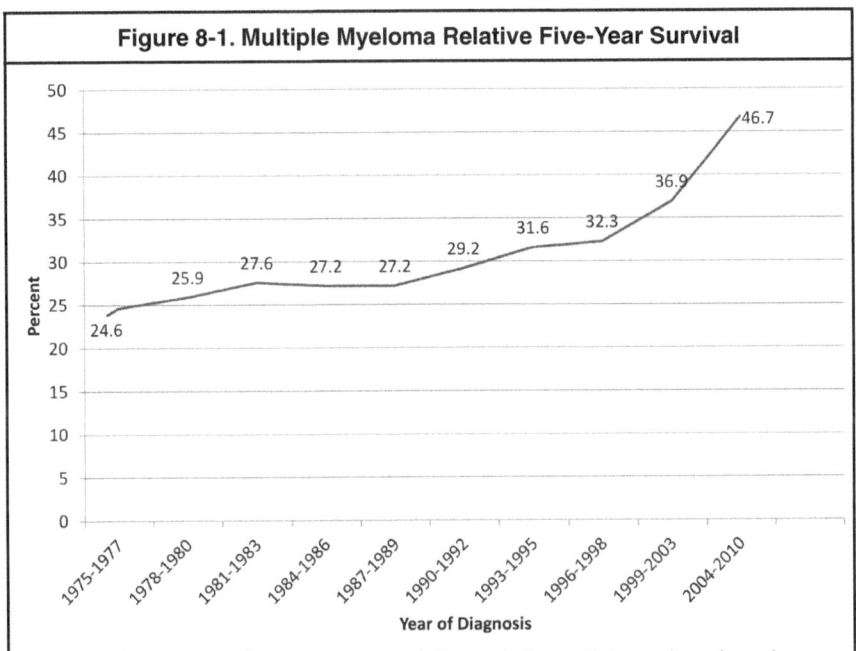

Figure 8-1. Multiple Myeloma Relative Five-Year Survival

Estimated five-year survival rates by year of diagnosis for multiple myeloma based on Surveillance, Epidemiology, and End Results (SEER) data from a series of hospital registries and one population-based registry. The difference between 1975–1977 and 2004–2010 is statistically significant ($p < 0.05$).

Note. Based on information from National Cancer Institute Surveillance, Epidemiology, and End Results Program, 2014.

of newly diagnosed patients with multiple myeloma are younger than age 65, an important consideration for hematopoietic stem cell transplant (HSCT) eligibility. For each age group diagnosed with myeloma, specific age, health, financial, and psychosocial factors must be considered in survivorship planning.

Importantly, clinical trials often exclude patients with more complex medical histories or uncontrolled comorbidities, and historically, enrollment of older patients in clinical trials has been very limited (Talarico, Chen, & Pazdur, 2004). Clinical trials conducted since 2005 have provided improved diagnostics, established risk-stratified treatment guidelines, introduced novel therapies, and refined supportive care strategies, resulting in improved overall response rates, overall survival, disease control, and quality of life for patients with multiple myeloma. However, barriers to participation in trials still exist. Some of these barriers include provider reluctance to recommend trials because of toxicity fears, limited expectation of benefit, or ageism and reluctance on the part of patients to participate in clinical trials for similar reasons, as well as concern regarding the cost of participation and the strain on caregivers. Limited representation of older adults in clinical trials impedes the development of evidence-based practice guidelines specific to the general older adult population (Kurtin, 2010b; Lichtman, Balducci, & Aapro, 2007). Familiarity with recent clinical trial data, including inclusion and exclusion criteria, will provide a sound basis for individualized care of multiple myeloma survivors (Kurtin, 2010b).

Survivorship: Historical Perspective and Future Directions

The National Cancer Institute (NCI) Office of Cancer Survivorship was established in 1996. It supports the definition of *cancer survivor* developed by the National Coalition for Cancer Survivorship, which includes any individual with cancer through the entire disease trajectory—survivorship begins at the time of diagnosis (NCI, 2014b). Importantly, NCI also recognized the effect a cancer diagnosis of a loved one may have on family members, friends, and caregivers and the essential role these individuals play in support of optimal outcomes for the cancer survivor. Welch-McCaffrey, Hoffman, Leigh, Loescher, and Meyskens (1989) recognized that the survivorship journey takes many paths. The potential paths described range anywhere from living many years free of disease to dying of a late recurrence, dying from a secondary cancer, living with periods of relapse and remission, living with persistent disease, or surviving after expecting imminent death.

This model provides a broader scope of application given the numerous cancers that remain incurable, including multiple myeloma.

The IOM report identified key elements of cancer survivorship care along with recommendations for practices and programs to support them (see Figure 8-2). Recommendations include development and implementation of interdisciplinary evidence-based clinical practice guidelines, multidisciplinary healthcare teams, and communication strategies that address cancer survivors' healthcare needs throughout the continuum of care and across providers and settings (Ganz, 2009; Kurtin, 2012; Stricker et al., 2011). Among the healthcare needs for cancer survivors are evaluation and management of treatment toxicities and late effects, continued cancer surveillance, and prevention and health promotion (Kurtin, 2012; Stricker et al., 2011). Most importantly, an individualized approach to survivorship care with a shared model of care among providers, patients, and caregivers is imperative to successful survivorship care. A shared model of care that promotes well-informed patients and caregivers who are engaged in their day-to-day care and participate in shared decision making will encourage self-management capabilities and adherence to the jointly derived treatment and survivorship plan.

Survivorship care plans (SCPs), including a treatment summary and follow-up plan, have been suggested as the primary tool to promote coordination of post-treatment cancer care among providers, particularly the oncologist and primary care provider (PCP) (Forsythe et al., 2013). A recent analysis of use of SCPs among medical oncologists (n = 1,130) and PCPs (n = 1,020) evaluating survivorship care of patients with breast and colon cancers identified factors associated with oncologist provision of treatment summaries and SCPs to PCPs. Oncologists who reported always or almost always providing treatment summaries (49.1%; 95% CI 46.4–51.8) or SCPs (20.2%; 95% CI 17.7–22.9) to PCPs were more likely to be knowledgeable about the long-term and late effects of treatment and were more likely to use electronic medical records ($p < 0.5$) (Forsythe et al., 2013). PCPs who reported always or almost always receiving treat-

---

Figure 8-2. Key Elements of Survivorship Care

- Prevention of recurrent and new cancers and other late effects
- Surveillance for cancer spread, recurrence, or second cancers
- Assessment of physical and psychosocial late effects
- Intervention for consequences of cancer and its treatment including physical, psychosocial, and financial concerns
- Coordination between specialists and primary care providers to ensure all aspects of the survivor's health needs are met

Note. Based on information from Hewitt et al., 2006.

ment summaries (22.9%) and SCPs (13.4%) reported better coordination, physician-to-physician communication, and confidence in survivorship care knowledge compared to PCPs who received neither treatment summaries nor SCPs ($p < 0.05$) (Forsythe et al., 2013). In a separate analysis of this study, 64% of the oncologists always/almost always discussed recommendations for follow-up care with their patients; however, only 32% offered specific recommendations for who should provide that care and less than 5% provided written SCPs to patients (Blanch-Hartigan et al., 2014). Similarly, survivorship care recommendations and provider responsibility were not regularly discussed by PCPs and survivors (12%). The same attributes of increased knowledge of long-term and late effects of treatment and access to an electronic medical record were associated with increased discussion between providers (oncologists and PCPs) and cancer survivors.

A similar study of 2,026 physicians including 938 PCPs and 1,088 oncologists evaluated preferences for survivorship models of care (Cheung et al., 2013). Similar to previous studies, there is discordance between oncologists, who preferred a specialist-based model of survivorship (59%), and PCPs, who preferred a shared model of survivorship (51%) (Cheung et al., 2013). The majority (87%) of oncologists in this study felt that PCPs were not adequately prepared to assume the primary role for cancer survivorship care, and 68% of PCPs indicated they were not willing to assume sole responsibility for survivorship management ($p < 0.001$). Less than 25% of PCPs or oncologists preferred specialized survivorship clinics. Analysis of psychosocial follow-up care for cancer survivors indicated that slightly more than half of the oncologists surveyed (52%) felt they were very involved in survivorship care and saw themselves as the primary providers of survivorship care as opposed to PCPs ($p < 0.001$), in particular cancer-related pain management (82.7%). The study underscores the need to better define survivorship care, identify which providers will take the primary role in coordinating individual aspects of care, and determining who will ultimately oversee and coordinate survivorship care. It is clear that all providers involved in the care of cancer survivors bear some responsibility in the coordination of survivorship care.

As mentioned previously, the majority of patients living with multiple myeloma are older than age 65, and these patients commonly have comorbid conditions that require ongoing management by PCPs and other specialists (Kurtin, 2010b). Although many patients remain under the primary care of their oncologist, PCPs have responded positively to the concept of improved communication about the ongoing needs of cancer survivors using treatment summaries and SCPs. Yet, multiple studies have shown that although oncology providers believe SCPs offer a positive tool for care coordination, barriers to full implementation of SCPs remain, including a lack of resources and the lack of evidence to support the use of SCPs in improving overall survival in patients with cancer (Forsythe et al., 2013; Salz et al., 2014). In fact, fewer than 50% of NCI-designated cancer centers consistently use SCPs for their survivors of breast or colorectal cancer (Salz, Oeffinger, McCabe, Layne, & Bach, 2012), and many recently diagnosed survivors have reported not receiving either a treatment summary (62%) or written follow-up instruction (42%) (Forsythe et al., 2013). Although the IOM report intended the SCP to be a patient-focused process and tool, 85% of oncology providers surveyed in one study perceived a greater benefit to PCPs than to cancer survivors (Forsythe et al., 2013). This emphasizes the need to develop SCPs that are relevant, are adaptable to individual patients, allow integration into the electronic medical record, and facilitate patient and caregiver involvement.

Despite the continued barriers to SCP implementation, SCPs are endorsed by survivorship experts and have now been recommended by multiple professional societies and accrediting agencies. The American College of Surgeons Commission on Cancer (CoC) has recommended that all cancer survivors receive a customized SCP at the time of completion of active cancer treatment. This will be a requirement for institutional reaccreditation starting in 2015. Although the CoC standards are primarily focused on cancer diagnoses with defined endpoints in treatment, the requirements imply application of survivorship principles and development of programs and processes to address all cancer survivors. Furthermore, studies surveying patient preferences for disease information, including a summary of the diagnosis, treatment, recommended ongoing care, and aspects of oncology care follow-up support, show a growing interest in patient and caregiver involvement, including use of electronic medical records and Internet-based resources (Cheung et al., 2009; Hill-Kayser et al., 2013; Husson et al., 2013). A study of 4,446 cancer survivors in the Netherlands between 1998 and 2008 participating in survivorship programs found that of the 3,080 responders (69%), patients with lymphoma and multiple myeloma received more information about their disease than other diagnostic groups ($p < 0.01$) and were the most satisfied with the information they received ($p < 0.01$) (Husson et al., 2013).

The Hybrid Survivorship Model for Myeloma

Multiple myeloma remains an incurable but highly treatable disease characterized by multiple relapses over the course of the illness. At the time of initial diagnosis and with each relapse, the goals of treatment are to achieve an early and deep response to effectively reverse disease-related complications and to maintain that response for as long as possible while maintaining quality of life for the patient (Lonial & Anderson, 2013). Risk-adapted treatment together with effective prevention and supportive care strategies are necessary to achieve these outcomes. Optimizing each phase of treatment through understanding of the individual regimen, toxicity profile, and best practice for clinical management will improve clinical outcomes and, perhaps more importantly, preserve future treatment options for patients who face inevitable relapses. These patients will need to meet treatment criteria for either clinical trials or the next available standard treatment option to continue their treatment (Kurtin, 2013).

The majority of multiple myeloma survivors will receive several treatment regimens over the course of their disease. For many, this will include one or more HSCT. A biopharmaceutical industry report estimated that of the 71,213 individuals living with multiple myeloma in 2009, 19,650 were receiving first-line therapy, 15,030 were receiving second-line therapy, and 10,220 were receiving third-line therapy. Registration trials for the four most recently U.S. Food and Drug Administration–approved agents for multiple myeloma (lenalidomide and bortezomib in the second-line setting and pomalidomide and carfilzomib in patients relapsed or refractory to both of these agents) demonstrate the ongoing treatment required for this disease and the challenge of continued treatment in a heavily pretreated population (Kurtin, 2013; Kurtin & Bilotti, 2013). The challenge for providers, patients, and caregivers is to minimize the potential progressive damage from the disease itself, prevent or minimize any cumulative treatment-related toxicity, and adequately address physical and psychosocial problems that may negatively impact HRQOL (Boland et al., 2013).

Sonneveld and colleagues (2013) summarized the HRQOL components of key registration and pivotal trials for thalidomide, bortezomib, and lenalidomide, including currently approved combination regimens. In general, HRQOL correlated to response to treatment with a temporary decline in HRQOL in the initial induction phase in several trials with gradual improvement as the patient responded to treatment. HRQOL declined in patients experiencing more severe adverse events. The authors noted the limitations in currently available HRQOL data relative to patients with multiple myeloma, including no comparative trials, varied trial design, heterogeneous populations, and HRQOL primarily as secondary endpoints only (Sonneveld et al., 2013). Strategies for the diagnosis, risk stratification, and treatment selection are addressed elsewhere in this book. However, a guiding principle for all clinicians working with multiple myeloma survivors is to consider the long-term view of treatment for patients diagnosed with myeloma, evaluate all available treatment options at each phase of the disease trajectory, and, in the absence of differences in treatment efficacy, select the option least likely to negatively impact HRQOL (Sonneveld et al., 2013).

Phases of Survivorship and Episodes of Care for the Multiple Myeloma Survivor: A Chronic Disease Model

Dr. Fitzhugh Mullan described three phases of survival based on his experience as a cancer survivor: acute survival, extended survival, and permanent survival (Mullan, 1985). The acute survival phase encompasses the time period from diagnosis through the completion of initial therapy. The extended survival phase is characterized by consolidation or intermittent therapy and periods of watchful waiting while the disease is monitored at intervals for recurrence. The final phase, permanent survivorship, implies a decreased emphasis on the cancer diagnosis and a lower perceived risk of recurrence. For most patients with multiple myeloma, treatment will continue indefinitely and relapses are inevitable; thus, they will remain in the extended survival phase. Working with patients facing an incurable disease requires time, compassion, clarity of message, and resilience on the part of healthcare providers, patients, and caregivers (Kurtin, 2010b). Survivorship care planning for multiple myeloma survivors and their caregivers requires that all healthcare providers maintain a current working knowledge of a variety of conditions and treatment standards, including risk-adapted treatment selection over the course of the disease, evidence-based interdisciplinary management strategies for prevention and management of disease- and treatment-related adverse events, principles of shared decision making and self-management to promote patient and caregiver engagement, recommendations for surveillance of myeloma recurrence or development of other cancers, and health promotion strategies (Kurtin, Demakos, Hayden, & Boglione, 2012; Litton et al., 2010; McCorkle et al., 2011).

The diagnostic phase of any disease is associated with a cadre of emotions including uncertainty, fear, anxiety, sadness, anger, and denial. Given the incurable nature of multiple myeloma, a diagnosis forces patients to confront their mortality. Strategies that may assist multiple myeloma survivors and their caregivers during this phase include clear explanations of each step in the process of the diagnostic workup, explanations for the implications of test results, provision of written results when possible, and continued reinforcement of all information provided.

Once the diagnosis of multiple myeloma is confirmed, patients generally are started immediately on induction therapy with the goal of obtaining a complete response as early in the treatment course as possible. For transplant-eligible patients, the next phase of survivorship represents an intensive treatment regimen with equally intensive follow-up requiring frequent clinic visits, continued supportive care, and vigilant surveillance of potential treatment-related adverse events (Miceli et al., 2013).

A percentage of patients do not respond to first-line novel agents, and many are not eligible for HSCT. Relapse or progression is inevitable for the majority of patients, including those who respond to first-line therapies. Patients who fail first-line proteasome inhibitors or immunomodulatory agents have been shown to have poor overall survival (6–9 months from the time of relapse) (Kumar et al., 2013). Patients with relapsed or relapsed refractory disease represent a heterogeneous population with unique clinical considerations. In a population of multiple myeloma survivors (N = 32) with a median age of 55 years who had undergone HSCT and at least one line of therapy for post-transplant progressive disease that had achieved a treatment plateau, fatigue and pain (primarily neuropathic) had a negative impact on physical functioning ($p < 0.001$) and were associated with progressive work disability and concerns about loss of independence ($p < 0.001$) (Boland et al., 2013). Emphasizing the need to maintain HRQOL while maximizing response to treatment and preserving future treatment options by preventing and managing disease- or treatment-related adverse events should be the goal for multiple myeloma survivors. Each phase of survivorship will require adaptation of the information provided to patients and caregivers and reinforcement of previous learning.

Living While Surviving Multiple Myeloma

All of the current standards for survivorship emphasize improving or maintaining quality of life and promoting wellness. Living with multiple myeloma is a challenge for most patients. Surviving multiple myeloma requires ongoing integration of the key elements of survivorship mentioned earlier in this chapter, namely the most effective therapy to achieve the best and most durable response with the least amount of toxicity. To "live" while surviving multiple myeloma is the ultimate goal. This requires an interdisciplinary approach to both treatment and wellness strategies and the engagement of patients and their caregivers as partners in their care. Figure 8-3 outlines the strategies for improving survivorship care of patients with multiple myeloma.

Shared Decision Making and Self-Management

Patients living with multiple myeloma face complex decisions throughout their journey relative to their diagnosis, options for treatment, and how their disease and treatment choices may affect them physically, emotionally, financially, and spiritually. Currently, the majority of clinical management is episodic and provided in the outpatient setting. Therefore, the bulk of care for patients living with multiple myeloma is managed by the patient together with his or her caregivers, who face similar challenges to those faced by the patient living with myeloma (Kurtin, Lilleby,

> **Figure 8-3. Strategies to Improve Survivorship Care for Patients With Multiple Myeloma**
>
> - Understand the disease state.
> - Understand risk-adapted treatment selection.
> - Develop evidence-based guidelines for management of common disease- or treatment-related adverse events.
> - Preserve future treatment options by promoting wellness and limiting the severity of adverse events.
> - Encourage clinical trial participation.
> - Adopt an interdisciplinary team approach to care.
> - Consistently communicate with all members of the interdisciplinary team.
> - Form a partnership with the patient and caregiver(s).
> - Individualize the survivorship plan for each patient.
> - Focus should be on *living* while surviving multiple myeloma.

& Spong, 2013). Caregivers are required to take in complex information, perform often complicated or technical procedures such as line care or injections, assist patients with activities of daily living, and attend the myriad of appointments required.

Communication strategies are critical to effectively engage patients and caregivers in shared decision making and self-management strategies. A systematic review of nine randomized trials and eight systematic reviews conducted by Rodin and colleagues (2009) focused on patient and clinician communication styles. Results of this investigation found increased patient and caregiver satisfaction to be associated with consultations that were patient-centered and incorporated key elements of effective communications and patient-caregiver engagement. Understanding the dynamics of the patient-caregiver relationship, the strengths and weaknesses unique to that relationship, common elements of patient and caregiver stress or strain, and available tools and strategies to promote a sense of control and enhance self-management skills may improve the HRQOL for both patients with multiple myeloma and their caregivers (Kurtin, 2013).

Staying Well: Health Promotion and Prevention

Health promotion and prevention are key elements of survivorship care. Health promotion includes risk avoidance (modifiable risk factors) and integration of elements of a healthy lifestyle including diet and exercise. These same principles apply to cancer survivors regardless of prognosis, yet they require realistic adaptation for each patient (Kurtin, 2012).

Risk factors for multiple myeloma include advanced age, male gender, obesity, and African American descent (Perrotta et al., 2013). Thus, some risk factors provide an opportunity for modification (e.g., obesity), and others are nonmodifiable (e.g., age, gender, ethnicity) (Kurtin & Faiman, 2013). The incidence of multiple myeloma in African American males in 2013 was estimated at 14.4 per 100,000, more than double the 6.6 per 100,000 for Caucasian males (NCI, 2014a). Similarly, African American females are more likely to develop multiple myeloma compared to Caucasian females (9.8 per 100,000 versus 4.1 per 100,000). The cause of the increased incidence in the African American population has not been determined and emphasizes the need for continued investigation into genetic predisposition. Survivorship planning for African American patients should incorporate genetic counseling and inclusion in epidemiologic studies if possible. Exposure to chemicals including pesticides, arsenic, cadmium, lead, and various cleaning solutions also has been linked to an increased risk of multiple myeloma (Perrotta et al., 2013). Once diagnosed, there are no clear data to suggest continued exposure will change the course of the disease.

Nutrition and Physical Activity

The American Cancer Society has proposed guidelines for nutrition and exercise based on the phase of cancer survivorship. The phases identified include active treatment, the immediate post-treatment phase (recovery), the post-recovery phase, and patients living with advanced cancer (Rock et al., 2012). Patients (N = 152) participating in an Internet-based SCP integrating health and lifestyle recommendations from the Livestrong Care Plan (www.livestrongcareplan.org) were most likely to make changes in their diet (33%) or exercise plan (44%), with fewer indicating plans to decrease alcohol intake (4%), stop smoking (7%), change use of vitamins or supplements (7%), or lose weight (5%) (Hill-Kayser et al., 2013).

More than 50% of newly diagnosed patients with cancer exhibit symptoms of nutritional deficits (Doyle et al., 2006). Significant weight loss (> 10%) within the six months prior to diagnosis is considered a high-risk attribute and often is indicative of more aggressive or advanced disease (Kurtin, 2012). All cancer survivors are likely to benefit from a nutritional analysis and recommendations tailored to their specific needs including their disease, the treatment plan, and any comorbidities. A registered dietitian will be able to calculate the caloric needs for the patient and the necessary balance of fat, protein, and carbohydrates and, together with the patient, assess existing eating habits, preferred foods and food intolerances, and any special dietary restrictions (Bratton & Kurtin, 2010). Inclusion of the family and caregivers in this education will promote consistency and adherence to any special recommended dietary regimens. For example, renal compromise is common in patients with multiple myeloma, and these patients will require modified intake of proteins and may need adjustment of other nutrients such as potassium, sodium, or calcium. Patients with multiple myeloma may be at increased risk for hyperglycemia as a result of the common use of corticosteroids, inactivity due to bone pain, or exercise limitations (Faiman,

Bilotti, Mangan, Rogers, & the IMF Nurse Leadership Board, 2008). Poorly controlled blood glucose places multiple myeloma survivors at increased risk for certain complications including neuropathy, nephropathy, retinopathy, cardiovascular disease, and infection. Patients with preexisting diabetes may be at greater risk for these complications. Aggressive management of treatment- or disease-related symptoms, such as nausea, vomiting, gastroesophageal reflux disease, constipation, diarrhea, pain, and depression, will improve nutritional intake. In severe cases of malnutrition, enteral or parenteral nutrition may be required (Bratton & Kurtin, 2010).

The use of dietary supplements, vitamins, minerals, and herbal compounds should be avoided during active treatment because of unclear effects on treatment outcomes in most instances (Velicer & Ulrich, 2008). Some supplements are safe and have no known interactions with cancer therapies; however, patients should be instructed to discuss any supplement use in detail with their providers. Providers must familiarize themselves with the current literature for use of supplements and herbal compounds during treatment (Kurtin, 2012).

Cancer survivors often struggle with nutrition, particularly if dietary restrictions are in place. Families and caregivers often feel this is an area that they can support, but it often leads to a daily struggle to get the patient to eat the recommended diet. Aversion or intolerance to certain foods during active treatment is not uncommon, and although this may resolve with time, it presents another challenge for patients and their caregivers. Reinforcement of nutrition goals at each visit will promote continued patient involvement and identify those patients who may require more focused interventions. Simplifying the regimen, avoiding unnecessary restrictions, and allowing "forbidden foods" in small quantities now and then will make the diet seem less like work and more natural for the patient (Kurtin, 2012).

Maintaining a healthy weight is a primary goal for all cancer survivors. Obesity is a known risk factor for a number of cancers, including multiple myeloma (Wallin & Larsson, 2011). Obesity has been shown to increase the risk of recurrence and decrease survival for several tumors types, including breast, colorectal, liver, gallbladder, pancreatic, kidney, uterine, and advanced prostate (Doyle et al., 2006; Eheman et al., 2012). Integration of a healthy diet and exercise plan as part of the approach to overall wellness and improved tolerance to treatment should be part of any survivorship plan and should be introduced at the time of diagnosis with ongoing reinforcement at each provider visit. The basic balanced diet together with a program for strengthening and endurance exercises remains the preferred strategy for sustained effective weight control and can provide positive effects on common comorbidities in cancer survivors, such as diabetes, hypertension, arthritis, and cardiovascular disease.

Physical activity is critical to maintaining independence, avoiding injury and falls, and reducing the risk of complications of immobility, including thrombosis, osteoporosis, fractures, fatigue, insomnia, depression, infections, and skin breakdown (Doyle et al., 2006). Evaluation of a 12-month home-based diet and exercise program targeted at older adult cancer survivors found several positive outcomes, including increased quality of life, improved dietary behaviors, and increased physical activity ($p < 0.001$) (Morey et al., 2009). The U.S. Preventive Services Task Force (USPSTF) and the American Cancer Society recommend 30–60 minutes of moderate to vigorous exercise three to five days per week (Eheman et al., 2012; U.S. Department of Health and Human Services, 2014). Patients with multiple myeloma may face several potential barriers to regular exercise including vertebral fractures, neuropathy, stroke, pain, and steroid myopathy, and they may be at increased risk for fractures and further mobility limitations. Physical therapy or sports medicine consultation will assist in developing a safe, effective, and realistic exercise plan to avoid injury and promote continued adherence to the exercise plan (Rome, Jenkins, Lilleby, & International Myeloma Foundation Nurse Leadership Board, 2011). Tailoring the instructions for patients undergoing active therapy is recommended, including (1) avoidance of infections during at-risk periods (e.g., avoiding public gyms and swimming pools), (2) adaption for underlying anemia, and (3) activity restrictions for patients at risk such as those in the immediate postoperative period, those with the presence or increased risk of pathologic fractures, or those who have had recent cardiac, pulmonary, or neurologic events (Kurtin, 2012).

Tobacco and Alcohol Use

Tobacco and alcohol are leading risk factors for most cancers and contribute to other chronic health problems such as chronic obstructive lung disease and cardiovascular disease. Tobacco use represents the single greatest cause of morbidity and mortality. Smoking cessation is a key goal for health promotion and prevention based on the risks associated with tobacco use over time and the potential for immediate and long-term health benefits of quitting (Kurtin, 2012). Up to 70% of smokers have expressed a desire to quit smoking (Fiore et al., 2008). The U.S. Department of Health and Human Services (2014) recommends a combined strategy of counseling and pharmacotherapy where appropriate, inquiry about tobacco use at each patient visit, reinforcement of the potential risks of tobacco use and the benefits of smoking cessation, and referral to smoking cessation programs.

Alcohol misuse or abuse places the cancer survivor at an increased risk for falls, malnutrition, and social, psychological, and socioeconomic consequences and may increase the risk of treatment-related adverse events (Ganz, 2009). Similar to smoking cessation, evaluating alcohol use and instituting counseling and referral strategies will promote effective discussion with patients and caregivers and increase the potential for successful abstinence (Willenbring, Massey, & Gardner, 2009).

Managing Comorbid Conditions and Late Effects of Treatment

Given the average age of 69 years at diagnosis, comorbid conditions are common in multiple myeloma survivors. The most common chronic diseases in this primarily older population include cardiovascular disease (coronary artery disease, hyperlipidemia, and hypertension), chronic lung disease, endocrine disorders including diabetes, and arthritis. Kleber et al. (2013) evaluated the effect of comorbidities on a population of 466 multiple myeloma survivors using the Frieburg Comorbidity Index (FCI) in combination with the International Staging System (ISS). The FCI incorporated measures for performance status; age; pain; liver, heart, or lung disease; hypertension; diabetes; renal impairment; and secondary malignancies. Overall survival (OS) differed by FCI score (FCI = 0, Not reached; FCI = 2, 89 months; FCI = 3, 39 months) ($p < 0.0001$). When combined with the ISS stages, three distinct groups emerged with differing probabilities of OS at five years: low-risk (FCI 0, ISS I–II, 85% OS); intermediate-risk (all remaining, 74% OS), and high-risk (FCI 1–3, ISS I–III, 42% OS) ($p < 0.0001$).

Cancer survivors are at increased risk for exacerbation of these underlying diseases throughout the cancer survivorship continuum. Many of these illnesses will precede the cancer diagnosis, and these patients may have well-established relationships with their PCPs or other medical specialists. Effective management of existing or treatment-related adverse events including inducing or exacerbating comorbid conditions will increase the potential for continued treatment and limit the severity of the adverse events (Kurtin, 2012). The threshold for symptoms may need to be adjusted depending on the prognosis, treatment plan, patient adherence to the medical regimen, and cost of therapies. Late effects of cancer treatment contribute to the symptom profile for multiple myeloma survivors. Familiarity with common late effects is essential to long-term follow-up of multiple myeloma survivors (see Table 8-1).

Cancer Surveillance

Screening patients for secondary malignancies as well as continuing general cancer screening should be incorporated into every survivorship plan. The American Cancer Society publishes guidelines for cancer screening of asymptomatic patients at average risk (Smith et al., 2014). Cancer survivors, including patients with multiple myeloma, are at higher risk because of a number of factors including their myeloma diagnosis, treatment with antineoplastic or targeted therapies, genetic instability, hereditary predisposition, and continued at-risk behaviors. An individualized risk-adapted model

Table 8-1. Common Late Effects of Cancer Treatment and Implications for Survivorship Care

Organ System	Common Late Effects of Cancer Treatment	Risk Factors	Implications for Primary Care of the Cancer Survivor
Head and neck	Xerostomia	Radiation to the head and neck Surgical reconstruction Graft-versus-host disease	Dental follow-up because of increased risk of dental caries Nutrition consult to avoid weight loss
	Osteonecrosis of the jaw	Bisphosphonate administration Dental procedures	Baseline dental exam Patient and dental professional education regarding risks associated with dental procedures
	Hearing loss	Cisplatin Cranial radiation	Baseline audiology exam Referral to ear, nose, and throat specialist with any changes Referral to neuro-otolaryngologist as indicated
	Visual changes Cataracts Retinopathy	Cranial irradiation Chronic steroids Optic neuritis	Baseline eye exam with repeat evaluation as clinically indicated Consideration of referral to retinal specialist or neuro-ophthalmologist as clinically indicated
Cardiovascular	Congestive heart failure Cardiomyopathy Coronary artery disease Atherosclerosis	Cumulative dose and combinations of cardiotoxic drugs (e.g., anthracyclines) Concurrent or prior chest irradiation Preexisting cardiovascular disease Longer duration of survival	Baseline and periodic evaluation of ejection fraction based on symptoms Coordination of care with cardiologist and primary care provider Patient education for modifiable risk factors: tobacco use, obesity, and sedentary lifestyle

(Continued on next page)

Table 8-1. Common Late Effects of Cancer Treatment and Implications for Survivorship Care (Continued)

Organ System	Common Late Effects of Cancer Treatment	Risk Factors	Implications for Primary Care of the Cancer Survivor
Cardiovascular (cont.)	Hypertension	Vascular endothelial growth factor inhibitors Small molecule tyrosine kinase inhibitors Family history Obesity, sedentary lifestyle, tobacco use	Baseline evaluation of blood pressure, repeated at each visit Possible need for dose modifications for medications known to contribute to hypertension Coordination of care with cardiologist and primary care provider Patient education for modifiable risk factors: tobacco use, obesity, sedentary lifestyle
	Thromboembolism	Active cancer Obesity, tobacco use Diabetes Vascular endothelial growth factor inhibitors, immunomodulatory agents	Identification of at-risk patients Institution of anticoagulation therapy as indicated Coordination of care with cardiologist, primary care provider, and anticoagulation clinic Patient education for modifiable risk factors: tobacco use, obesity, sedentary lifestyle
Endocrine	Hypothyroidism	Radiation to the thyroid gland Preexisting hypothyroidism Stem cell transplantation Radioimmunotherapy Systemic therapies: vascular endothelial growth factor inhibitors, immunomodulatory agents, retinoid inhibitors	Baseline testing for thyroid function, repeated as clinically indicated Thyroid replacement therapy
	Adrenal insufficiency	Chronic steroid use Adrenalectomy	Baseline testing for adrenal gland function, repeated as clinically indicated Mineralocorticoid replacement therapy

(Continued on next page)

Table 8-1. Common Late Effects of Cancer Treatment and Implications for Survivorship Care *(Continued)*

Organ System	Common Late Effects of Cancer Treatment	Risk Factors	Implications for Primary Care of the Cancer Survivor
Pulmonary	Pneumonitis Pulmonary fibrosis Restrictive lung disease	Preexisting pulmonary disease: asthma, chronic obstructive pulmonary disease, bronchitis Radiation to the thorax/lungs Tobacco use	Baseline assessment of risk Avoidance of aggravating factors: treatment- or lifestyle-related Coordination of care with pulmonologist and primary care provider
Genitourinary/renal	Chronic renal insufficiency Nephrotic syndrome Incontinence	High-dose chemotherapy Radiation to the renal bed Chronic graft-versus-host disease Nephrotoxic drugs	Close monitoring of renal function Avoidance of aggravating factors: medications, dehydration, IV contrast Referral to urologist for urinary incontinence treatment
Gastrointestinal	Strictures Malabsorption syndrome Chronic diarrhea Incontinence Pancreatic insufficiency	Surgery Radiation to the abdomen or pelvis Bypass surgery Whipple procedure	Referral to dietitian for modified diet Review of bowel regimen for chronic constipation or diarrhea, including medications and diet Endoscopy/colonoscopy for persistent symptoms
Gonadal	Infertility Testosterone deficiency	Radiation to the pelvis High-dose chemotherapy Surgical removal of the ovaries or testes Immunomodulatory agents Age	Counseling of patients of childbearing age Baseline testing, repeated as clinically indicated Hormone replacement after careful consideration of risks versus benefits

(Continued on next page)

Table 8-1. Common Late Effects of Cancer Treatment and Implications for Survivorship Care (Continued)

Organ System	Common Late Effects of Cancer Treatment	Risk Factors	Implications for Primary Care of the Cancer Survivor
Nervous system	Peripheral neuropathy	Preexisting neuropathy: diabetes, drug-induced, nerve damage, myeloma Cumulative doses of neurotoxic drugs: platinum compounds, thalidomide, vinca alkaloids, bortezomib, protein-bound paclitaxel, taxanes	Careful history based on patient's daily activities for employment and enjoyment; focused neurologic exam based on reported symptoms or clinical findings Avoidance of aggravating factors: control of diabetes, smoking cessation, neurotoxic drugs Treatment of neuropathic pain Evaluation of central nervous system disease as indicated Safety evaluation
Musculoskeletal	Osteonecrosis (joints) Avascular necrosis Osteoporosis	Preexisting bone disease: metastases, osteopenia, osteoporosis, fracture Chronic steroid use Tobacco use	Baseline evaluation of bone disease, preexisting conditions Coordination of care with orthopedic specialist and primary care provider as indicated Patient education for modifiable risk factors: exercise, tobacco and alcohol, safety guidelines
Hematologic	Cytopenias Secondary malignancies • Acute myeloid leukemia (AML) • Therapy-related myelodysplastic syndrome (tMDS)	Tobacco use Ionizing radiation exposure (therapeutic and diagnostic) Early-onset tMDS/AML (3 years after primary therapy): • Agents: topoisomerase II inhibitors—etoposide, teniposide, topotecan, doxorubicin • Cytogenetics: *MLL* gene (11q23) most common, t(8;21), t(15;17), *AML1* (21q;22)	Smoking cessation Monitoring of cumulative dosing of agents with potential for tMDS/AML Incorporation of monitoring for tMDS/AML into routine screening: • Complete blood count, differential, platelets, to include mean corpuscular volume • Lactate dehydrogenase, comprehensive metabolic panel at each visit

(Continued on next page)

Table 8-1. Common Late Effects of Cancer Treatment and Implications for Survivorship Care *(Continued)*

Organ System	Common Late Effects of Cancer Treatment	Risk Factors	Implications for Primary Care of the Cancer Survivor
Hematologic *(cont.)*		Late-onset tMDS/AML (5–10 years after primary therapy): • Agents: therapeutic alkylators—cyclophosphamide, melphalan, or radiation • Cytogenetics: chromosome 5 or 7 abnormalities most common, 17p, del(3p) Immunomodulatory agents in multiple myeloma: Association between lenalidomide and secondary malignancies has not been established.	Repeat of bone marrow biopsy for any unresolved cytopenias, elevated lactate dehydrogenase or mean corpuscular volume with analysis of fluorescence in situ hybridization for AML, tMDS, cytogenetics, and standard hematopathology

Note. Based on Information from Bertoia et al., 2011; Bilotti et al., 2011; Dokken & Kurtin, 2010; Fadol & Lech, 2011; Felicetti et al., 2011; Ganz, 2009; Kurtin, 2010a; Mohty & Apperley, 2010; Oeffinger & Tonorezos, 2011; Oeffinger et al., 2011; Stricker & Jacobs, 2008; Wenger, 2011.

From "Primary Care of the Cancer Survivor: A Collaborative Continuum-Based Model for Care" (pp. 203–205), by S. Kurtin in J.K. Payne (Ed.), *Current Trends in Oncology Nursing*, 2012, Pittsburgh, PA: Oncology Nursing Society. Copyright 2012 by Oncology Nursing Society. Adapted with permission.

for cancer screening is required for all cancer survivors, including patients living with multiple myeloma.

Key Supportive Care Issues

Multiple myeloma survivors often have pronounced symptoms and substantially reduced HRQOL (Sonneveld et al., 2013). The most common disease-related symptoms at the time of diagnosis include skeletal-related events (80%), anemia (73%), and renal insufficiency (30%) (Sonneveld et al., 2013). Impaired immune function is also an important characteristic of the disease that increases the risk of infections (Palumbo et al., 2014). These symptoms correlate to the presence of myeloma-related end-organ dysfunction, commonly described by the CRAB criteria (hyperCalcemia, Renal impairment, Anemia, and Bone disease), and indicates the need for active treatment of the disease (Palumbo et al., 2014). Symptoms experienced over the course of the survivorship journey will vary for patients based on the characteristics of their disease, personal characteristics, treatment history, and adverse event profile and can range from troublesome to severe and life threatening and may be associated with specific treatments (see Table 8-1). Familiarity with these common, life-threatening, and bothersome treatment-associated adverse events will allow implementation of prevention strategies and prompt intervention to reduce the severity and improve the HRQOL for patients with multiple myeloma. Integrating prevention, monitoring, and self-management strategies into the SCP with education tailored for the individual multiple myeloma survivor will provide an effective tool and will encourage patient and caregiver involvement.

Fatigue, neuropathy, and pain are common symptoms identified by cancer survivors as having a negative effect on HRQOL (Pachman, Barton, Swetz, & Loprinzi, 2012), and these symptoms also are common in multiple myeloma survivors. The National Comprehensive Cancer Network® issued survivorship guidelines that include suggested prevention, assessment, and management guidelines for symptoms thought to pose potential risks to cancer survivors due to long-term and late effects of treatment (Denlinger & Ligibel, 2014; Kvale & Urba, 2014). The scope of these guidelines is intended to address symptoms that may negatively affect HRQOL. Elements of these guidelines have been incorporated into the recommendations for adjunctive and supportive care (see Table 8-2) and have been added to the template for the Multiple Myeloma Survivorship Care Plan (see Figure 8-4).

The International Myeloma Working Group, the National Comprehensive Cancer Network, and the International Myeloma Foundation Nurse Leadership Board have issued recommendations for prevention and management of common treatment-associated adverse events, including recom-

Table 8-2. Recommendations for Adjunctive Treatments and Supportive Care for Common Disease- or Treatment-Related Symptoms

Symptom	Clinical Management Strategies
Anemia	Consider erythropoiesis-stimulating agent. Provide transfusion support to target hemoglobin based on individual factors.
Asthenia/fatigue	Counsel patient. Avoid concurrent medications causing asthenia. Encourage activity/exercise with consideration of any bone disease, myopathy.
Bone disease	Bisphosphonate therapy • Monitor renal function. • Obtain dental evaluation prior to start if possible. • Monitor for osteonecrosis of the jaw. Radiation therapy (low dose) • Impending fracture, cord compression, plasmacytomas Physical therapy/sports medicine consult Obtain orthopedic consultation. Perform vertebroplasty or kyphoplasty. Perform home safety evaluation. Provide pain management. Use of spinal support (braces) may be indicated. Recommend calcium and vitamin D supplements. Encourage weight-bearing exercise as tolerated.
Constipation	Ensure adequate hydration. Modify diet. Increase fluids. Recommend use of laxatives and stool softeners.
Diarrhea	Ensure adequate hydration. Monitor electrolytes. Modify diet to avoid aggravating foods/beverages. Recommend use of antidiarrheal agents. Perform perineal care if indicated. In more severe cases, treatment dose modification may be needed.
Hypercalcemia	Ensure adequate hydration. Administer steroids, furosemide. Zoledronic acid is preferred for reduction of calcium. Provide antiemetics for nausea/vomiting. Perform home safety evaluation if severe.
Hyperviscosity	Plasmapheresis Provide tumor lysis prophylaxis when instituting treatment.

(Continued on next page)

Table 8-2. Recommendations for Adjunctive Treatments and Supportive Care for Common Disease- or Treatment-Related Symptoms *(Continued)*

Symptom	Clinical Management Strategies
Hypotension (proteasome inhibitors)	Perform baseline evaluation of risk factors. Antihypertensive medications may need to be adjusted. Increase oral fluids; additional IV hydration may reduce severity.
Infection	Administer IV immunoglobulin for recurrent infections. Administer pneumococcal and influenza vaccines. Patients with multiple myeloma should NOT receive the live herpes zoster vaccine. Provide pneumocystis pneumonia, herpes, and antifungal prophylaxis for high-dose or long-term steroids. Provide herpes zoster prophylaxis with bortezomib. Obtain baseline chest x-ray; repeat if respiratory symptoms.
Neuropathy	Instruct patient on early detection. Monitor at each visit. Dose adjustment may be needed for selected agents. Perform home safety evaluation. Obtain symptom control with pharmacologic interventions.
Rash (immunomodulatory drugs)	Symptoms generally are self-limiting. Treat symptomatically with antihistamines. Provide careful evaluation for potential severe drug reactions (rare).
Renal dysfunction	Avoid aggravating factors: contrast dye, nonsteroidal anti-inflammatory drugs, dehydration. Renal dysfunction is not a contraindication to hematopoietic cell transplant. Monitor bisphosphonates closely.
Steroid-related symptoms	Immunosuppression • Symptoms may require pneumocystis pneumonia and antiviral prophylaxis. • Provide careful monitoring for atypical infections. Weight gain, cushingoid appearance • Obtain nutrition consultation. • Counsel patient that symptoms are reversible once steroids are discontinued but may require several weeks/months. Constitutional symptoms: "let down" effect, flushing, sweating, sleep disturbance • Taper schedule may reduce severity of "let down" effect. • Taking the medication in the morning with food may improve tolerance. Personality/mood alterations • Monitor carefully. • Provide counseling for patient and family as needed. • Discontinue for any signs of suicidal or homicidal ideation.

(Continued on next page)

Table 8-2. Recommendations for Adjunctive Treatments and Supportive Care for Common Disease- or Treatment-Related Symptoms *(Continued)*

Symptom	Clinical Management Strategies
Steroid-related symptoms *(cont.)*	Dyspepsia • Take with food. • Use of H_2 blocker or proton pump inhibitor may reduce symptoms of gastritis. Myopathy • Perform baseline and ongoing assessment. • Differentiate lower extremity weakness due to steroid myopathy versus spinal cord compression. • Obtain physical therapy consultation. • Encourage strengthening exercises. Blurred vision, cataracts • Perform baseline evaluation. • Obtain regular ophthalmic evaluation. Hyperglycemia • Perform baseline and ongoing evaluation, particularly in patients who are diabetic or who have a strong family history of diabetes. • Initiate antidiabetic medication or adjust existing regimen if needed. • Obtain nutrition consultation. Acneform rash: Recommend antibacterial wash. Oral candidiasis • Perform regular oral assessment. • Institute oral care regimen including mucolytic and neutralizing rinses. • Provide antifungal agent if needed.
Thrombocytopenia	Implement bleeding precautions. Provide transfusion support based on bleeding risk. Monitor complete blood count, differential, and platelet count every 1–2 weeks for the first 12 weeks of treatment and as clinically indicated thereafter. Dose adjustment may be needed for selected agents.
Thrombosis	Prophylactic anticoagulation with immunomodulatory drugs based on risk factors (prior clot, erythropoiesis-stimulating agents, obesity, sedentary lifestyle, surgery, inherent genetics, hypertension, diabetes, high-dose steroids with immunomodulatory drugs) Hold anticoagulation if platelets < 50,000/mm^3.

Note. Based on information from Faiman et al., 2011; Miceli et al., 2011; National Comprehensive Cancer Network®, 2014; Niesvizky & Badros, 2010.

Figure 8-4. Key Components of a Multiple Myeloma Survivorship Care Plan

Organizing Health History and Personal History
- Medical and surgical history—Listing of all healthcare providers
- Personal history—Listing of key contacts, caregivers, advocates
- Healthcare and legal profile—Insurance information, power of attorney, advance directives

Myeloma History and Treatment Summary
- Diagnostic profile—Dates, International Staging System stage, cytogenetic and molecular profile, presence of bone disease, creatinine clearance
- Treatment summary—Dates, regimen or procedures, outcomes and key events, providers, treatment center
- Supportive care/adjunctive therapy—Dates, transfusion history, bisphosphonates, dialysis, providers, treatment center

Health Maintenance Referrals and Follow-Up
- Infection prophylaxis—General infection prevention guidelines
- See Centers for Disease Control and Prevention guidelines (www.cdc.gov/mmwr/preview/mmwrhtml/rr4910a1.htm; note caution for use of live vaccines)
  - Flu vaccine
  - Pneumonia vaccine
  - Antiviral prophylaxis

Bone Health
- Bisphosphonate therapy—See Figure 8-5.
- Activity/mobility—Physical therapy, exercise physiologist/sports medicine
- Safety—Home safety evaluation, "Get Up and Go" test
- Cancer surveillance—Modified surveillance recommendations for patients at increased risk (American Cancer Society screening guidelines available at www.cancer.org/healthy/findcancerearly/cancerscreeningguidelines/index); referral to genetic counselor if indicated
- Routine physical exam—Performed by primary care provider at least yearly
- Myeloma-specific evaluation—Individualized for each patient based on current disease and treatment status
- Management of comorbidities—Primary care provider and specialists as indicated
- Management of late effects—See Table 8-2.

Healthy Lifestyle Referrals and Follow-Up
- Dietary recommendations—Clinical dietitian, diabetes specialist if indicated
- Exercise/activity recommendations—Individualized for each patient based on disease- and treatment-specific attributes
- Sleep
  - Consider sleep study in patients with poor sleep patterns.
  - Review bedtime rituals.
  - Perform medication review.
- Smoking cessation—Referral to smoking cessation programs (reinforcement by all healthcare providers)
- Reduce alcohol intake—Referral to alcohol cessation/reduction programs if needed (reinforcement by all healthcare providers)

Psychosocial and Financial Health Referrals and Follow-Up
- Family/interpersonal dynamics—Family counselor, social worker
- Financial concerns—Financial counselor, social worker (counseling for return to work), referral to assistance programs (counseling for return to work, tips on maintaining insurance coverage)
- Anxiety/depression—Should be addressed by all healthcare providers; referral to psychologist/psychiatrist as indicated; referral to support groups

mendations for adjunctive and supportive care. Table 8-2 provides a summary of these recommendations with integration of evidence-based/best practice standards of care. Bone disease, renal damage, hematologic toxicities, infections, thromboembolism, and peripheral neuropathy are the most frequent disabling events requiring prompt and active supportive care (Palumbo et al., 2014). Bone health, mobility, and fatigue pose particular risks for multiple myeloma survivors and will be discussed in greater detail.

The underlying pathobiology of multiple myeloma is inherently linked to the common findings of osteolytic lesions, bone pain (at times severe), and pathologic fractures. Skeletal-related events affect nearly 85% of multiple myeloma survivors over the course of their disease and have a major impact on both patient morbidity and mortality (Terpos & Dimopoulos, 2005). Comprehensive skeletal imaging, first using plain radiographs and then more advanced modalities if necessary, is critical both at the time of diagnosis and throughout the course of therapy to assess the skeletal impact of the disease. Treatment of the underlying disease can prevent further bone destruction or skeletal-related events (Terpos & Dimopoulos, 2005). Bisphosphonate therapy (see Figure 8-5) is an important standard of care for all patients with multiple myeloma (Palumbo et al., 2014). The use of bisphosphonate therapy in smoldering multiple myeloma should be considered only in the setting of a clinical trial. IV bisphosphonate therapy has significantly improved the quality of life of patients with myeloma by limiting the amount of osteolytic destruction that occurs, and the use of zoledronic acid has been shown to improve OS when compared to clodronate (Morgan et al., 2011). However, bisphosphonate therapy does not lead to repair of bone damage that has already occurred. Bisphosphonate therapy is generally well tolerated, but strategies should be adopted to avoid renal impairment or osteonecrosis of the jaw. Local radiotherapy should be considered for painful bone lesions or solitary plasmacytomas (Palumbo et al., 2014). Therefore, it is critical to adequately assess each patient at the time of diagnosis, at regular intervals based on established standards for monitoring, and in the event they develop new symptoms suspicious for skeletal-related events.

Maintaining independence, both in activities of daily living and independent activities of daily living, is a primary goal for multiple myeloma survivors. Functional decline is associated with a loss of independence and decreased quality of life (Carreca & Balducci, 2009). Preservation of quality of life and independent function should remain a priority. This requires mobility, which for the multiple myeloma survivor may be jeopardized by bone disease, fractures, proximal muscle weakness, neuropathy, fatigue, and pain. Immobility, in turn, predisposes the patient to further weakness, depression, thromboembolism, and falls. Effective pain control, prevention strategies for neuropathy, a tailored activity program, and assessment of fall risk can reduce further disability. Fall risk can be effectively evaluated

Figure 8-5. Recommendations for IV Bisphosphonate Therapy in Multiple Myeloma

Indications
1. All patients with myeloma-related bone disease should be started on zoledronic acid or pamidronate IV.
2. Symptomatic patients without documented bone disease should be considered for zoledronic acid.
3. Patients with age-related osteoporosis and smoldering multiple myeloma can be treated using the appropriate dose for osteoporosis.
4. Bisphosphonates are not recommended for patients with smoldering multiple myeloma except in a clinical trial.

Duration of Therapy
1. Recommend that patients on primary multiple myeloma therapy receive bisphosphonates for up to two years.
2. Patient with active disease may continue beyond two years on zoledronic acid with close monitoring for skeletal-related events or osteonecrosis of the jaw.
3. Upon relapse and evidence of new bone involvement, additional bisphosphonate use is recommended.
4. In patients with renal impairment, bisphosphonates may be administered with dose adjustment, close monitoring, and discontinuation for severe impairment.

Clinical Management
1. Bisphosphorate infusion–related symptoms
   a. Fever, myalgias, and arthralgias may occur 12–48 hours after the infusion and may last 6–24 hours.
   b. Reactions occur in minority of patients (10%–20%).
   c. Symptoms generally are reduced with continued dosing.
   d. Slow rate of infusion and use of steroids and antihistamines may help reduce intensity.
2. Osteonecrosis of the jaw
   a. Excellent oral hygiene is the best prophylaxis.
   b. Limit alcohol and tobacco use.
   c. Dental evaluation is recommended prior to starting IV bisphosphonates and dental procedures (extensive) should be done prior to starting IV bisphosphonates if possible.
   d. Avoid unnecessary dental procedures once IV bisphosphonates start.
   e. If dental procedures are required, hold IV bisphosphonates two weeks prior to and after the procedure.
   f. There is no standard treatment.
   g. Consider supplementation with calcium 1,000 mg/day (avoid in patients with hypercalcemia) and vitamin D 400 IU/day.
3. Renal dosing: Monitor serum creatinine clearance before each dose.

Pamidronate Dosing
- Creatinine clearance > 30: 90 mg/500 ml IV over 2–4 hours
- Creatinine clearance < 30: Not recommended

Zoledronic Acid Dosing
- Creatinine clearance > 60: 4 mg IV over 15 minutes
- Creatinine clearance 50–60: 3.5 mg IV over 15 minutes
- Creatinine clearance 40–49: 3.3 mg IV over 15 minutes
- Creatinine clearance 30–39: 3 mg IV over 15 minutes
- Creatinine clearance < 30: Not recommended

Note. Based on information from Miceli et al., 2011; National Comprehensive Cancer Network®, 2014; Palumbo et al., 2014; Rome et al., 2011.

using the Hendrich II Fall Risk Model, which assigns a score to factors that have been correlated to an increased risk of falling and then uses a simple "Get Up and Go" test to evaluate patients' ability to rise in a single movement from a sitting position without a loss of balance (Hendrich, Bender, & Nyhuis, 2003). Home safety evaluation, particularity for older patients or those with significantly impaired mobility, is also recommended. Assessment of sleep disturbances, nutrition, medications, and other possible contributing factors is recommended.

The kidneys play an important role in the health of each individual. Their main function is to clear toxins and waste from our bodies. Approximately 25% of individuals with multiple myeloma have temporary or permanent renal damage at some point during their illness. This damage may be a result of the disease itself due to free light-chain damage of proximal tubules that must be filtered by the kidneys (Palumbo et al., 2014). Additional factors may impair renal function for patients with multiple myeloma, including both disease-related factors (e.g., hypercalcemia, hyperviscosity, amyloidosis) and individual patient factors (e.g., dehydration, loop diuretics, nonsteroidal anti-inflammatory drugs, contrast media) (Faiman, Mangan, Spong, Tariman, & the IMF Nurse Leadership Board, 2011). The general approach to improving renal health for patients with multiple myeloma is to effectively treat the myeloma to reduce the M-protein load, treat any metabolic processes (e.g., hypercalcemia, hyperuricemia, hyperviscosity syndrome), avoid aggravating factors, and coordinate care with the nephrology and dialysis team if indicated (Dimopoulos et al., 2013). Many patients who present with acute renal failure requiring dialysis may have improved renal function with effective treatment of their disease, and some will be able to discontinue dialysis.

Care for the Family Unit: Caregivers and Households

The impact of a cancer diagnosis is broad, affecting not only the individual diagnosed with cancer but the family, friends, acquaintances, and caregivers associated with the cancer survivor. Physical, social, emotional, and financial problems are among the challenges faced by cancer survivors and their caregivers. Maintaining relationships and meaningful connections can be difficult with the frequent appointments and treatment schedules that may continue for months or years. Social isolation is a potential risk. Sexual dysfunction, including decreased libido, is a potential disease- or treatment-related sequela that may place additional stress on the patient–partner relationship. Financial hardship, including loss of wages, difficulty in paying bills, lack of sick leave, managing health claims and bills, premature use of retirement funds (often with penalty), and the inability to contribute to a 401(k) with loss of employer-matched contributions, may create further stress for patients, their families, and their caregivers. The culmination of these stressors will increase the risk of anxiety, fear, depression, uncertainty, and feelings of despair (Kurtin, 2013). Taking the time to get to know patient, family, and caregiver dynamics and perceived stressors will provide a framework for pursuing available resources for support (see Figure 8-6). An integrated interdisciplinary approach to management is imperative to address the multifaceted stressors and dynamics for multiple myeloma survivors.

Figure 8-6. Resources for Multiple Myeloma Survivors

American Association for Cancer Research
www.aacr.org; www.crmagazine.org/archive/Crpodcasts/Pages/SurvivingThriving.aspx
Offers a six-part podcast series, Surviving and Thriving: Life With Cancer, in partnership with *CR* magazine and The Wellness Community

American Cancer Society
www.cancer.org
Help Line: 800-227-2345
Offers and funds research, education, patient services, advocacy, and rehabilitation resources

American Psychosocial Oncology Society
www.apos-society.org
Help Line: 866-276-7443
Offers a number of publications to support the psychosocial needs of cancer survivors

American Society of Clinical Oncology
www.cancer.net/survivorship
Provides extensive survivorship information, including a survivorship care plan template, information on rehabilitation and healthy living, and links to additional resources

Cancer*Care*
www.cancercare.org
Provides support services to anyone affected by cancer through counseling, support groups, education, financial assistance, and practical help

Good Days (formerly Chronic Disease Fund)
www.gooddaysfromcdf.org
Helps underinsured patients with chronic diseases, life-altering conditions, and cancer obtain the medications they need

International Myeloma Foundation
www.myeloma.org
International organization that supports research and provides education, advocacy, and support for patients with myeloma, families, researchers, and physicians

(Continued on next page)

> **Figure 8-6. Resources for Multiple Myeloma Survivors *(Continued)***
>
> **Leukemia and Lymphoma Society**
> www.leukemia-lymphoma.org
> Supports funding for blood cancer research, education, and patient services to search for a cure and improve quality of life
>
> **Livestrong Foundation**
> www.livestrong.org
> Help Line: 855-220-777
> Focuses on prevention, access to care, screening, improvement in quality of life, and funding research
>
> **Multiple Myeloma Research Foundation**
> www.themmrf.org
> Educates patients and raises funds to provide support for research
>
> **National Cancer Institute Office of Cancer Survivorship**
> http://cancercontrol.cancer.gov/ocs
> Help Line: 800-4-CANCER
> Conducts and supports research, training, and health information dissemination with respect to all aspects of cancer from etiology to treatment and beyond; offers the Facing Forward publication series addressing challenges associated with the diagnosis of cancer
>
> **National Coalition for Cancer Survivorship**
> www.canceradvocacy.org
> Survivor-led cancer advocacy organization that helps bring about changes at the federal level to ensure the delivery of quality cancer care
>
> **National Marrow Donor Program**
> www.marrow.org
> Dedicated to assisting individuals who require a bone marrow or umbilical cord blood transplant with finding a donor
>
> **Partnership for Prescription Assistance**
> www.pparx.com
> Provides access to numerous public and private patient assistance programs for qualifying patients without prescription coverage

Conclusion

Improvement in OS for patients with multiple myeloma has been a welcome development. However, the challenges that multiple myeloma survivors will face over the course of their disease require an integrated interdisciplinary survivorship plan that should be implemented at the time of diagnosis. Unlike patients who are expected to complete their therapy, patients with multiple myeloma are likely to continue treatment from the time of diagnosis until their death. A hybrid model of survivorship using an

SCP as a working document that is modified over time to reflect the patient's individual multiple myeloma journey will provide a useful tool for structuring support for the multiple myeloma survivor.

References

Bertoia, M.L., Waring, M.E., Gupta, P.S., Roberts, M.B., & Eaton, C.B. (2011). Implications of new hypertension guidelines in the United States. *Hypertension, 58,* 361–366. doi:10.1161/HYPERTENSIONAHA.111.175463

Bilotti, E., Faiman, B.M., Richards, T.A., Tariman, J.D., Miceli, T.S., & Rome, S.I. (2011). Survivorship care guidelines for patients living with multiple myeloma: Consensus statements of the International Myeloma Foundation Nurse Leadership Board. *Clinical Journal of Oncology Nursing, 15*(Suppl. 4), 5–8. doi:10.1188/11.S1.CJON.5-8

Blanch-Hartigan, D., Forsythe, L.P., Alfano, C.M., Smith, T., Nekhlyudov, L., Ganz, P.A., & Rowland, J.H. (2014). Provision and discussion of survivorship care plans among cancer survivors: Results of a nationally representative survey of oncologists and primary care physicians. *Journal of Clinical Oncology, 32,* 1578–1585. doi:10.1200/JCO.2013.51.7540

Boland, E., Eiser, C., Ezaydi, Y., Greenfield, D.M., Ahmedzai, S.H., & Snowden, J.A. (2013). Living with advanced but stable multiple myeloma: A study of the symptom burden and cumulative effects of disease and intensive (hematopoietic stem cell transplant-based) treatment on health-related quality of life. *Journal of Pain and Symptom Management, 46,* 671–680. doi:10.1016/j.jpainsymman.2012.11.003

Bratton, M., & Kurtin, S.E. (2010). Collaborative approach to managing a 59-year-old woman with stage IIB pancreatic cancer and diabetes. *Journal of the Advanced Practitioner in Oncology, 1,* 257–265.

Carreca, I., & Balducci, L. (2009). Cancer chemotherapy in the older cancer patient. *Urologic Oncology, 27,* 633–642. doi:10.1016/j.urolonc.2009.08.006

Cheung, W.Y., Aziz, N., Noone, A.M., Rowland, J.H., Potosky, A.L., Ayanian, J.Z., ... Earle, C.C. (2013). Physician preferences and attitudes regarding different models of cancer survivorship care: A comparison of primary care providers and oncologists. *Journal of Cancer Survivorship, 7,* 343–354. doi:10.1007/s11764-013-0281-y

Cheung, W.Y., Neville, B.A., Cameron, D.B., Cook, E.F., & Earle, C.C. (2009). Comparisons of patient and physician expectations for cancer survivorship care. *Journal of Clinical Oncology, 27,* 2489–2495. doi:10.1200/JCO.2008.20.3232

Denlinger, C.S., & Ligibel, J. (2014). A work in progress: Developing the new NCCN guidelines for survivorship. *Journal of the National Comprehensive Cancer Network, 12,* 1–4.

Dimopoulos, M.A., Roussou, M., Gkotzamanidou, M., Nikitas, N., Psimenou, E., Mparmparoussi, D., ... Kastritis, E. (2013). The role of novel agents on the reversibility of renal impairment in newly diagnosed symptomatic patients with multiple myeloma. *Leukemia, 27,* 423–429. doi:10.1038/leu.2012.182

Dokken, B., & Kurtin, S.E. (2010). Collaborative approach to managing a 47-year-old male with stage IIB rectosigmoid colon cancer and new onset of diabetes. *Journal of the Advanced Practitioner in Oncology, 1,* 184–194.

Doyle, C., Kushi, L.H., Byers, T., Courneya, K.S., Demark-Wahnefried, W., Grant, B., ... American Cancer Society. (2006). Nutrition and physical activity during and after cancer treatment: An American Cancer Society guide for informed choices. *CA: A Cancer Journal for Clinicians, 56,* 323–353. doi:10.3322/canjclin.56.6.323

Eheman, C., Henley, S.J., Ballard-Barbash, R., Jacobs, E.J., Schymura, M.J., Noone, A.M., ... Edwards, B.K. (2012). Annual Report to the Nation on the status of cancer, 1975–2008, featuring cancers associated with excess weight and lack of sufficient physical activity. *Cancer, 118,* 2338–2366. doi:10.1002/cncr.27514

Fadol, A., & Lech, T. (2011). Cardiovascular adverse events associated with cancer therapy. *Journal of the Advanced Practitioner in Oncology, 2,* 229–242.

Faiman, B., Bilotti, E., Mangan, P.A., Rogers, K., & the IMF Nurse Leadership Board. (2008). Steroid-associated side effects in patients with multiple myeloma: Consensus statement of the IMF Nurse Leadership Board. *Clinical Journal of Oncology Nursing, 12*(Suppl. 3), 53–63. doi:10.1188/08.CJON.S1.53-62

Faiman, B.M., Mangan, P., Spong, J., Tariman, J.D., & the IMF Nurse Leadership Board. (2011). Renal complications in multiple myeloma and related disorders: Survivorship care plan of the International Myeloma Foundation Nurse Leadership Board. *Clinical Journal of Oncology Nursing, 15*(Suppl. 4), 66–76. doi:10.1188/11.CJON.S1.66-76

Felicetti, F., Manicone, R., Corrias, A., Manieri, C., Biasin, E., Bini, I., ... Brignardello, E. (2011). Endocrine late effects after total body irradiation in patients who received hematopoietic cell transplantation during childhood: A retrospective study from a single institution. *Journal of Cancer Research and Clinical Oncology, 137,* 1343–1348. doi:10.1007/s00432-011-1004-2

Fiore, M.C., Jaen, C.R., Baker, T.B., Bailey, W.C., Benowitz, N.L., Curry, S.J., ... Wewers, M.E. (2008). *Treating tobacco use and dependence: 2008 update. Clinical practice guideline.* Retrieved from http://bphc.hrsa.gov/buckets/treatingtobacco.pdf

Forsythe, L.P., Parry, C., Alfano, C.M., Kent, E.E., Leach, C.R., Haggstrom, D.A., ... Rowland, J.H. (2013). Use of survivorship care plans in the United States: Associations with survivorship care. *Journal of the National Cancer Institute, 105,* 1579–1587. doi:10.1093/jnci/djt258

Ganz, P.A. (2009). Survivorship: Adult cancer survivors. *Primary Care: Clinics in Office Practice, 36,* 721–741. doi:10.1016/j.pop.2009.08.001

Hendrich, A.L., Bender, P.S., & Nyhuis, A. (2003). Validation of the Hendrich II Fall Risk Model: A large concurrent case/control study of hospitalized patients. *Applied Nursing Research, 16,* 9–21. doi:10.1053/apnr.2003.016009

Hewitt, M., Greenfield, S., & Stovall, E. (Eds.). (2006). *From cancer patient to cancer survivor: Lost in transition.* Retrieved from http://www.iom.edu/Reports/2005/From-Cancer-Patient-to-Cancer-Survivor-Lost-in-Transition.aspx

Hill-Kayser, C.E., Vachani, C.C., Hampshire, M.K., Di Lullo, G., Jacobs, L.A., & Metz, J.M. (2013). Impact of internet-based cancer survivorship care plans on health care and lifestyle behaviors. *Cancer, 119,* 3854–3860. doi:10.1002/cncr.28286

Husson, O., Thong, M.S., Mols, F., Oerlemans, S., Kaptein, A.A., & van de Poll-Franse, L.V. (2013). Illness perceptions in cancer survivors: What is the role of information provision? *Psycho-Oncology, 22,* 490–498. doi:10.1002/pon.3042

Kleber, M., Ihorst, G., Gross, B., Koch, B., Reinhardt, H., Wäsch, R., & Engelhardt, M. (2013). Validation of the Freiburg Comorbidity Index in 466 multiple myeloma patients and combination with the International Staging System are highly predictive for outcome. *Clinical Lymphoma, Myeloma and Leukemia, 13,* 541–551. doi:10.1016/j.clml.2013.03.013

Kumar, S.K., Dispenzieri, A., Lacy, M.Q., Gertz, M.A., Buadi, F.K., Pandey, S., ... Rajkumar, S.V. (2013). Continued improvement in survival in multiple myeloma: Changes in early mortality and outcomes in older patients. *Leukemia, 28,* 1122–1128. doi:10.1038/leu.2013.313

Kurtin, S. (2010a). Leukemia and myelodysplastic syndromes. In C.H. Yarbro, B.H. Gobel, & D. Wujcik (Eds.), *Cancer nursing: Principles and practice* (7th ed., pp. 1370–1396). Burlington, MA: Jones & Bartlett Learning.

Kurtin, S. (2010b). Risk analysis of hematologic malignancies in the elderly. *Journal of the Advanced Practitioner in Oncology, 1,* 19–30.

Kurtin, S. (2012). Primary care of the cancer survivor: A collaborative continuum-based model for care. In J.K. Payne (Ed.), *Current trends in oncology nursing* (pp. 191–209). Pittsburgh, PA: Oncology Nursing Society.

Kurtin, S.E. (2013). Relapsed or relapsed/refractory multiple myeloma. *Journal of the Advanced Practitioner in Oncology, 4*(Suppl. 1), 5–14.

Kurtin, S.E., & Bilotti, E. (2013). Novel agents for the treatment of multiple myeloma: Proteasome inhibitors and immunomodulatory agents. *Journal of the Advanced Practitioner in Oncology, 4*, 307–321.

Kurtin, S.E., Demakos, E.P., Hayden, J., & Boglione, C. (2012). Treatment of myelodysplastic syndromes: Practical tools for effective management. *Clinical Journal of Oncology Nursing, 16*(Suppl. 1), 23–35. doi:10.1188/12.CJON.S1.23-35

Kurtin, S., & Faiman, B. (2013). The changing landscape of multiple myeloma: Implications for oncology nurses. *Clinical Journal of Oncology Nursing, 17*(Suppl. 6), 7–11. doi:10.1188/13.CJON.S2.7-11

Kurtin, S., Lilleby, K., & Spong, J. (2013). Caregivers of multiple myeloma survivors. *Clinical Journal of Oncology Nursing, 17*(Suppl. 6), 25–32. doi:10.1188/13.CJON.S2.25-32

Kvale, E., & Urba, S.G. (2014). NCCN guidelines for survivorship expanded to address two common conditions. *Journal of the National Comprehensive Cancer Network, 12*(Suppl. 5), 825–827.

Lichtman, S.M., Balducci, L., & Aapro, M. (2007). Geriatric oncology: A field coming of age. *Journal of Clinical Oncology, 25*, 1821–1823. doi:10.1200/JCO.2007.10.6567

Litton, G., Kane, D., Clay, G., Kruger, P., Belnap, T., & Parkinson, B. (2010). Multidisciplinary cancer care with a patient and physician satisfaction focus. *Journal of Oncology Practice, 6*, e35–e37. doi:10.1200/JOP.2010.000028

Lonial, S., & Anderson, K.C. (2013). Association of response endpoints with survival outcomes in multiple myeloma. *Leukemia, 28*, 258–268. doi:10.1038/leu.2013.220

McCorkle, R., Ercolano, E., Lazenby, M., Schulman-Green, D., Schilling, L.S., Lorig, K., & Wagner, E.H. (2011). Self-management: Enabling and empowering patients living with cancer as a chronic illness. *CA: A Cancer Journal for Clinicians, 61*, 50–62. doi:10.3322/caac.20093

Miceli, T.S., Colson, K., Faiman, B.M., Miller, K., & Tariman, J.D. (2011). Maintaining bone health in patients with multiple myeloma: Survivorship care plan of the International Myeloma Foundation Nurse Leadership Board. *Clinical Journal of Oncology Nursing, 15*(Suppl. 4), 9–23. doi:10.1188/11.S1.CJON.9-23

Miceli, T., Lilleby, K., Noonan, K., Kurtin, S., Faiman, B., & Mangan, P.A. (2013). Autologous hematopoietic stem cell transplantation for patients with multiple myeloma: An overview for nurses in community practice. *Clinical Journal of Oncology Nursing, 17*(Suppl. 6), 13–24. doi:10.1188/13.CJON.S2.13-24

Mohty, M., & Apperley, J.F. (2010). Long-term physiological side effects after allogeneic bone marrow transplantation. *Hematology, the ASH Education Program, 2010*, 229–236. doi:10.1182/asheducation-2010.1.229

Morey, M.C., Snyder, D.C., Sloane, R., Cohen, H.J., Peterson, B., Hartman, T.J., ... Demark-Wahnefried, W. (2009). Effects of home-based diet and exercise on functional outcomes among older, overweight long-term cancer survivors: RENEW: A randomized controlled trial. *JAMA, 301*, 1883–1891. doi:10.1001/jama.2009.643

Morgan, G.J., Child, J.A., Gregory, W.M., Szubert, A.J., Cocks, K., Bell, S.E., ... Davies, F.E. (2011). Effects of zoledronic acid versus clodronic acid on skeletal morbidity in patients with newly diagnosed multiple myeloma (MRC Myeloma IX): Secondary outcomes from a randomised controlled trial. *Lancet Oncology, 12*, 743–752. doi:10.1016/S1470-2045(11)70157-7

Mullan, F. (1985). Seasons of survival: Reflections of a physician with cancer. *New England Journal of Medicine, 313*, 270–273. doi:10.1056/NEJM198507253130421

National Cancer Institute. (2014a). SEER stat fact sheets: Myeloma. Retrieved from http://seer.cancer.gov/statfacts/html/mulmy.html

National Cancer Institute. (2014b). Survivorship definitions. Retrieved from http://cancercontrol.cancer.gov/ocs/statistics/definitions.html

National Cancer Institute Surveillance, Epidemiology, and End Results Program. (2014). SEER cancer statistics review, 1975–2011. Retrieved from http://seer.cancer.gov/csr/1975_2011/browse_csr.php?sectionSEL=18&pageSEL=sect_18_table.08.html

National Comprehensive Cancer Network. (2014). *NCCN Clinical Practice Guidelines in Oncology (NCCN Guidelines®): Multiple myeloma* [v.2.2014]. Retrieved from http://www.nccn.org/professionals/physician_gls/pdf/myeloma.pdf

Niesvizky, R., & Badros, A.Z. (2010). Complications of multiple myeloma therapy, part 2: Risk reduction and management of venous thromboembolism, osteonecrosis of the jaw, renal complications, and anemia. *Journal of the National Comprehensive Cancer Network, 8*(Suppl. 1), S13–S20.

Oeffinger, K.C., & Tonorezos, E.S. (2011). The cancer is over, now what?: Understanding risk, changing outcomes. *Cancer, 117*(Suppl. 10), 2250–2257. doi:10.1002/cncr.26051

Oeffinger, K.C., van Leeuwen, F.E., & Hodgson, D.C. (2011). Methods to assess adverse health-related outcomes in cancer survivors. *Cancer Epidemiology, Biomarkers and Prevention, 20,* 2022–2034. doi:10.1158/1055-9965.EPI-11-0674

Pachman, D.R., Barton, D.L., Swetz, K.M., & Loprinzi, C.L. (2012). Troublesome symptoms in cancer survivors: Fatigue, insomnia, neuropathy, and pain. *Journal of Clinical Oncology, 30,* 3687–3696. doi:10.1200/JCO.2012.41.7238

Palumbo, A., & Anderson, K. (2011). Multiple myeloma. *New England Journal of Medicine, 364,* 1046–1060. doi:10.1056/NEJMra1011442

Palumbo, A., Rajkumar, S.V., San Miguel, J.F., Larocca, A., Niesvizky, R., Morgan, G., ... Orlowski, R.Z. (2014). International Myeloma Working Group consensus statement for the management, treatment, and supportive care of patients with myeloma not eligible for standard autologous stem-cell transplantation. *Journal of Clinical Oncology, 32,* 587–600. doi:10.1200/JCO.2013.48.7934

Perrotta, C., Kleefeld, S., Staines, A., Tewari, P., De Roos, A.J., Baris, D., ... Cocco, P. (2013). Multiple myeloma and occupation: A pooled analysis by the International Multiple Myeloma Consortium. *Cancer Epidemiology, 37,* 300–305. doi:10.1016/j.canep.2013.01.008

Rock, C.L., Doyle, C., Demark-Wahnefried, W., Meyerhardt, J., Courneya, K.S., Schwartz, A.L., ... Gansler, T. (2012). Nutrition and physical activity guidelines for cancer survivors. *CA: A Cancer Journal for Clinicians, 62,* 242–274. doi:10.3322/caac.21142

Rodin, G., Mackay, J.A., Zimmermann, C., Mayer, C., Howell, D., Katz, M., ... Brouwers, M. (2009). Clinician-patient communication: A systematic review. *Supportive Care in Cancer, 17,* 627–644. doi:10.1007/s00520-009-0601-y

Rome, S.I., Jenkins, B.S., Lilleby, K.E., & International Myeloma Foundation Nurse Leadership Board. (2011). Mobility and safety in the multiple myeloma survivor: Survivorship care plan of the International Myeloma Foundation Nurse Leadership Board. *Clinical Journal of Oncology Nursing, 15*(Suppl. 4), 41–52. doi:10.1188/11.S1.CJON.41-52

Salz, T., McCabe, M.S., Onstad, E.E., Baxi, S.S., Deming, R.L., Franco, R.A., ... Oeffinger, K.C. (2014). Survivorship care plans: Is there buy-in from community oncology providers? *Cancer, 120,* 722–730. doi:10.1002/cncr.28472

Salz, T., Oeffinger, K.C., McCabe, M.S., Layne, T.M., & Bach, P.B. (2012). Survivorship care plans in research and practice. *CA: A Cancer Journal for Clinicians, 62,* 101–117. doi:10.3322/caac.20142

Siegel, D.S., & Bilotti, E. (2009). New directions in therapy for multiple myeloma. *Community Oncology, 6*(Suppl. 3), 22–30.

Siegel, R.L., Miller, K.D., & Jemal, A. (2015). Cancer statistics, 2015. *CA: A Cancer Journal for Clinicians, 65,* 5–29. doi:10.3322/caac.21254

Smith, R.A., Manassaram-Baptiste, D., Brooks, D., Cokkinides, V., Doroshenk, M., Saslow, D., ... Brawley, O.W. (2014). Cancer screening in the United States, 2014: A review of current American Cancer Society guidelines and current issues in cancer screening. *CA: A Cancer Journal for Clinicians, 64,* 30–51. doi:10.3322/caac.21212

Sonneveld, P., Verelst, S.G., Lewis, P., Gray-Schopfer, V., Hutchings, A., Nixon, A., & Petrucci, M.T. (2013). Review of health-related quality of life data in multiple myeloma patients treated with novel agents. *Leukemia, 27*, 1959–1969. doi:10.1038/leu.2013.185

Stricker, C.T., & Jacobs, L.A. (2008). Physical late effects in adult cancer survivors. *Oncology (Williston Park), 22*(Suppl. 8, Nurse Ed.), 33–41.

Stricker, C.T., Jacobs, L.A., Risendal, B., Jones, A., Panzer, S., Ganz, P.A., ... Palmer, S.C. (2011). Survivorship care planning after the institute of medicine recommendations: How are we faring? *Journal of Cancer Survivorship, 5*, 358–370. doi:10.1007/s11764-011-0196-4

Talarico, L., Chen, G., & Pazdur, R. (2004). Enrollment of elderly patients in clinical trials for cancer drug registration: A 7-year experience by the US Food and Drug Administration. *Journal of Clinical Oncology, 22*, 4626–4631. doi:10.1200/JCO.2004.02.175

Terpos, E., & Dimopoulos, M.A. (2005). Myeloma bone disease: Pathophysiology and management. *Annals of Oncology, 16*, 1223–1231. doi:10.1093/annonc/mdi235

U.S. Department of Health and Human Services. (2014). Agency for Healthcare Research and Quality's guide to clinical preventive services, 2014. Retrieved from http://www.ahrq.gov/professionals/clinicians-providers/guidelines-recommendations/guide/index.html

Velicer, C.M., & Ulrich, C.M. (2008). Vitamin and mineral supplement use among US adults after cancer diagnosis: A systematic review. *Journal of Clinical Oncology, 26*, 665–673. doi:10.1200/JCO.2007.13.5905

Wallin, A., & Larsson, S.C. (2011). Body mass index and risk of multiple myeloma: A meta-analysis of prospective studies. *European Journal of Cancer, 47*, 1606–1615. doi:10.1016/j.ejca.2011.01.020

Welch-McCaffrey, D., Hoffman, B., Leigh, S.A., Loescher, L.J., & Meyskens, F.L., Jr. (1989). Surviving adult cancers. Part 2: Psychosocial implications. *Annals of Internal Medicine, 111*, 517–524. doi:10.7326/0003-4819-111-6-517

Wenger, N.K. (2011). What do the 2011 American Heart Association guidelines tell us about prevention of cardiovascular disease in women? *Clinical Cardiology, 34*, 520–523. doi:10.1002/clc.20940

Willenbring, M.L., Massey, S.H., & Gardner, M.B. (2009). Helping patients who drink too much: An evidence-based guide for primary care clinicians. *American Family Physician, 80*, 44–50.

CHAPTER **9**

Nursing Research

Tiffany Richards, MS, ANP-BC, AOCNP®

Introduction

Multiple myeloma is expected to be diagnosed in nearly 27,000 patients in the United States over the next year, with more than 11,000 dying from the disease (Siegel, Miller, & Jemal, 2015). Most patients present with disease complications such as anemia, lytic bone lesions, renal failure, or hypercalcemia. These symptomatic patients will receive therapy with novel agents such as thalidomide, lenalidomide, bortezomib, liposomal doxorubicin, pomalidomide, or carfilzomib either as single agents or in combination with other chemotherapeutic agents and dexamethasone. Although the five-year survival rates for patients with myeloma have increased in the past decade, these patients remain on long-term therapy and may experience both acute and chronic side effects as a result (Kumar et al., 2008; Pulte, Redaniel, Brenner, Jansen, & Jeffreys, 2013).

Oncology nurses play an important role in identifying disease- and treatment-related complications and in the management of common side effects from treatment. Because of the paucity of nursing research specifically addressing the management of disease- and treatment-related complications, interventions predominantly have been adapted from research in other malignancies. Few nurse-led myeloma-related studies in the area of symptom management during and after chemotherapy or in the supportive care arena have been conducted, but a wealth of opportunities exists for well-designed nursing studies to evaluate problems related to complications of myeloma and chemotherapy effects. In the era of novel agents, oncology nurses must be cognizant of the results from current nursing research studies (2000–2013) and continue to explore research areas that need clarification.

A literature review was performed to identify published nursing research related to multiple myeloma. PubMed (2000 to January 2014), CINAHL® (2000 to January 2014), and Google databases were searched to access relevant myeloma-related nursing literature using search terms such as *nursing research, multiple myeloma, nursing, pain, peripheral neuropathy, myelosuppression, autologous stem cell transplantation, diagnosis, fatigue, exercise, supportive care, psychosocial care, adherence, chemotherapy,* and *symptom management.*

Nursing Research Topics in Multiple Myeloma

Early Diagnosis

Timely diagnosis is critical to prevent serious complications from myeloma. Nurses have a unique opportunity to contribute to early diagnosis of patients because of differences in interactions between patients and various healthcare professionals. The National Cancer Institute developed the Surveillance, Epidemiology, and End Results (SEER) Program to collect incidence and survival data from regional and state cancer registries, including patient demographics, tumor site, date of treatment initiation, and patient survival (http://seer.cancer.gov). To determine the time from initial symptom presentation to diagnosis, a nurse-led study identified 5,483 eligible patients with myeloma diagnosed between 1992 and 2002 from the SEER-Medicare data set (Friese et al., 2009).

Frequent signs and symptoms of multiple myeloma were matched with the ninth edition of the International Classification of Diseases and current procedural terminology codes (Friese et al., 2009). Researchers found that 70% of the patients had a sign or symptom of the disease within six months prior to diagnosis. The median time from onset of a symptom to diagnosis was 99 days, and in those patients with a delayed diagnosis, 66% had a delay that exceeded 30 days. Factors that correlated with delayed diagnosis included higher frequency of physician visits or hospital visits, non-Caucasian ethnicity, female sex, increased age, and the presence of one comorbid condition in combination with anemia and back pain. Male patients who were diagnosed during an inpatient stay were less likely to have a delay in their diagnosis compared to female patients. Investigators reported that being diagnosed with myeloma while hospitalized (odds ratio [OR] 2.5, 95% confidence interval [CI] 2.2–2.9) and receiving chemotherapy treatment within six months of diagnosis (OR 1.4, 95% CI 1.2–1.6) were significant predictors of complications; diagnostic delay was not (OR 0.9, 95% CI 0.8–1.1). The researchers concluded that myeloma complications were more strongly associated with health status and disease severity than with diagnostic delays (Friese et al., 2009). These findings may be explained by the need for prompt diagnosis in symptomatic patients and unnecessary early interventions in asymptomatic patients. Furthermore, the findings demonstrate the importance of assessing patients' health status and stage of myeloma during the diagnostic workup to identify patients who are at a higher risk for complications.

Psychosocial Impact of Myeloma Diagnosis

Nurse researchers have investigated the psychosocial impact of receiving a diagnosis of multiple myeloma (Vlossak & Fitch, 2008). The purpose of this qualitative study was to explore the impact that the diagnosis had on patients and their families. Patients were evaluated by telephone interviews lasting 30–90 minutes. Twenty patients were interviewed, and several themes were identified: shock, few treatment options, concern and worry, complex treatment, fatigue, loss of independence, change in self-image, obsession on when life will end, fear of recurrence, and rationalizing their hopes for the future (Vlossak & Fitch, 2008).

All patients expressed the shock of receiving a diagnosis of myeloma. Additionally, many expressed disbelief at the negative information on the Internet and the lack of treatment options. Interestingly, many expressed that they had entertained the thought of cancer because of frequent physician visits related to chronic pain, infections, and fractures before they received their diagnosis. Although patients expressed surprise at the lack of treatment options, they felt overwhelmed by the urgency for treatment. In patients older than 65 years of age, health issues of other family members were important when making treatment-related decisions, particularly when it came to autologous stem cell transplantation (ASCT). One thing the authors of the study noted was that once patients had made a treatment decision, they did not deviate from the plan of care (Vlossak & Fitch, 2008).

The concern about family was voiced among both men and women and included a sense of inadequacy, guilt, and uselessness. Patients voiced that the responsibility of appointments and recording of information typically was performed by another family member. In patients with young children, discussing issues surrounding the cancer diagnosis was difficult regardless of the child's age. Patients described the treatment for the disease as long, complex, and requiring frequent office visits. Further complicating the treatment regimens were the multiple modalities used to treat the disease and its complications, including chemotherapy, radiation therapy, and pain medications (Vlossak & Fitch, 2008).

One important aspect that researchers noted was the concept of hope, defined as "living well for as long as possible" (Vlossak & Fitch, 2008). This study demonstrated the importance of not only providing patients with written treatment plans, coordinating physician visits, and providing patient education, but also supporting the goals and hopes of each individual patient.

Additionally, nurses should consider complex family dynamics that influence patients when they are making treatment decisions.

In a hermeneutical phenomenology study, researchers explored the lived experience of being diagnosed with myeloma among 11 patients (Kelly & Dowling, 2011). The median time since diagnosis ranged from one to four years, with a mean age of 63 years (range 42–83). Interviews lasted 60–90 minutes and were conducted either in the home or at the cancer center. Researchers identified 4 themes and 11 subthemes. The four main themes were Lived Body: a changed body; Lived Space: living in limbo; Lived Time: time is precious; and Lived Relations: significance of support.

Lived Body: A Changed Body

Participants in the study voiced concerns on the impact of body and physical appearance on their relationships and how others viewed them. They also discussed how those changes prevented them from concealing their diagnosis from others. The inability of participants to be able to conceal their diagnosis had a psychosocial impact. While none of the participants were on active treatment, they voiced the impact of alopecia on their lives. Fatigue also affected participants, and they indicated in the interview that it was the most debilitating symptom they experienced (Kelly & Dowling, 2011).

Lived Space: Living in Limbo

Participants voiced that the diagnosis of cancer was difficult because they, and the general public, were unfamiliar with multiple myeloma. The three subthemes under Lived Space included stigma of cancer, loss, and feeling lucky. The participants voiced the recurrent sense of loss they experienced throughout their diagnosis; in particular they noted the sense of sadness they experienced with the lifestyle changes they had to make since their diagnosis. Despite their sense of loss, participants voiced that they felt lucky compared to others with myeloma as well as to those who were diagnosed with other types of cancer (Kelly & Dowling, 2011).

Lived Time: Time Is Precious

Participants voiced the sense of fear they experienced around the time they had a physician appointment to review their myeloma status and when they heard of another disease progression. Interestingly, some participants expressed that their appreciation for life increased. Participants also expressed frustration with the lack of time with their physicians and nurses (Kelly & Dowling, 2011).

Lived Relations: Significance of Support

Patients expressed the importance of family members in their ability to cope with their illness. For many of the patients, their families and intimate partners provided strength and comfort to them. They also expressed distress at the thought of dying and leaving behind family. Patients also voiced the need to protect their family from bad news and would refrain from discussing their fears. They also mentioned the importance of talking to others with myeloma even if they had never had the opportunity to do so (Kelly & Dowling, 2011).

This study describes the life experience of patients living with myeloma and the emotional needs they may have during their disease. Providing patients with educational materials and referring them to reliable patient advocacy groups such as the International Myeloma Foundation, Multiple Myeloma Research Foundation, and Leukemia and Lymphoma Society enables them to obtain information for themselves and for their families and friends. Encouraging patients to either talk to other patients or attend a local myeloma support group permits patients to discuss their disease and fears with people who are going through a similar experience. Additionally, recognizing and acknowledging the multiple losses patients may experience as a result of their disease is an important component of nursing care.

Symptom Management and Quality of Life

Patients with multiple myeloma may experience a variety of symptoms either from the disease or from treatment, including pain, neuropathy, bone disease, anemia, fatigue, gastrointestinal symptoms, and myelosuppression. Recommendations for symptom management often come from anecdotal information or single case reports, thus making evidence-based interventions difficult. One study has addressed the potential link between the development of symptoms and subsequent need for hospitalizations.

Most patients, during the course of their disease, will proceed into ASCT either during induction therapy or at first relapse. To determine reasons for unplanned admissions during ASCT, Coleman, Coon, Mattox, and O'Sullivan (2002) conducted a retrospective study of patients who required an unplanned admission and those who completed ASCT without hospitalization. The researchers analyzed symptom development and management in 87 patients with myeloma who were undergoing outpatient ASCT. Of these, 16% required hospitalization during their outpatient treatment. The average length of hospital stay for all 14 patients was 7.3 days with no pattern for admission diagnosis identified (Coleman et al., 2002).

Pain

Lytic bone lesions are present in 67% of patients diagnosed with symptomatic multiple myeloma and may result in somatic or neuropathic pain (Melton, Kyle, Achenbach, Oberg, & Rajkumar, 2005). Stimulation of nociceptive receptors in the musculoskeletal system results in pain, which patients often describe as a localized, dull, achy pain that may radiate to another part of the body (Levy, Chwistek, & Mehta, 2008). Neuropathic pain may result from nerve root compression or as a complication of treatment (Ludwig & Zojer, 2007). Patients with myeloma may develop fractures of vertebral bodies, long bones, and ribs, resulting in decreased mobility and chronic pain (Ludwig & Zojer, 2007). There is a great need to study pain in patients with myeloma, especially in regard to how narcotic and non-narcotic interventions work specifically among the patients who are experiencing treatment-related pain.

A descriptive study by Poulos, Gertz, Pankratz, and Post-White (2001) conducted among patients with myeloma was performed to examine pain intensity, pain interference, mood, and quality of life. A convenience sample of 346 participants, whose names were located in a myeloma database, were mailed a cover letter as well as the study instruments. The response rate was 64% for a total sample size of 206, with the majority being males (67% versus 33%) and Caucasians (97%). The mean time from diagnosis was three years (range 0.1–20.6). The mean pain score was 2.7 (range 0–10) with a pain interference score of 1.9 (range 0–10). However, 30% of participants rated their pain as a five or higher. A correlation was found between pain interference and mood (Spearman's $r = 0.45$, $p < 0.0001$). The mean quality of life score was 6.2 (range 1.6–9.4) for the overall group. On univariate analysis, age was found to be a predictor of higher quality-of-life scores ($p = 0.017$), whereas total pain, pain interference, and mood disturbance were associated with a lower quality of life ($p < 0.0001$).

Psychological Aspects of Self-Administration of Bisphosphonates

Researchers have evaluated the psychological effects of ambulatory infusion of pamidronate in patients with myeloma. They evaluated the psychological benefits of self-administration of pamidronate in 21 patients who received ambulatory pamidronate via a programmable infusion pump (Johansson, Langius-Eklof, Engervall, & Wredling, 2005). Patients who participated in the study received information related to the drug, step-by-step instruction on disconnection of the pump, removal of the access line, potential complications, staff contact information, and relevant references. After three doses, 12 patients were interviewed about their experiences. While the patients reported a positive experience, they thought that self-administration was not ideal at the time of initial diagnosis, but over time would become a consideration. Many of the participants worked either part-time or full-time, indicating that self-administration is a feasible option for people with limited time schedules. Patients also reported that the program provided not only a greater sense of freedom but also additional time to spend with family (Johansson et al., 2005).

The negatives associated with the self-administration program included lack of written materials/group education and patients' concern regarding their venous access device. However, over time, patients felt they had acquired sufficient knowledge to proceed with self-administration (Johansson et al., 2005).

The results of this study indicate that patients may require verbal, or preferably written, educational materials as well as group instruction or return demonstration prior to starting a self-administration program. Additionally, a self-administration program should be avoided in the first few months after diagnosis because of the overwhelming nature of diagnosis and initiation of chemotherapy. Taken further, this study suggests that patient education is most beneficial when repeated and evaluated at each patient encounter.

Home Administration of Bortezomib

In a pilot and feasibility study performed in Ireland, 23 patients with newly diagnosed myeloma were enrolled in a study to evaluate the feasibility of administering bortezomib intravenously within the home setting (Meenaghan et al., 2010). The inclusion criteria included the following: willing to provide consent, good performance status, able to verbalize understanding of the treatment program, good venous access, and adequate score on a nine-item risk assessment tool. On day 0, a hematology clinical nurse specialist met with each patient to review bortezomib side effects, provide educational materials, and review whom to contact in case of an emergency or side effect. All patients provided blood samples for blood count and chemistry on day 8 of each cycle. Of the 23 people enrolled on the study, 5 patients had treatment discontinued, with 3 from other medical conditions (cardiac complications and Parkinson disease), 1 from disease progression, and 1 death from pneumonia. In this study, no complications or problems arose from the home administration of bortezomib. Additionally, patients voiced satisfaction with the home administration. This study suggests that administering bortezomib within the home is safe and feasible. This is an exciting potential option for patients who have transportation problems and do not have a contraindication to home administration of bortezomib.

Peripheral Neuropathy and Neuropathic Pain

Another source of pain in patients with multiple myeloma is chemotherapy-induced neuropathy from bortezomib, thalidomide, vincristine, and, less often, lenalidomide. Approximately 80% of previously treated patients with myeloma report some degree of peripheral neuropathy (Richardson et al., 2009). Unfortunately, no studies have evaluated either pharmacologic or nonpharmacologic agents in relieving or preventing treatment-related neuropathy in this patient population. Although case reports have noted the benefit of supplemental agents such as acetyl L-carnitine, vitamin B complex, or alpha-lipoic acid, no formal studies have been conducted in patients with multiple myeloma (Tariman, Love, McCullagh, Sandifer, & the IMF Nurse Leadership Board, 2008). The role of nurses in recognizing and reporting peripheral neuropathy makes this an ideal topic for nursing research, particularly in evaluating the benefit of nonpharmacologic therapies.

Fatigue

Fatigue in patients with myeloma may be attributed to a variety of factors, including anemia and the secretion of proinflammatory cytokines such as interleukin-6 (IL-6) and nuclear factor–kappa-B. IL-6 is expressed by the bone marrow stromal cells and stimulates myeloma cell growth (Booker, Olson, Pilarski, Noon, & Bahlis, 2009). C-reactive protein (CRP) is synthesized by liver hepatocytes and is reflective of IL-6 concentration (Bataille, Boccadoro, Klein, Durie, & Pileri, 1992; San Miguel, Garcia-Sanz, & Gutierrez, 2008). Studies utilizing an IL-6 monoclonal antibody have found decreased CRP levels and reduction in fever, pain, and cachexia (Booker et al., 2009). Patients with myeloma have described fatigue as a constantly present "inner" tiredness (Vlossak & Fitch, 2008, p. 143).

In a study of 56 patients with multiple myeloma, nurse and physician investigators analyzed the impact of hemoglobin and CRP on fatigue and quality of life (Booker et al., 2009). Patients received a 30-item questionnaire that measured quality of life and a 28-item questionnaire that measured fatigue levels at a single point in time. Additionally, CRP levels were measured at the time of study entry. Although anemia often is thought to be the cause of fatigue in patients with cancer, the median hemoglobin level of patients was 129 g/L, whereas the median fatigue level was 31 (range 7–52) in the Functional Assessment of Cancer Therapy–Fatigue (FACT-F) scale, and the median quality-of-life score was 4 (range 1–7) in the European Organization for Research and Treatment of Cancer QLQ-C30 scale. The researchers found that CRP was a predictor of fatigue ($p = 0.003$) and quality of life ($p = 0.020$), but hemoglobin level was not predictive of fatigue ($p = 0.237$) or quality of life ($p = 0.412$), as it was codependent with CRP (Booker et al., 2009).

Coleman et al. (2002) measured fatigue in admitted patients compared to outpatients by using the percentage of usual energy. The researchers assessed study participants three days before transplant, on the day of transplant, and on either the day of admission or day 20 for patients not admitted. Both groups of patients exhibited a decline in energy. The average percentage of usual energy for admitted patients before transplant was 84%, compared with 80% for those not admitted. The percentage of usual energy significantly declined the day of transplantation, with both groups reporting a mean of 66%. Following the transplant, the admitted group continued to decline more than the outpatient group: 39% for the admitted group versus 51% for the outpatients. However, in the group of patients admitted to the hospital, energy levels significantly declined when compared with those patients not admitted ($p = 0.017$). Another factor affecting hospital admission was the level of hydration ($p < 0.001$). In those patients who were admitted to the hospital, the level of hydration decreased from 1.2 L/day to 0.73 L/day on the day of transplant to 0.59 L/day on the day of admission. In patients who were not admitted to the hospital, a slight decrease occurred in the amount of oral intake from 1 L/day pretransplant to 0.99 L/day on the day of transplant, but hydration remained fairly consistent at 0.99 L/day for day 20. Interestingly, age was not found to influence whether a person was admitted, which is important given that the median age at diagnosis for patients with myeloma is 69 (Coleman et al., 2002; Howlader et al., 2015). Although this study was based on a small number of patients, it raises some interesting points, including the importance of educating patients on oral hydration during treatment and of managing fatigue before, during, and after stem cell transplantation.

A systematic review of research in cancer-related fatigue found that exercise and psychosocial methods (e.g., counseling, yoga, massage) were equally effective in reducing fatigue in patients with cancer ($p > 0.05$) (Kangas, Bovbjerg, & Montgomery, 2008). However, fatigue was reduced by 40%–43% in studies that included a multimodal exercise program. Programs lasting eight weeks or more (effect size = 0.67) had a greater effect in reducing fatigue than those lasting six to eight weeks (effect size = 0.75). Interestingly, exercise demonstrated a greater impact on fatigue during cancer treatment, whereas psychosocial interventions had a greater impact on post-treatment fatigue (Kangas et al., 2008).

Several studies have demonstrated the benefit of exercise in improving fatigue levels in patients with myeloma who were undergoing induction therapy. In a study of 24 patients, patients were randomized to an exercise group and a usual care group (Coleman et al., 2003). The exercise program included six months of aerobic activity (walking, cycling, or running) and resistance training (using stretch bands). Prior to the start of the study, patients in the exercise arm met with an exercise physiologist to determine their body mass index and fitness level using the Balke protocol (a method used to measure cardiovascular health on a graded treadmill), and they subsequently received a personal exercise program based on their health history. The only statistically significant difference between the two groups was the degree of change in lean body mass (+0.40 kg/month in the exercise group versus –0.44 kg/month in the nonexercise group, $p < 0.01$) (Coleman et al., 2003). Differences between the groups in level of fatigue, daytime sleepiness, and total minutes of sleep were not statistically significant; however, a trend toward improved scores may indicate that aerobic exercise and resistance training may be more significant in a larger patient sample.

In a study of 135 patients with multiple myeloma who were undergoing induction therapy followed by tandem ASCT, patients were randomized to receive erythropoietin alfa with or without exercise (Coleman et al., 2008). In the exercise group, patients received an individualized exercise plan, exercise stretch bands, and a videotape illustrating the exercises. The usual care group was advised to follow exercise recommendations provided by their physicians. The exercise group had better exercise performance and less aerobic capacity loss compared to the usual care group. Interestingly, the exercise group demonstrated a decrease in the number of days required for stem cell collection (p < 0.025) and the number of blood or platelet transfusions (p < 0.025) compared to the usual care group (Coleman et al., 2008).

In an attempt to determine patients' feelings, beliefs, and experiences related to exercise, researchers interviewed 21 patients participating in the Coleman et al. (2003) study (Coon & Coleman, 2004). Three themes were identified: beliefs, social context (culture), and experience. The belief theme included the following ideas: exercise as beneficial, associations between exercise and decreased fatigue, active participants in treatment, and their commitment to keeping their word. The theme of social context included the following: life before cancer, social support (accountability), caregivers' and participants' congruence regarding exercise, and the impact of the social environment on participants' ability to exercise. Regarding experience, many patients reported that they would recommend an exercise program to other patients with multiple myeloma for management of fatigue. Researchers identified factors that created barriers to exercise, including disease and treatment complications, such as fatigue, nausea, vomiting, pain, and chemotherapy administration. However, the investigators found that patients' ability to exercise increased as their disease improved. Weather and schedule demands created barriers to exercise as well (Coon & Coleman, 2004).

Coleman et al. (2012) conducted a repeated measures experimental study among 187 patients with newly diagnosed multiple myeloma. Patients were randomized to receive either a home-based exercise program with aerobic and strength training or to usual care consisting of walking 20 minutes three times a week. No statistically significant difference was observed in level of fatigue or insomnia between the two groups. Researchers also reported in a separate analysis the baseline fatigue, mood, sleep, pain, performance status, and muscle strength. The mean fatigue score on the FACT-F was 32.1 (standard deviation [SD] = 9.6) for females and 38.7 (SD = 12.8) for males (p = 0.000) (Coleman et al., 2011). Severe fatigue was present in 19.3% of participants as determined by a FACT-F score less than 25. The mean pain rating showed no statistically significant difference between males and females (1.4 versus 1.8). Pain correlated with fatigue (Spearman rho $[r_s]$ = –0.33), total mood disturbance (r_s = 0.25), six-minute walk test (r_s = –0.36), and muscle strength (r_s = –0.37). The mean total mood disturbance score was 31.3 in females and 18.4 in males (p = 0.008). Fatigue and total mood disturbance correlated in the current study (Pearson's r = –0.70) (Coleman et al., 2011).

In a subset analysis of 18 of the patients enrolled on the Coleman et al. (2011) study, researchers sought to describe the sleep quality of patients with myeloma undergoing stem cell mobilization (Enderlin et al., 2013). Patients underwent a polysomnography (PSG) prior to the second cycle of chemotherapy for stem cell mobilization (PSG 1) and a second one prior to stem cell transplantation (PSG 2). A total of 12 patients completed both PSG 1 and PSG 2; the remainder were unable to complete PSG 2 because of other medical problems that developed. The mean wake time after onset of sleep was lower than normal for both PSG 1 and PSG 2, 118.6 minutes and 97.5 minutes, respectively. The total sleep time (360 minutes versus 395.6 minutes) and sleep efficiency (360 minutes versus 395.6 minutes) were lower than normal for age at both time points. Although non–rapid eye movement (NREM) 1 and NREM 2 remained in the normal range for both PSG 1 and PSG 2, patients spent less time in NREM 3 and 4 (26.9 minutes versus 33.7 minutes) at both time points (8% versus 7%). Additionally, patients spent less than the expected percentage of sleep in REM at PSG 1 and PSG 2 (13% versus 8%). The mean periodic limb movement (PLM) was elevated at both time points; they doubled in the second time point (8 PLMs, SD = 11.68 versus 16 PLMs, SD = 17.1). Upon completion of a chart review to determine if patients were on known causative agents or if they had additional factors predisposing them to PLMs, researchers did not find gender, age, known medications, anemia, or renal function as being causative factors for PLMs in this sample.

In a repeat measures pilot study of 19 patients undergoing ASCT or allogeneic stem cell transplant, patients were randomized to receive either a strength training intervention or to a usual care group. Eight of the 19 patients had a diagnosis of myeloma, and all participants underwent testing prior to admission for stem cell transplant, eight days following transplant, and six weeks following discharge from hospital. In this current study, the intervention arm received strength training supervised/unsupervised three to four times a week for a total of six weeks. The usual care group received exercise and physical activity recommendations from the research team. While no interaction effect was observed, a time effect was noted among the three time points in the level of fatigue, physical activity, health status perceptions, and quality of life. Participants had a decrease in physical activity after stem cell transplant that increased by 116% in the physical activity group and 88% in the usual care group. Similar findings were noted in the level of fatigue, muscle strength, and health status perceptions. The only significant difference observed between the exercise group (22.6) and usual care group (34.4) was found in fatigue level ($p < 0.01$) at the third time point (Hacker et al., 2011).

Fatigue affects patients' quality of life and interpersonal relationships. The previously discussed studies demonstrate that the etiology of fatigue may be related to multiple factors, including lack of oral hydration, decreased sleep quality, pain, and mood disturbance. Prior to initiating interventions for fatigue, it is important to perform a thorough assessment of fatigue to determine the potential etiology. Nurses are in an ideal position to develop nursing interventions that address the multiple causes of fatigue in patients with myeloma. If pain or mood disturbance is the underlying issue, the physician should be notified of the patient's pain level and mood disturbance prior to initiating an exercise regimen. Furthermore, nurses are in a position to discuss the potential benefits of exercise and sleep hygiene with patients.

Treatment Decision Making and Information Need Priorities

A recent study on patient and physician factors influencing treatment decision making (TDM) in older adults newly diagnosed with symptomatic myeloma uncovered several patient- and physician-specific factors that influence eventual treatment choice (Tariman, Doorenbos, Schepp, Becker, & Berry, 2014). The researchers found patient-specific factors that included age, opinions of others (e.g., physician, family members, other patients with myeloma), past health-related experience, personal beliefs and values (e.g., valuing autonomy, being a burden to family and others), faith in higher power, social support, insurance coverage, transportation issues/convenience of pills versus IV medications, geographic barriers, finances (e.g., co-pays, out-of-pocket expenses), and significant events in patients' families. Physicians' influential factors in TDM included patients' comorbidities, functional status, and supportive care requirements; physicians' beliefs and values (e.g., physicians' personal beliefs on patient-physician relationship or dynamics during TDM); patients' medical and clinical factors; physicians' expertise and type of practice; patients' age; patients' treatment preferences; family opinions; and clinical trials as an option. The study researchers noted that although there are similarities in both patient- and physician-specific influential factors, some patient-specific factors merit consideration in actual TDM to improve decision outcomes such as higher patient decision satisfaction and lower decisional regret (Tariman, Doorenbos, Schepp, Becker, et al., 2014). Unless there is an unequivocal randomized controlled trial result that supports one therapy over others, physicians must listen to their patients' personal and contextual factors and incorporate them in the TDM process. Additionally, researchers reported that older adults newly diagnosed with symptomatic myeloma want to participate in the treatment decision (Tariman, Doorenbos, Schepp, Singhal, & Berry, 2014). This finding is contrary to the most recent finding from a systematic review of the preferences of older adult patients with cancer, which indicated that they preferred a passive role during the TDM process (Singh et al., 2010).

A study on priority of information needs in older adults newly diagnosed with symptomatic multiple myeloma found that these patients have different priorities of information needs as compared to younger patients diagnosed with various types of cancer. The top three information priorities for patients with multiple myeloma are information related to treatment, prognosis, and self-care, respectively (Tariman, Doorenbos, Schepp, Singhal, & Berry, 2015). No sociodemographic variable was found to have any relationship to the priorities of information needs among older adults with symptomatic multiple myeloma. The study researchers also reported that the Internet, physicians, and family and friends were among the top sources of information for patients with myeloma. The findings of this study could be used as a starting point in developing Internet-based patient education programs.

Gaps in the Literature

Overall, myeloma-related nursing studies are few when compared to other cancer specialties. The studies reviewed in this chapter were predominantly in fatigue management, exercise, diagnosis delay, psychosocial aspects of quality of life, information needs, and TDM and unexpected admissions during ASCT. Currently, nursing interventions for treatment-related toxicities are based on studies conducted in other malignancies, including pain management and supportive care in patients receiving novel agents, particularly thalidomide and bortezomib. Research studies in the areas of emotional and cognitive dysfunction, end-of-life care, and survivorship issues, as well as interventional studies related to treatment- and disease-related complications, also are direly needed.

As discussed earlier, 80% of previously treated patients with multiple myeloma report some form of neuropathy that is reversible (Richardson et al., 2009). Studies conducted among patients with neuropathy related to diabetes or other chemotherapy-induced neuropathies indicate that vitamin and mineral supplements may alleviate or prevent neuropathy. Drugs such as bortezomib and thalidomide exert different mechanisms of action than taxanes or platinum-based chemotherapy, and the mechanism by which neuropathy develops may differ between agents or diabetic neuropathy. Therefore, prospective studies evaluating these regimens among patients with multiple myeloma are needed.

The life expectancy of patients with multiple myeloma has nearly doubled over the past decade (Kumar et al., 2008, 2013). This increase in life expectancy has led to consideration of multiple myeloma as a chronic disease. Therefore, survivorship issues associated with disease and long-term treatment-related toxicities such as neuropathy, fatigue, bone health, sexual dysfunction, and renal complications, as well as health maintenance, will need to be addressed in this patient population. Additionally, although patients are living longer with myeloma, they will still require end-of-life care at some point during their care continuum. Studies evaluating the needs of patients at the end of life, as well as symptom management during this period, are needed in order to relieve pain, psychological distress, anticipated bereavement, and caregiver stress that may be experienced by patients and their families.

Culture, religious beliefs, and values influence the way individuals view their lives and the meaning of disease. Therefore, studies should include a broad examination of the cultural influences on diagnosis, treatment, management of side effects, and the end of life to provide personalized care.

Future Scenario of Nursing Research in Myeloma

A huge gap exists in the multiple myeloma literature when it comes to evidence-based nursing care. Additional nursing research is needed to shape the delivery of nursing care, including chemotherapy administration in patients with this disease. In particular, research on adherence to the prescribed chemotherapy, whether it is given through the oral, subcutaneous, or IV route, is very much needed. Furthermore, the impact of treatment adherence or nonadherence to the clinical outcomes also is critically needed to guide the development of effective nursing interventions and practice policy. Oncology nurses can change the current status of nursing research in multiple myeloma and contribute to the currently established evidence-based nursing interventions. Specifically, nursing research effort in the area of disease- and treatment-related symptom management, psychosocial interventions, patient and caregiver education, decision- making aids, health maintenance, survivorship care, and end-of-life care needs continued support from all stakeholders, including multiple myeloma patient advocacy groups and philanthropic foundations. The future nursing research scenario in multiple myeloma could be one that is full of research activities or one that remains unstudied or understudied.

Conclusion

Although some studies have been conducted in patients with multiple myeloma, more research is needed to better address symptoms and quality of life both during treatment and at the end of life. Oncology nurses must continue to perform literature searches to look for studies that provide the evidence supporting current nursing practice. Oncology nurses are in an excellent position to design and conduct clinical trials that evaluate the impact of nursing interventions on patient care and clinical outcomes.

References

Bataille, R., Boccadoro, M., Klein, B., Durie, B., & Pileri, A. (1992). C-reactive protein and beta-2 microglobulin produce a simple and powerful myeloma staging system. *Blood, 80,* 733–737.

Booker, R., Olson, K., Pilarski, L.M., Noon, J.P., & Bahlis, N.J. (2009). The relationships among physiologic variables, quality of life, and fatigue in patients with multiple myeloma. *Oncology Nursing Forum, 36,* 209–216. doi:10.1188/09.ONF.209-216

Coleman, E.A., Coon, S.K., Hall-Barrow, J., Richards, K., Gaylor, D., & Stewart, B. (2003). Feasibility of exercise during treatment for multiple myeloma. *Cancer Nursing, 26,* 410–419. doi:10.1097/00002820-200310000-00012

Coleman, E.A., Coon, S.K., Kennedy, R.L., Lockhart, K.D., Stewart, C.B., Anaissie, E.J., & Barlogie, B. (2008). Effects of exercise in combination with epoetin alfa during high-dose chemotherapy and autologous peripheral blood stem cell transplantation for multiple myeloma [Online exclusive]. *Oncology Nursing Forum, 35,* E53–E61. doi:10.1188/08.ONF.E53-E61

Coleman, E.A., Coon, S.K., Mattox, S.G., & O'Sullivan, P. (2002). Symptom management and successful outpatient transplantation for patients with multiple myeloma. *Cancer Nursing, 25,* 452–460. doi:10.1097/00002820-200212000-00009

Coleman, E.A., Goodwin, J.A., Coon, S.K., Richards, K., Enderlin, C., Kennedy, R., ... Barlogie, B. (2011). Fatigue, sleep, pain, mood and performance status in patients with multiple myeloma. *Cancer Nursing, 34,* 219–227. doi:10.1097/NCC.0b013e3181f9904d

Coleman, E.A., Goodwin, J.A., Kennedy, R., Coon, S.K., Richards, K., Enderlin, C., ... Anaissie, E.J. (2012). Effects of exercise on fatigue, sleep, and performance: A randomized trial. *Oncology Nursing Forum, 39,* 468–477. doi:10.1188/12.ONF.468-477

Coon, S.K., & Coleman, E.A. (2004). Exercise decisions within the context of multiple myeloma, transplant, and fatigue. *Cancer Nursing, 27,* 108–118. doi:10.1097/00002820-200403000-00003

Enderlin, C.A., Coleman, E.A., Davila, D., Richards, K., Jegley, S.M., Kennedy, R., ... Reed, P.J. (2013). Sleep measured by polysomnography in patients receiving high-dose chemotherapy for multiple myeloma prior to stem cell transplantation. *Oncology Nursing Forum, 40,* 73–81. doi:10.1188/13.ONF.73-81

Friese, C.R., Abel, G.A., Magazu, L.S., Neville, B.A., Richardson, L.C., & Earle, C.C. (2009). Diagnostic delay and complications for older adults with multiple myeloma. *Leukemia and Lymphoma, 50,* 392–400. doi:10.1080/10428190902741471

Hacker, E.D., Larson, J., Kujath, A., Peace, D., Rondelli, D., & Gaston, L. (2011). Strength training following hematopoietic stem cell transplant. *Cancer Nursing, 34,* 238–249. doi:10.1097/NCC.0b013e3181fb3686

Howlader, N., Noone, A.M., Krapcho, M., Garshell, J., Miller, D., Altekruse, S.F., ... Cronin, K.A. (Eds.). (2015). SEER cancer statistics review, 1975–2012. Retrieved from http://seer.cancer.gov/csr/1975_2012

Johansson, E., Langius-Eklof, A., Engervall, P., & Wredling, R. (2005). Patients' experience of ambulatory self-administration of pamidronate in multiple myeloma. *Cancer Nursing, 28,* 158–165. doi:10.1097/00002820-200503000-00011

Kangas, M., Bovbjerg, D.H., & Montgomery, G.H. (2008). Cancer-related fatigue: A systematic and meta-analytic review of non-pharmacological therapies for cancer patients. *Psychology Bulletin, 134,* 700–741. doi:10.1037/a0012825

Kelly, M., & Dowling, M. (2011). Patients' lived experience of myeloma. *Nursing Standard, 25,* 38–44. doi:10.7748/ns2011.03.25.28.38.c8397

Kumar, S.K., Dispenzieri, A., Lacy, M.Q., Gertz, M.A., Buadi, F.K., Pandey, S., ... Rajkumar, S.V. (2013). Continued improvement in survival in multiple myeloma: Changes in early mortality and outcomes in older patients. *Leukemia, 28,* 1122–1128. doi:10.1038/leu.2013.313

Kumar, S.K., Rajkumar, S.V., Dispenzieri, A., Lacy, M.Q., Hayman, S.R., Buadi, F.K., ... Gertz, M.A. (2008). Improved survival in multiple myeloma and the impact of novel therapies. *Blood, 111,* 2516–2520. doi:10.1182/blood-2007-10-116129

Levy, M.H., Chwistek, M., & Mehta, R.S. (2008). Management of chronic pain in cancer survivors. *Cancer Journal, 14,* 401–409. doi:10.1097/PPO.0b013e31818f5aa7

Ludwig, H., & Zojer, N. (2007). Supportive care in multiple myeloma. *Best Practice and Research Clinical Haematology, 20,* 817–835. doi:10.1016/j.beha.2007.10.001

Meenaghan, T., O'Dwyer, M., Hayden, P., Hayat, A., Murray, M., & Dowling, M. (2010). Home administration of bortezomib: Making a difference to myeloma patients' lives. *European Journal of Oncology Nursing, 14,* 134–136. doi:10.1016/j.ejon.2009.09.003

Melton, L.J., III, Kyle, R.A., Achenbach, S.J., Oberg, A.L., & Rajkumar, S.V. (2005). Fracture risk with multiple myeloma: A population-based study. *Journal of Bone and Mineral Research, 20,* 487–493. doi:10.1359/JBMR.041131

Poulos, A.R., Gertz, M.A., Pankratz, V.S., & Post-White, J. (2001). Pain, mood disturbance, and quality of life in patients with multiple myeloma. *Oncology Nursing Forum, 28,* 1163–1171.

Pulte, D., Redaniel, M.T., Brenner, H., Jansen, L., & Jeffreys, M. (2013). Recent improvement in survival of patients with multiple myeloma: Variation by ethnicity. *Leukemia and Lymphoma, 55,* 1083–1089. doi:10.3109/10428194.2013.827188

Richardson, P.G., Sonneveld, P., Schuster, M., Stadtmauer, E., Facon, T., Harousseau, J.-L., ... San Miguel, J. (2009). Reversibility of symptomatic peripheral neuropathy with bortezomib in the phase III APEX trial in relapsed multiple myeloma: Impact of a dose-modification guideline. *British Journal of Haematology, 144,* 895–903. doi:10.1111/j.1365-2141.2008.07573.x

San Miguel, J., Garcia-Sanz, R., & Gutierrez, N. (2008). Prognostic factors and classification in multiple myeloma. In K.C. Anderson & I. Ghobrial (Eds.), *Multiple myeloma: Translational and emerging therapies* (pp. 115–139). New York, NY: Informa Healthcare.

Siegel, R.L., Miller, K.D., & Jemal, A. (2015). Cancer statistics, 2015. *CA: A Cancer Journal for Clinicians, 65,* 5–29. doi:10.3322/caac.21254

Singh, J.A., Sloan, J.A., Atherton, P.J., Smith, T., Hack, T.F., Huschka, M.M., ... Degner, L.F. (2010). Preferred roles in treatment decision making among patients with cancer: A pooled analysis of studies using the Control Preferences Scale. *American Journal of Managed Care, 16,* 688–696.

Tariman, J.D., Doorenbos, A., Schepp, K.G., Becker, P., & Berry, D.L. (2014). Patient, physician and contextual factors are influential in the treatment decision making of older adults newly diagnosed with symptomatic myeloma. *Cancer Treatment Communications, 2*(2–3), 34–47. doi:10.1016/j.ctrc.2014.08.003

Tariman, J.D., Doorenbos, A., Schepp, K.G., Singhal, S., & Berry, D.L. (2014). Older adults newly diagnosed with symptomatic myeloma and treatment decision making. *Oncology Nursing Forum, 41,* 411–419. doi:10.1188/14.ONF.411-419

Tariman, J.D., Doorenbos, A., Schepp, K.G., Singhal, S., & Berry, D.L. (2015). Top information need priorities of older adults diagnosed with active myeloma. *Journal of the Advanced Practitioner in Oncology, 6,* 14–21.

Tariman, J.D., Love, G., McCullagh, E., Sandifer, S., & the IMF Nurse Leadership Board. (2008). Peripheral neuropathy associated with novel therapies in patients with multiple myeloma: Consensus statement of the IMF Nurse Leadership Board. *Clinical Journal of Oncology Nursing, 12*(Suppl. 3), 29–36. doi:10.1188/08.CJON.S1.29-35

Vlossak, D., & Fitch, M.I. (2008). Multiple myeloma: The patient's perspective. *Canadian Oncology Nursing Journal, 18,* 141–151. doi:10.5737/1181912x183141145

CHAPTER **10**

On the Horizon: Advances in Genomics and Biomarkers

Beth Faiman, PhD, APRN-BC, AOCN®, and Joseph D. Tariman, PhD, ANP-BC

Introduction

Significant advances in the diagnosis and management of patients with multiple myeloma have occurred in the last 20 years. New insights into the genetic characteristics and bone marrow microenvironment have allowed oncology clinicians to stratify patients' disease risk status (Rajkumar, 2013). The techniques used to stratify one's genomic risk include conventional bone marrow chromosomal and cytogenetics analysis, fluorescence in situ hybridization (FISH) analysis, and gene expression profiling (GEP). The combined use of biomarkers such as beta-2 microglobulin (β2M) and albumin has been reported as a strong predictor of overall survival, providing the framework for the International Staging System (ISS) for myeloma (Greipp et al., 2005). Most recently, the use of multiparameter flow cytometry (MFC) provides newer information on plasma cell labeling index (PCLI) at S phase, myeloma cells ploidy, and minimal residual disease detection by immunophenotyping, which also provide overall survival prognostic value for clinical use (Paiva, Gutierrez, et al., 2012; Paiva, Vidriales, et al., 2012; Pessoa de Magalhaes et al., 2013).

Despite increased knowledge of myeloma disease at the molecular level, much remains unknown in multiple myeloma genomics from the time of diagnosis to the late stage of the disease (Egan et al., 2012). Moreover, the state of the science of myeloma genomics is rapidly changing, and newer predictive models using genomic data are being proposed by various myeloma research centers around the world (Avet-Loiseau et al., 2013; Kumar et al., 2012; Mikhael et al., 2013; Shaughnessy et al., 2007; Stephens et al., 2012). Hence, the purpose of this chapter is to review what is known about the concepts and advances of genomics and biomarkers in multiple myeloma and identify how these new data are used in the treatment decision-making process. Additionally, this chapter will discuss how these advances in biomarkers and genomics will affect myeloma nursing practice in the future.

Overview of Multiple Myeloma Biomarkers and Genomics

A biomarker is a distinctive biologic characteristic that can be objectively measured to diagnose disease, determine response to medications, or estimate prognosis (Jain, 2010). There are many ways of classifying biomarkers in health and research, and numerous biomarkers in multiple myeloma exist. Biomarkers are commonly used in the diagnosis and disease monitoring of multiple myeloma and are integral to management of the disease. Common laboratory biomarkers used to assess patients' disease status include serum protein electrophoresis (SPEP), urine protein electrophoresis (UPEP), and serum free light chains (kappa or lambda) (Landgren, 2013). Many multiple myeloma biomarkers and genomic tests are performed on blood, urine, or bone marrow aspirate samples depending on the type of information requested by the oncology clinician. For genomic studies, bone aspirate samples commonly are analyzed using conventional cytogenetics, FISH, DNA microarrays, MFC, or GEP techniques (Landgren & Morgan, 2013). A list of disease monitoring and prognostic multiple myeloma biomarkers is presented in Table 10-1.

Genomics is a discipline concerned with mapping the genes ("gen-") and chromosomes ("-ome") of an organism as well as the identification of dysregulated genes (Biemar & Foti, 2013). Genomics as a science has gained popularity thanks to the Human Genome Project (HGP). The HGP was an international, collaborative research program completed in 2003. Over several years, researchers were able to map the human genome and develop a "blueprint" of human genetic material. The HGP revealed there are approximately 20,500 human genes, 99% of which humans share (International Human Genome Sequencing Consortium, 2004).

Integral to the identification of the human genome was an understanding of the coiled double helix structure known as DNA (Brown, 2002). Genetic information is contained in cells, which forms a sequence. A DNA molecule consists of four nucleotide base pairs of DNA: adenine (A), thymine (T), guanine (G), and cytosine (C). Each base pair develops a sequence that can be followed and replicated. For example, the purine adenine always pairs with the pyrimidine thymine ("A with T"), while the pyrimidine cytosine always pairs with the purine guanine ("C with G") (Brown, 2002). All individ-

Table 10-1. Examples of Biomarkers in Multiple Myeloma*

Name	Origin	Use	Notes
Serum protein electrophoresis with immunofixation (SPEP + IFE)	Serum	To diagnose, monitor multiple myeloma	The presence of a monoclonal protein is not definitive for diagnosis.
Urine protein electrophoresis with immunofixation (UPEP + IFE)	Urine	To diagnose, monitor multiple myeloma	The presence of a monoclonal protein is not definitive for diagnosis.
Kappa/lambda free light chain	Serum	To diagnose, monitor multiple myeloma	The presence of a monoclonal protein is not definitive for diagnosis.
Beta-2 microglobulin (β2M)	Serum	Prognosis	β2M is a nonspecific biomarker; higher levels mean the individual is at risk for poorer prognosis.
del(13)	Bone marrow aspirate	Prognosis	The presence of del(13) on cytogenetics is a poor prognostic factor.
del(17p) t(14;16) t(14;20)	Bone marrow/fluorescence in situ hybridization (FISH)	Prognosis	High-risk disease with associated poor survival outcomes/25% of patients
t(4;14)	Bone marrow/FISH	Prognosis	Intermediate risk
t(11;14) t(6;14)	Bone marrow/FISH	Prognosis	Standard risk/75% of patients
del(1)	Bone marrow/FISH	Prognosis	Del(1) confers a poor prognosis in post-transplant patients.
Gene expression profiling (GEP)/MyPRS	Bone marrow	Prognosis	High-risk GEP is associated with shorter durations of complete remissions, event-free survival, and overall survival.

*The list is not inclusive of all biomarkers in multiple myeloma.

Note. Based on information from Avet-Loiseau et al., 2007; Faiman, 2014; Rajkumar et al., 2014; Segges & Braggio, 2011.

uals are born with DNA that expresses genes and represents opportunities for variability from one human to the next (International Human Genome Consortium, 2004).

Each human cell contains 23 pairs of chromosomes. Genes are situated on each chromosome and found within the nucleus of a cell. The genome is the absolute complete genetic material found within a chromosome. Alleles are alternate forms of paired genes, which encode for proteins (see Figure 10-1). Different combinations of aberrant alleles can predispose an individual to certain diseases. For example, when three copies of chromosome 21 (trisomy 21) are found in the gene analysis of an individual, this confirms the presence of Down syndrome, a congenital disease characterized by moderate to severe mental retardation and other associated disease features (National Down Syndrome Society, 2014).

Genetic expression occurs with the activation of a gene, which, in turn, forms a protein. Two steps to gene expression involve RNA molecules and include (1) transcription and (2) translation. Transcription is the process of creating a complementary RNA copy of the DNA sequence to produce a complementary RNA strand. Transcription is different from DNA replication where RNA is not involved. Translation occurs when the messen-

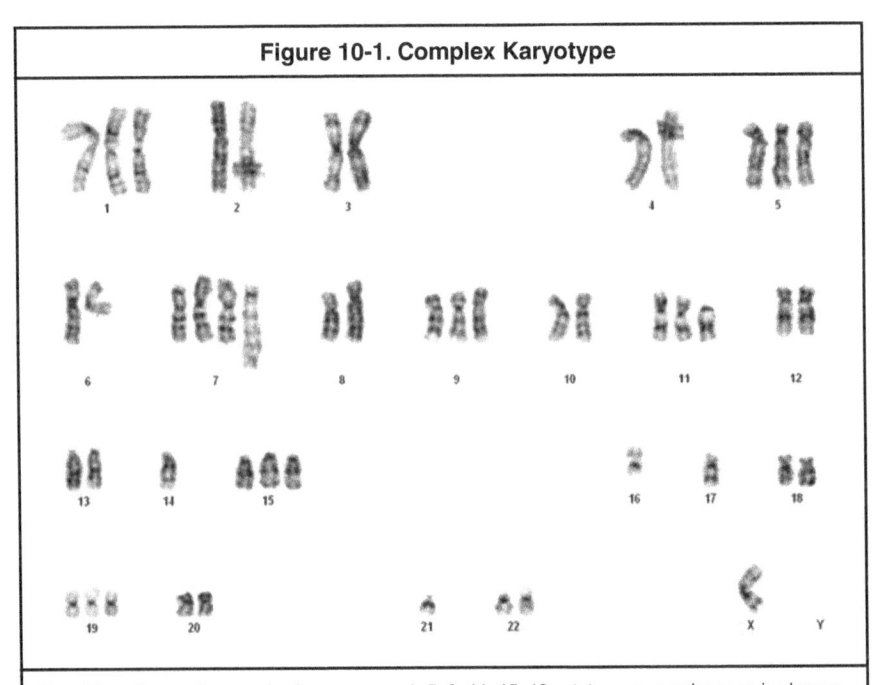

Figure 10-1. Complex Karyotype

Note. Trisomies can be seen in chromosomes 1, 5, 9, 11, 15, 19; a tetrasomy can be seen in chromosome 7; and deletions can be seen in chromosomes 14, 16, 17, and 21.

ger RNA sequence is read and used as a template to assemble the chain of amino acids (Brown, 2002).

DNA methylation occurs when a strand of DNA following replication is modified. DNA methylation is one of the main processes used to regulate gene expression, which occurs when a methyl (CH_3) group is added to a cytosine molecule. Methylation of cytosines can alter gene expression. It is important to remember one is born with DNA and one's DNA will never change, but genetic expression can be altered through a variety of mechanisms either intrinsic (within the individual) or extrinsic (external, environmental) (Jain, 2010).

A major area of research in genomics involves single nucleotide polymorphisms (SNPs). SNPs (pronounced "snips") are DNA sequence variations and occur when a single nucleotide (A, T, G, or C) in the genome sequence is altered within a particular region. Variations in genetic sequences may underlie differences in health. More than 1.42 million SNPs have been identified in the human genome (International SNP Map Working Group, 2001).

Specific SNPs have been evaluated in patients with multiple myeloma by peripheral blood analysis to identify risks in developing multiple myeloma itself or for disease-related complications (International SNP Map Working Group, 2001; Munshi et al., 2011). One case control study identified a variant allele of the interleukin (IL)-6 promoter SNP-572 to be associated with a twofold increased risk of development of plasma cell neoplasms (Cozen et al., 2006). Two additional SNPs have been associated with an increased risk of myeloma in previous studies: the insulin receptor substrate type 1 (IRS1) and the IL-6 receptor (IL6R). When tested in a cohort of participants from the Nurses' Health Study and the Health Professionals Follow-Up Study, researchers found a 42% increase in multiple myeloma risk per copy of the variant IRS1 allele (Rand et al., 2013). RNA and SNP targeted sequencing techniques have been identified, and it is hoped that they will improve our understanding of myeloma disease progression and response to treatment (Newman et al., 2013).

Genomics has been used in multiple myeloma to improve the outcome of patients with relapsed or refractory disease and to identify patients at risk for complications of the disease. A main focus of the research is to identify mechanisms of drug resistance toward available therapies and immune surveillance. Several classes of drugs are under study to address heritable changes to gene expression (*epigenetic changes*) that can lead to disease progression. Highly alkaline proteins (*histones*) are responsible to package and order DNA nucleosomes. Removal of acetyl groups from an N-acetyl-lysine amino acid allows the histones to rewrap and package DNA more tightly. To target the defect, the use of drugs such as demethylating agents and histone deacetylase (HDAC) inhibitors is under study (Heuck et al., 2013; Manning, Whyte, Martinez, Hunter, & Sudarsanam, 2002). The initiation of tumorigenesis and onset of disease-related complications results from a complex interplay between oncogenes, tumor suppressors, and unknown agents. Each of these changes has the opportunity to produce significant effects within a cell.

To understand the pathogenesis and the molecular basis of multiple myeloma, whole genome sequencing was performed. In one study, several unexpected oncogenetic mechanisms were suggested, which included the mutation of genes critical to protein translation, histone methylation, and blood coagulation (Bergsagel & Kuehl, 2005; Chapman et al., 2011). Genetic alterations and mutations responsible for translation of proteins, such as histone methylation and *BRAF* (a human gene that creates a protein called b-raf), have been noted. Each of these biomarkers represents an opportunity to develop targeted therapies to halt myeloma disease progression (Chapman et al., 2011).

The current state of the science of myeloma genomics is getting closer to identifying the significant genetic changes and designing of drugs that can modify adverse genetic changes and disrupt the communication among the bone marrow microenvironment, signaling pathways, cytokines, and cellular proteins. Many newer agents were developed from an improved understanding of multiple myeloma cell development and genomics. The process of drug development to target changes to genes and chromosomes is called *pharmacogenomics*. A major goal of pharmacogenomic research is to gain understanding into illness and develop drugs to prevent or reverse changes to aberrant pathways. Pharmacogenomics holds the promise of individualized treatment approaches in the future, where a patient will have higher probability of treatment success based on known genomic data and their corresponding treatment responses.

Genomic-Based Risk Stratification Techniques

Bone marrow aspirate and biopsy are obtained in patients with multiple myeloma to determine the percentage of plasma cells present in one's bone marrow and to evaluate the genes, chromosomes, and their aberrations. An estimated 40% of patients with newly diagnosed multiple myeloma will have chromosomal translocations on genetic testing (Dispenzieri et al., 2007). A conventional chromosomal analysis and FISH studies can be performed on liquid bone marrow aspirate to evaluate cytogenetic changes that can occur in myeloma cells. These cytogenetic changes include additions, deletions, and translocations of chromosomes. FISH tests for specific immunoglobulin (IgH) translocations on bone marrow aspirate of monoclonal plasma cells. Cytogenetics and FISH are performed on abnormal plasma cells and therefore reflect actual tumor characteristics. One of the most common myeloma disease risk stratifications using genomic data, called mSMART (Mayo Stratification for Myeloma and Risk-Adapted Therapy), was developed by the

Mayo Clinic researchers. Based on consensus among Mayo Clinic researchers, the negative prognostic impact of specific IgH translocations such as t(4;14), t(14;16), t(14;20), metaphase chromosome 13 deletion by conventional cytogenetics, loss of 17p13 by interphase FISH, high-risk GEP signature, hypodiploidy, high plasma cells S-phase labeling index, and complex karyotype has been established (Mikhael et al., 2013).

In general, the characteristics of most tumors can be divided into hyperdiploid and nonhyperdiploid (Fonseca et al., 2009). Approximately 50% of tumors are considered nonhyperdiploid and include one of the following IgH translocations: 11q13 (CCN D1), 6p21 (CCN D3), 16q23 (MAF), 20q12 (MAFB), or 4p16 (FGFR3 and MMSET). Other types of hyperdiploid tumors affect the odd-numbered chromosomes: 3, 5, 7, 9, 11, 15, 19, and 21 (Bergsagel & Kuehl, 2005; Fonseca et al., 2009). These hyperdiploid myeloma cells could be seen as trisomies (e.g., three copies of chromosome 9) or tetrasomies (e.g., four copies of chromosome 15) either in conventional cytogenetic testing as seen in Figure 10-1 or by FISH technique. Nonhyperdiploidy and complex karyotype seen in myeloma cells are considered high-risk disease features (Mikhael et al., 2013).

A third genomic test known as *gene expression profiling*, or *GEP*, is now commercially available. Researchers at the University of Arkansas for Medical Sciences have identified 70 signatures of genes, which can be also substituted with a 17-gene model that is capable of prognostic significance using microarray technology (Shaughnessy et al., 2007). Signal Genetics is a company that developed the Myeloma Prognostic Risk Signature (MyPRS®), which analyzes the whole-genome expression profile of the patient's myeloma cells to provide a molecular characterization of the disease. The results are reported in low-, standard-, or high-risk groups; the high-risk group had shorter durations of complete remission, event-free survival, and overall survival. To perform the test, 3–5 ml of bone marrow aspirate is collected in a heparinized, lavender-top tube and sent to Signal Genetics (Signal Genetics, 2014). Insurance coverage for the MyPRS test varies depending on the patient's insurance policy. Given that the test is relatively new and universal insurance coverage for the test is not seen in practice, oncology clinicians must explain to patients that the cost of GEP testing may not be covered by health insurance. It is important to inform patients because ultimately they will be responsible for paying the cost of GEP testing if their insurance denies coverage.

Additional Biologically Based Prognostic Factors

A high burden of disease is associated with a poor prognosis and may be evaluated by looking at bone marrow plasmacytosis, the presence of circulating plasma cells in peripheral blood (> 20% absolute plasma cells in the peripheral blood is considered plasma cell leukemia), as well as serum beta-2 microglobulin (β2M) (Avet-Loiseau, 2010; Dispenzieri et al., 2007). Elevated lactic dehydrogenase and high S-phase plasma cell labeling index also are indicative of high tumor burden, suggesting a worse outcome (Kumar et al., 2012). Serum β2M also is useful for assessing renal function, and the presence of renal dysfunction at the time of diagnosis confers a poor prognosis (Dimopoulos et al., 2011). It is critical that both patient- and disease-related prognostic factors are considered when recommending therapeutic options to patients.

Implications for Treatment Decision Making

Currently, the National Comprehensive Cancer Network® (NCCN®) does not recommend one single best therapy for newly diagnosed symptomatic patients with multiple myeloma (NCCN, 2014). NCCN recommends clinical trials at all stages of the myeloma treatment continuum. Autologous hematopoietic stem cell transplantation (HSCT) remains an important treatment option for patients with multiple myeloma younger than age 65. However, autologous HSCT now is being challenged through historical control studies and randomized controlled trials (RCTs) comparing outcomes from high-dose therapy (HDT) followed by autologous HSCT versus nonintensive therapy using novel therapies such as thalidomide, bortezomib, lenalidomide, and carfilzomib (Bladé, Rosiñol, Cibeira, Rovira, & Carreras, 2010; Rajkumar, 2013).

At the time of this writing, an RCT comparing lenalidomide with bortezomib plus or minus HDT followed by autologous HSCT is ongoing at Dana-Farber Cancer Institute and other participating clinical trial sites (Richardson, 2014). The findings of this trial will provide essential information to oncology clinicians as to whether HDT followed by autologous HSCT is still relevant to multiple myeloma care in this new era of novel agents. Novel agents offer convenience; oral chemotherapies such as thalidomide, lenalidomide, and pomalidomide can be taken by patients at home, and bortezomib can be easily administered subcutaneously in an outpatient clinic. IV chemotherapies such as carfilzomib also are administered in an outpatient setting twice a week, requiring only 10 minutes maximum infusion time. On the other hand, HDT followed by autologous HSCT is time intensive (up to three months, which necessitates time off from work for patients who are not retired) and requires significant supportive care during stem cell collection, stem cell transplant admission, and post-transplant periods.

Although the science of myeloma genomics still needs further development, some academic practice institutions have begun using institutional guidelines, which recommend treatment based on disease risk using genomic data. One of the commonly recognized algorithms for treatment decision making (TDM) in newly diagnosed symptomatic myeloma is the mSMART protocol mentioned previously. Mayo Clinic researchers, using stratification of myeloma disease risk status based on genomic and biomarkers data and patients' disease risk status (high, intermediate, or low), created an adapted therapy for each risk category. The mSMART classification system assesses patient and tumor characteristics to take a standardized approach to multiple myeloma patient care within the Mayo Clinic health systems, which are located in many places across the United States (Mikhael et al., 2013). An illustration of mSMART protocol is located in Figure 10-2.

A recent study on TDM in adults age 60 and older with symptomatic myeloma showed there are many influential factors that affect the actual treatment choice for a patient with myeloma (Tariman, Doorenbos, Schepp, Becker, & Berry, 2014). These factors include patient-specific factors such as age; opinions of others including family members and physicians; past health-related experiences; faith in a higher power; social support; insurance coverage; transportation issues/convenience of pills; geographic barriers; finances; and significant events in the family. This study also showed that similarly, physicians considered patients' age, family opinion, context, and treatment preference during TDM. However, the physicians in this study shared their perspectives that primarily they considered patients' comorbidities, functional status, and supportive care requirements as their top influential factors in the treatment recommendations they have offered to patients with multiple myeloma (Tariman et al., 2014). Based on the findings of this study, the role of genomics as an influential factor in actual treatment choice was not evident. The researchers of this study concluded that there is a need for oncology clinicians to integrate genomic data into the TDM process along with patients' personal and contextual factors. Further research studies on how patient-, physician-, health system-, and disease-related factors (including genomics) interplay with each other during TDM are still needed.

Implications for Nursing Practice

The science of multiple myeloma biomarkers and genomics is evolving. The general purpose of this chapter is to provide a basic overview of multiple myeloma biomarkers and genomics and to familiarize oncology clinicians with the importance of biomarkers and genomics in the diagnosis and management of myeloma. All oncology clinicians must stay abreast of the most recent advances in biomarkers and genomics and utilize them during TDM and disease monitoring to eventually improve patients' overall survival outcomes and quality of life. Oncology nurses must continue to provide

Figure 10-2. Cytogenetic Risk and Treatment Recommendations According to mSMART

Standard Risk[a,b]	Intermediate Risk[a]	High Risk

• All others
  – Hyperdiploidy
  – t(11;14)[b]
  – t(6;14)
	• FISH[c]
	  – t(4;14)
	• Cytogenetic deletion 13 or hypodiploidy
	  – PCLI ≥ 3%
		• FISH
		  – del(17p)
		  – t(14;16)
		  – t(14;20)
		• GEP
		  – High risk signature

Treatment Recommendations

• Rd[d] or CyBorD × 4 cycles
• Collect stem cells[e]
  – Autologous stem cell transplantation and consideration of lenalidomide maintenance
OR
  – Continue Rd[f].
	• CyBorD × 4 cycles
	• Autologous stem cell transplantation
	• Followed by bortezomib-based therapy for a minimum of one year
		• VRd × 4 cycles
		• Autologous stem cell transplantation
		• Followed by VRd for a minimum of one year

[a] A subset of patients with these features will be defined as high risk by GEP.

[b] Lactate dehydrogenase > upper limit of normal and beta-2 microglobulin > 5.5 may indicate worse prognosis.

[c] Prognosis is worse when associated with high beta-2 microglobulin and anemia.

[d] Bortezomib-containing regimens preferred in renal failure or if rapid response is needed.

[e] If age > 65 or > 4 cycles of Rd, consider granulocyte–colony-stimulating factor plus cyclophosphamide or plerixafor.

[f] Continuing Rd is option for patients responding to Rd with low toxicities; dexamethasone is usually discontinued after first year.

CyBorD—cyclophosphamide-bortezomib-dexamethasone; FISH—fluorescence in situ hybridization; GEP—gene expression profiling; PCLI—plasma cell labeling index; Rd—lenalidomide-dexamethasone; VRd—bortezomib-lenalidomide-dexamethasone

Note. From "Management of Newly Diagnosed Symptomatic Multiple Myeloma: Updated Mayo Stratification of Myeloma and Risk-Adapted Therapy (mSMART) Consensus Guidelines 2013," by J.R. Mikhael, D. Dingli, V. Roy, C.B. Reeder, F.K. Buadi, S.R. Hayman, ... M.Q. Lacy, 2013, *Mayo Clinic Proceedings, 88*, pp. 364–365. doi:10.1016/j.mayocp.2013.01.019. Copyright 2013 by Elsevier. Adapted with permission.

patient education and deliver much-needed information related to multiple myeloma including biomarkers and genomics, treatment options, and treatment-related side effects.

Survival and quality-of-life outcomes have significantly improved in the past decade thanks to our improved understanding of myeloma leading to the development of effective therapies. Patients with multiple myeloma and their families are hopeful that someday a cure will be found for the disease.

Oncology nurses and advanced oncology clinicians such as nurse practitioners are capable of designing and implementing clinical studies that can improve the current state of the science of myeloma care from diagnosis to end-of-life care. Future studies are essential for more biomarker discoveries and genomic breakthroughs, which eventually will further enhance multiple myeloma knowledge and understanding at the molecular level. The future advances that will be achieved in the field of genomics and therapeutics will be the key to improve patient outcomes, and these advances could potentially lead us to the path for myeloma cure.

Conclusion

There are many steps involved in DNA synthesis, chromosomal morphology, and transcription and translation of proteins. Each step provides opportunities in which genetic changes to cells can occur and lead to oncogenesis. Malignancies such as multiple myeloma occur through a series of genetic changes, mutations, and alterations to the bone marrow microenvironment. The complex interplay between altered genetic expression, cytokines, and the bone marrow stroma produce genetic changes that can lead to development of disease and poorer prognosis. Prognostic information based on biomarkers and genomic data should guide TDM. Advances in diagnostics, therapeutics, genomics, and pharcogenomics must be utilized in clinical practice, and every oncology clinician must value evidence-based practice.

References

Avet-Loiseau, H. (2010). Ultra high-risk myeloma. *Hematology, 2010*, 489–493. doi:10.1182/asheducation-2010.1.489

Avet-Loiseau, H., Attal, M., Moreau, P., Charbonnel, C., Garban, F., Hulin, C., ... Mathiot, C. (2007). Genetic abnormalities and survival in multiple myeloma: The experience of the Intergroupe Francophone du Myélome. *Blood, 109*, 3489–3495. doi:10.1182/blood-2006-08-040410

Avet-Loiseau, H., Durie, B.G., Cavo, M., Attal, M., Gutierrez, N., Haessler, J., ... Morgan, G. (2013). Combining fluorescent in situ hybridization data with ISS staging improves risk assessment in myeloma: An International Myeloma Working Group collaborative project. *Leukemia, 2*, 711–717. doi:10.1038/leu.2012.282

Bergsagel, P.L., & Kuehl, W.M. (2005). Molecular pathogenesis and a consequent classification of multiple myeloma. *Journal of Clinical Oncology, 23*, 6333–6338. doi:10.1200/JCO.2005.05.021

Biemar, F., & Foti, M. (2013). Global progress against cancer—Challenges and opportunities. *Cancer Biology and Medicine, 10*, 183–186. doi:10.7497/j.issn.2095-3941.2013.04.001

Bladé, J., Rosiñol, L., Cibeira, M.T., Rovira, M., & Carreras, E. (2010). Hematopoietic stem cell transplantation for multiple myeloma beyond 2010. *Blood, 115,* 3655–3663. doi:10.1182/blood-2009-08-238196

Brown, T.A. (2002). *Genomes* (2nd ed.). Retrieved from http://www.ncbi.nlm.nih.gov/books/NBK21128

Chapman, M.A., Lawrence, M.S., Keats, J.J., Cibulskis, K., Sougnez, C., Schinzel, A.C., & Golub, T.R. (2011). Initial genome sequencing and analysis of multiple myeloma. *Nature, 471,* 467–472. doi:10.1038/nature09837

Cozen, W., Gebregziabher, M., Conti, D.V., Van Den Berg, D.J., Coetzee, G.A., Wang, S.S., ... Ingles, S.A. (2006). Interleukin-6-related genotypes, body mass index, and risk of multiple myeloma and plasmacytoma. *Cancer Epidemiology, Biomarkers and Prevention, 15,* 2285–2291. doi:10.1158/1055-9965.EPI-06-0446

Dimopoulos, M.A., Kastritis, E., Michalis, E., Tsatalas, C., Michael, M., Pouli, A., ... Terpos, E. (2011). The International Scoring System (ISS) for multiple myeloma remains a robust prognostic tool independently of patients' renal function. *Annals of Oncology, 23,* 722–729. doi:10.1093/annonc/mdr276

Dispenzieri, A., Rajkumar, S.V., Gertz, M.A., Lacy, M.Q., Kyle, R.A., Greipp, P.R., ... Dalton, R.J. (2007). Treatment of newly diagnosed multiple myeloma based on Mayo Stratification of Myeloma and Risk-Adapted Therapy (mSMART): Consensus statement. *Mayo Clinic Proceedings, 82,* 323–341. doi:10.4065/82.3.323

Egan, J.B., Shi, C.X., Tembe, W., Christoforides, A., Kurdoglu, A., Sinari, S., ... Stewart, A.K. (2012). Whole-genome sequencing of multiple myeloma from diagnosis to plasma cell leukemia reveals genomic initiating events, evolution, and clonal tides. *Blood, 120,* 1060–1066. doi:10.1182/blood-2012-01-405977

Faiman, B. (2014). Myeloma genetics and genomics: Practice implications and future directions. *Clinical Lymphoma, Myeloma and Leukemia, 14,* 436–440. doi:10.1016/j.clml.2014.07.008

Fonseca, R., Bergsagel, P.L., Drach, J., Shaughnessy, J., Gutierrez, N., Stewart, A.K., ... Avet-Loiseau, H. (2009). International Myeloma Working Group molecular classification of multiple myeloma: Spotlight review. *Leukemia, 23,* 2210–2221. doi:10.1038/leu.2009.174

Greipp, P.R., San Miguel, J., Durie, B.G., Crowley, J.J., Barlogie, B., Bladé, J., ... Westin, J. (2005). International Staging System for multiple myeloma. *Journal of Clinical Oncology, 23,* 3412–3420. doi:10.1200/JCO.2005.04.242

Heuck, C.J., Mehta, J., Bhagat, T., Gundabolu, K., Yu, Y., Khan, S., ... Singhal, S.B. (2013). Myeloma is characterized by stage-specific alterations in DNA methylation that occur early during myelomagenesis. *Journal of Immunology, 190,* 2966–2975. doi:10.4049/jimmunol.1202493

International Human Genome Sequencing Consortium. (2004). Finishing the euchromatic sequence of the human genome. *Nature, 431,* 931–945. doi:10.1038/nature03001

International SNP Map Working Group. (2001). A map of human genome sequence variation containing 1.42 million single nucleotide polymorphisms. *Nature, 409,* 928–933. doi:10.1038/35057149

Jain, K.K. (2010). *The handbook of biomarkers.* doi:10.1007/978-1-60761-685-6_1

Kumar, S., Fonseca, R., Ketterling, R.P., Dispenzieri, A., Lacy, M.Q., Gertz, M.A., ... Rajkumar, S.V. (2012). Trisomies in multiple myeloma: Impact on survival in patients with high-risk cytogenetics. *Blood, 119,* 2100–2105. doi:10.1182/blood-2011-11-390658

Landgren, O. (2013). Monoclonal gammopathy of undetermined significance and smoldering multiple myeloma: Biological insights and early treatment strategies. *ASH Education Program Book, 2013,* 478–487. doi:10.1182/asheducation-2013.1.478

Landgren, O., & Morgan, G.J. (2013). Biological frontiers in multiple myeloma: From biomarker identification to clinical practice. *Clinical Cancer Research, 20,* 804-813. doi:10.1158/1078-0432.CCR-13-2159

CHAPTER 10. ON THE HORIZON: ADVANCES IN GENOMICS AND BIOMARKERS 243

Manning, G., Whyte, D.B., Martinez, R., Hunter, T., & Sudarsanam, S. (2002). The protein kinase complement of the human genome. *Science, 298,* 1912–1934. doi:10.1126/science.1075762

Mikhael, J.R., Dingli, D., Roy, V., Reeder, C.B., Buadi, F.K., Hayman, S.R., ... Lacy, M.Q. (2013). Management of newly diagnosed symptomatic multiple myeloma: Updated Mayo Stratification of Myeloma and Risk-Adapted Therapy (mSMART) consensus guidelines 2013. *Mayo Clinic Proceedings, 88,* 360–376. doi:10.1016/j.mayocp.2013.01.019

Munshi, N.C., Avet-Loiseau, H., Stephens, P.J., Bignell, G.R., Tai, Y.-T., Shammas, M., ... Futreal, A. (2011). *Whole genome sequencing defines the clonal architecture and genomic evolution in myeloma: Tumor heterogeneity with continued acquisition of new mutational change.* Paper presented at the 53rd Annual American Society of Hematology Meeting and Exposition, San Diego, CA. Abstract retrieved from https://ash.confex.com/ash/2011/webprogram/Paper43718.html

National Comprehensive Cancer Network. (2014, February). *NCCN Guidelines for Patients®: Multiple myeloma* [v.1.2014]. Retrieved from http://www.nccn.org/patients/guidelines/myeloma/#47/z

National Down Syndrome Society. (2014, February). Down syndrome. Retrieved from http://www.ndss.org/Down-Syndrome

Newman, S., Nooka, A.K., Kaufman, J.L., Bahlis, N.J., Neri, P., Matulis, S.M., ... Lonial, S. (2013). *Using RNA-Seq, SNP-CN and targeted deep sequencing to improve the diagnostic paradigm in multiple myeloma.* Poster presented at the 55th Annual American Society of Hematology Meeting and Exposition, New Orleans, LA. Abstract retrieved from https://ash.confex.com/ash/2013/webprogram/Paper65582.html

Paiva, B., Gutiérrez, N.C., Rosiñol, L., Vídriales, M.B., Montalbán, M.A., Martínez-López, J., ... San Miguel, J.F. (2012). High-risk cytogenetics and persistent minimal residual disease by multiparameter flow cytometry predict unsustained complete response after autologous stem cell transplantation in multiple myeloma. *Blood, 119,* 687–691. doi:10.1182/blood-2011-07-370460

Paiva, B., Vidríales, M.B., Montalbán, M.A., Pérez, J.J., Gutiérrez, N.C., Rosiñol, L., ... San Miguel, J.F. (2012). Multiparameter flow cytometry evaluation of plasma cell DNA content and proliferation in 595 transplant-eligible patients with myeloma included in the Spanish GEM2000 and GEM2005<65y trials. *American Journal of Pathology, 181,* 1870–1878. doi:10.1016/j.ajpath.2012.07.020

Pessoa de Magalhaes, R.J., Vidriales, M.B., Paiva, B., Fernandez-Gimenez, C., Garcia-Sanz, R., Mateos, M.V., ... Orfao, A. (2013). Analysis of the immune system of multiple myeloma patients achieving long-term disease control by multidimensional flow cytometry. *Haematologica, 98,* 79–86. doi:10.3324/haematol.2012.067272

Rajkumar, S.V. (2013). Multiple myeloma: 2013 update on diagnosis, risk-stratification, and management. *American Journal of Hematology, 88,* 226–235. doi:10.1002/ajh.23390

Rajkumar, S.V., Dimopoulos, M.A., Palumbo, A., Blade, J., Merlini, G., Mateos, M.V., ... Miguel, J.F. (2014). International Myeloma Working Group updated criteria for the diagnosis of multiple myeloma. *Lancet Oncology, 15,* e538–e548. doi:10.1016/s1470-2045(14)70442-5

Rand, K.A., Conti, D.V., Van Den Berg, D.J., Haiman, C.A., De Roos, A.J., Severson, R.K., ... Cozen, W. (2013). *Polymorphisms in IRS1 and IL6R and susceptibility to multiple myeloma.* Poster presented at the 55th Annual American Society of Hematology Meeting and Exposition, New Orleans, LA. Abstract retrieved from https://ash.confex.com/ash/2013/webprogram/Paper62843.html

Richardson, P.G. (2014, February). Randomized trial of lenalidomide, bortezomib, dexamethasone vs. high-dose treatment with SCT in MM patients up to age 65 (DFCI 10-106). Retrieved from http://clinicaltrials.gov/show/NCT01208662

Segges, P., & Braggio, E. (2011). Genetic markers used for risk stratification in multiple myeloma. *Genetics Research International, 2011.* doi:10.4061/2011/798089

Shaughnessy, J.D., Jr., Zhan, F., Burington, B.E., Huang, Y., Colla, S., Hanamura, I., ... Barlogie, B. (2007). A validated gene expression model of high-risk multiple myeloma is defined by deregulated expression of genes mapping to chromosome 1. *Blood, 109,* 2276–2284. doi:10.1182/blood-2006-07-038430

Signal Genetics. (2014, February). MyPRS overview. Retrieved from https://www.signalgenetics.com/myprsOverview.html

Stephens, O.W., Zhang, Q., Qu, P., Zhou, Y., Chavan, S., Tian, E., ... Shaughnessy, J.D., Jr. (2012). An intermediate-risk multiple myeloma subgroup is defined by sIL-6r: Levels synergistically increase with incidence of SNP rs2228145 and 1q21 amplification. *Blood, 119,* 503–512. doi:10.1182/blood-2011-07-367052

Tariman, J.D., Doorenbos, A., Schepp, K.G., Becker, P., & Berry, D.L. (2014). Patient, physician and contextual factors are influential in the treatment decision making of older adults newly diagnosed with symptomatic myeloma. *Cancer Treatment Communications, 2*(2–3), 34–47. doi:10.1016/j.ctrc.2014.08.003

CHAPTER 11

Patient Teaching

Sandra Rome, RN, MN, AOCN®, CNS

Introduction

Patient education begins at diagnosis and should continue along the entire cancer care trajectory. Because multiple myeloma is a complex disease and involves a variety of treatments and supportive care over time, patients may either feel not adequately informed or be susceptible to information overload (Spinks et al., 2012). Oncology nurses have the opportunity to influence clinical outcomes by teaching throughout the care continuum. Nurses are rated the highest among professionals in honesty and ethical standards (Gallup, Inc., 2014). Thus, it is by our ability to build trusting relationships that we can positively influence patient outcomes and quality of life.

As noted by Bartlett (1985),
> *Patient education* is defined as a planned learning experience using a combination of methods such as teaching, counseling, and behavior modification techniques that influence patients' knowledge and health and illness behavior. *Patient counseling* is an individualized process involving guidance and collaborative problem solving to help the patient to better manage the health problem. Patient education and counseling involve an interactive process that assists patients to participate actively in their health care. (p. 323)

Clinical health promotion can be considered a part of patient education and counseling. Thus, it would enable and reinforce patients to take greater control of the nonmedical determinants of their own health.

Multiple myeloma can now be considered a chronic disease, and there is hope for cure and long-term survival. The 5- and 10-year relative survival rates have improved over the past 20 years. For example, the 10-year survival rate for patients 66–79 years of age improved from 32% (1990–1999) to 41% (2000–2009). The 5-year survival rate for patients 51–65 years of age improved from 44% to 58% during those same time periods, and the 10-year survival rate for patients in this group diagnosed between 1990 and 1999 has reached 25% (Kristinsson, Anderson, & Landgren, 2014). The greatest improvements are in patients aged 15–44 years with 5- and 10-year survival rates reaching 70% and almost 50%, respectively (Pulte, Gondos, & Brenner, 2011). Unfortunately, patients may experience negative aspects of the disease at different times, thereby requiring the healthcare team to address and provide the appropriate education at each encounter. Furthermore, current and future novel therapies have their own potential side effects, and many are taken orally by patients at home, making oncology nurses' ongoing patient and family education essential.

Factors that affect patient teaching include the following (Bucher & Kotecki, 2014; Polovich, Olsen, & LeFebvre, 2014).
- The nurse's expertise regarding the subject
- The nurse's understanding of the individuals' learning styles
- The resources and strategies available to the nurse for patient education
- The nurse's ability to involve patients in the learning process
- The nurse matching appropriate strategies to specific content and learners' needs
- The learners' health literacy, language, and educational barriers
- The learners' physical or psychosocial barriers
  - Pain, fatigue, and visual, hearing, or cognitive impairment
  - Psychosocial or emotional issues (e.g., fear, denial)
  - Health beliefs, culture, and spiritual values (consistency with what will be taught)
  - Misconceptions already in place
- The ability of patients, significant others, and the healthcare team to share a clear vision of the goals of treatment and role expectations of each other

Matsuyama, Kuhn, Mosilani, and Wilson-Genderson (2012) examined the information needs of patients with cancer about disease, diagnostic tests, treatment, physical care, and psychosocial resources during treatment over a nine-month period. Although the authors found a significant reduction of needs over time, total information needs remained high throughout. Thus, patients actually may want a lot of information.

Husson et al. (2013) surveyed 4,446 survivors of lymphoma, multiple myeloma, or endometrial or colorectal cancer to examine the relationship between information provision and illness perception. Patients with lymphoma and multiple myeloma expressed greater satisfaction with the information they received and believed they had received more information about their treatment and other services compared with other cancer survivors. Patients with multiple myeloma reported the highest scores on the illness perception scales, indicating that they perceived their disease as very serious. More disease-specific information was associated with more personal and treatment control and a better understanding of their illness. However, the perceived receipt of more information on other services was associated with more negative consequences, less treatment control, and stronger emotional reactions.

They concluded that improving patients' illness perceptions by tailoring the information to their needs may help patients to better understand their disease, potentially leading to better health-related quality of life (Husson et al., 2013). In other words, the nurse should assess the desire for specific information at any given time, bearing in mind "need-to-know" safety information that must be imparted.

Assessment

Experienced clinicians respect the importance of the learning needs assessment phase: the assessment of the need to learn, motivation, and cultural, psychosocial, and other variables. These assessment-related activities must be performed before setting goals, performing interventions, and evaluating outcomes. The assessment phase of patient and caregiver education includes not only what is to be taught to the patient and caregiver but also patient and caregiver factors, adult learning principles, and nurse educator skills.

Although cognitive problems are increasingly apparent among cancer survivors, currently no evidence-based recommendations exist for the prevention or treatment of cognitive impairment. Practical solutions, however, have been proposed (Cheung et al., 2012; Polovich et al., 2014), including maintaining healthy lifestyle practices, ensuring adequate sleep and rest and a well-balanced diet, engaging in physical exercise, performing intellectual activities (reading, learning new skills, solving puzzles), participating in social activities (support groups), and employing practical management strategies (smartphones, voice recorders, daily planner, journal).

General open-ended screening questions should be a part of the nurse's initial assessment. The answers to an open-ended question, such as "Tell me your understanding of your diagnosis and the treatment plan you have discussed with your physician," can be very telling in terms of what the patient actually understands or remembers. Nurse behaviors can positively or negatively influence this interaction. Four principles the clinician should follow are reflective listening, asking open questions, affirming, and summarizing (Levensky, Forcehimes, O'Donohue, & Beitz, 2007). Figure 11-1 lists nurse behaviors for motivational interviewing.

Figure 11-1. Nurse Behaviors for Motivational Interviewing
• Create a quiet and calm environment; plan the interaction so that the time is uninterrupted. • Sit in a nonconfrontational, nonsuperior manner. • Listen rather than tell. • Take cues from the patient regarding the appropriateness of direct eye contact and other cultural behavior norms. • Adjust to, rather than oppose, patient resistance. • Express empathy through reflective listening. • Focus on the positive; do not criticize the patient or caregiver and avoid argument and direct confrontation. • Gently persuade with the understanding that change is up to the patient. • Focus on the patient's strengths to support the hope and optimism needed to make changes. • Help the patient to recognize the gap between where he or she is and where he or she hopes to be.
Note. Based on information from Bucher & Kotecki, 2014; Levensky et al., 2007; Oncology Nursing Society, 2009.

Assessment of motivation and readiness prior to educating patients and families is important in maintaining particular patient behaviors. The patient may have pain or cognitive changes that would require the need to be referred for more extensive evaluations (Jansen, 2013). Patient information such as primary caregiver, occupation, age, spirituality, culture, primary and secondary spoken and written languages, and highest education level achieved must be considered and assessed. According to the National Patient Safety Foundation (n.d.), "Literacy skills are a stronger predictor of an individual's health status than age, income, employment status, education level, or racial/ethnic group. One out of five American adults reads at the fifth grade level or below, and the average American reads at an eighth- to ninth-grade level. More than 66% of U.S. adults age 60 and older have either inadequate or marginal literacy skills" (p. 1). The impact of low literacy is that it affects compliance, patients may have fewer correct self-management skills and skills to navigate the healthcare system, and the risk of hospitalization increases (National Patient Safety Foundation, n.d.). Some studies demonstrate that overcoming barriers to informational needs may be less dependent on literacy consideration and more dependent on education level (Matsuyama et al., 2011). Nurses must assess patients and caregivers to the best of their ability. After the teaching has taken place, evaluation of the effectiveness (e.g., "teach-back") can allow nurses to then alter the educational strategy accordingly until a learner demonstrates the knowledge and behaviors necessary (Matsuyama et al., 2011). Figure 11-2 lists important aspects of a thorough patient and caregiver education needs assessment (Bucher & Kotecki, 2014).

Figure 11-2. Assessment of the Patient and Caregiver's Educational Needs

- Patient age and gender
- Current specific symptoms
- Current diagnosis and any other medical problems
- Current mental status and presence of any sensory or motor problems
- Current emotional state
- Current medications taken
- Current understanding and acceptance of the diagnosis
- Interest and motivation to learn
- Cultural values and health beliefs
- Educational background, occupational background, reading ability, and primary language
- Financial status
- Living situation and immediate support
- Understanding of disease and treatment
- Priorities of concern and interest in learning
- Preferred method of learning
- Caregiver's interest in learning and support of the patient
- Caregiver's involvement in patient teaching

Note. Based on information from Bucher & Kotecki, 2014.

Learning usually requires a change in beliefs and behavior. Prochaska and Velicer (1997) developed a transtheoretical model of health behavior change that has been used in health promotion programs. Their model proposes that stages of patient behavior occur, and clinicians can assess a patient's stage and intervene accordingly with the ultimate goal of an acquired new behavior (see Table 11-1). This model works well for nurses because they continually assess patients' learning needs and required behavior changes. For example, it might be easy for a patient to adapt to taking an oral treatment and seeing the provider monthly. However, if a treatment is suggested that requires the patient to come into the clinic more frequently for the treatment, blood work, or other reasons, the patient may have difficulty seeing the value in it.

Insufficient adaptation can hinder patients' ability to learn. Subsequently, clinicians may need to change their strategies at any given time in order to educate effectively. Education also can aid in modification of patient behavior for psychological adjustment to cancer. Thus, assistance with adaptation and education occur simultaneously. Legal aspects of patient and family education should not be ignored. Because much of the treatment and follow-up is done in an outpatient setting, more and more responsibility for safety relies on patients and families adhering to instructions. The healthcare team should verify and document reliable measures of patients' and families' understanding of the information given.

Table 11-1. Stages of Health Behavior Change—The Transtheoretical Model

Stage	Patient Behavior	Nursing Implications
1. Precontemplation	Is not considering a change; is not ready to learn	Provide support, increase awareness of condition, and describe benefits of change and risk of not changing.
2. Contemplation	Thinks about the change; may verbalize recognition of need to change: "I know I should," but identifies barriers	Introduce what is involved in changing the behavior. Reinforce the stated need to change.
3. Preparation	Starts planning the change, gathers information, sets a date to initiate change, shares decision to change with others	Reinforce the positive outcomes of change, provide information and encouragement, develop a plan, help to set priorities, and identify sources of support.
4. Action	Begins to change behavior through practice; tentative and may experience nonadherence	Reinforce behavior with reward, encourage self-reward, and discuss choices to help minimize nonadherence. Help patient plan to deal with potential changes in the plan.
5. Maintenance	Practices the behavior regularly; able to sustain the change	Continue to reinforce behavior. Provide additional teaching on the need to maintain change.
6. Termination	Change becomes part of lifestyle; behavior no longer considered a change	Evaluate effectiveness of the new behavior. No further intervention is needed until plan changes.

Note. Based on information from Bucher & Kotecki, 2014; Prochaska & Velicer, 1997.

Setting Goals and Desired Outcomes

Positive outcomes of patient education include the following (Polovich et al., 2014).
- Empowerment of active participation in healthcare and self-care behaviors
- Understanding of the diagnosis, treatment, goals, and duration of therapy and agreement with therapy
- Identification of all signs and symptoms that need to be reported
- Demonstration of the ability to perform self-care and/or adapt to potential limitations

- Promotion of adaptive coping skills
- Identification and appropriate use of resources (community, education, psychosocial)

Nurses play an important role in encouraging patients to help set their own goals by actively participating in their care. The Joint Commission's Speak Up™ program urges patients to take an active role in preventing healthcare errors by being involved in their care (Joint Commission, 2015). Brochures, posters, and videos are available on their website and can be used by nurses in all healthcare settings. The program is designed to encourage patients to do the following.

- **S**peak up if you have questions or concerns. If you still don't understand, ask again. It's your body and you have a right to know.
- **P**ay attention to the care you get. Always make sure you're getting the right treatments and medicines by the right healthcare professionals. Don't assume anything.
- **E**ducate yourself about your illness. Learn about the medical tests you get, and your treatment plan.
- **A**sk a trusted family member or friend to be your advocate (adviser or supporter).
- **K**now what medicines you take and why you take them. Medicine errors are the most common healthcare mistakes.
- **U**se a hospital, clinic, surgery center, or other type of healthcare organization that has been carefully checked out. For example, the Joint Commission visits hospitals to see if they are meeting the Joint Commission's quality standards.
- **P**articipate in all decisions about your treatment. You are the center of the healthcare team. (Joint Commission, 2015)

Clinicians need to clearly define the desired change in behavior (e.g., coming to the clinic three times a week for treatment and monitoring laboratory values), establish a baseline, and encourage patients to self-monitor their progress. Thus, general statements for expected behaviors such as "Monitor yourself for fever" or "Take your medication" need to be more specific: "Do you have a thermometer at home? Take your temperature once a day or if you feel warm or chilled. Call the clinic right away if your temperature is 100.5°F or higher." Patients can help in self-monitoring by learning to understand their laboratory values and keeping a notebook, symptom diary, or medication log to help to follow their clinical course and communicate with the healthcare team. The goals of patients with multiple myeloma may change as the disease or treatment changes.

Keeping abreast of how the disease and its ramifications are changing and why the treatment may be changing may help patients to cope by remaining engaged in the plan. Nurses must help learners set individual goals and provide feedback on progress toward these goals. Although patients and the healthcare team, along with patients' significant others, may make these goals together, clinicians need to ensure that priority is given to safety. Patients with multiple myeloma may be at high risk for sepsis and death from infection, have bleeding or clotting disorders, and have or be at risk for pathologic fractures, including spinal cord compression (Miceli et al., 2011; Miceli, Colson, Gavino, Lilleby, & the IMF Nurse Leadership Board, 2008). Weakness, fatigue, and uncontrolled pain, including neuropathies, can contribute to patients' fall risk, resulting in patient injury and possibly a delay in treatment (Rome et al., 2011; Tariman, Love, McCullagh, Sandifer, & the IMF Nurse Leadership Board, 2008). Safety always should be at the forefront of the education goals. If a nurse feels that a patient or family misunderstands the treatment plan or is concerned about patient behaviors that may affect safety, the nurse should immediately contact the physician.

Methods and Interventions

Application of adult learning theory, patient factors, the stages of health behavior change, and motivational interviewing can be seen as fluid; assessment is ongoing, and interventions need to be tailored to the situation at the time and then evaluated for effectiveness. For example, simple teaching with a handout on pain and pain medication may not be as effective if done without coaching (Thomas et al., 2012). Personalized and planned education sessions may be appropriate and feasible for some settings. In a quasiexperimental study, Mollaoglu and Erdogan (2014) compared patients who received planned education on chemotherapy to those who did not. The study demonstrated that there were statistically significant decreases in the frequencies of the following symptoms among patients attending the structured education sessions: nausea, vomiting, constipation, pain, infectious signs, problems of the mouth and throat, problems of the skin and nails, appetite changes, weight loss or gain, feeling distressed/anxious, feeling pessimistic and unhappy, unusual fatigue, and difficulty sleeping (Mollaoglu & Erdogan, 2014). Structured patient education sessions may not be feasible, but providing a standardized approach to patient education (e.g., nursing checklist, treatment-specific calendar, patient education assessment survey) may improve patient satisfaction with knowledge regarding what to expect during chemotherapy and knowledge of how to manage chemotherapy side effects (Dalby et al., 2013).

Visual media should be considered. Thompson, Silliman, and Clifford (2013) demonstrated that a 15-minute DVD on nutrition-related side effects from chemotherapy along with a handout increased short-term knowledge among patients with cancer. Although DVD media may be helpful, Fee-

Schroeder et al. (2013) showed that participants in their study liked being able to ask questions to the nursing staff in the group discussions that followed an 11-minute DVD on managing chemotherapy side effects. Thus, the DVD was a platform for further discussion and answering questions to meet individual needs. Additional results indicated this teaching method increased motivation and confidence to use self-management strategies and assimilation of new or different behaviors in managing side effects, such as maintaining fluid intake, eating small, frequent meals, increasing physical activity, communicating with the healthcare team, and employing psychological coping strategies (Fee-Schroeder et al., 2013).

The Internet and Other Resources

The concept of multiple myeloma may be difficult to understand, even for a well-educated and English-speaking adult. Because it constitutes only 1% of all cancers (Siegel, Miller, & Jemal, 2015), most Americans likely have not heard of the disease. A recent national survey from the Pew Research Center (2014) found that 7 in 10 adult Internet users indicated that they have conducted Internet searches for health-related information. One in four adult Internet users have read about or observed another person's health-related experience during the prior 12 months, and 16% went online to find people with the same health concerns. The survey found that "caregivers and those living with chronic conditions, such as diabetes, heart disease and cancer, are more likely than other Internet users to do all of these things. . . . Twitter, Facebook, blogs, and other platforms seem uniquely suited to adapt to the changing needs of people living with chronic health conditions, particularly as patients move from the shock of a new diagnosis to long-term management" (Pew Research Center, 2014, paras. 7 and 12).

Clinicians cannot assume that patients and families are computer savvy and should direct them to reputable and up-to-date online resources. Imprudent, often conflicting information could potentially be overwhelming for patients and add to ambivalence and anxiety toward treatment decisions. Lawrentschuk et al. (2011) did an Internet search of oncology information using the Google search engine to access 10,200 websites. They concluded that most oncologic sites lack validation in terms of quality. Thus, concerns regarding misinformation should be addressed with patients. The use of online support (and, thus, education) by patients and survivors can be influenced by multiple factors, including disease, background, culture, need, and Internet use, so clinicians should identify factors that may influence patients' use of online resources before recommending them (Im, 2011). Additionally, providing Internet information alone does not guarantee better patient outcomes. Existing studies of online cancer support and resources have demonstrated preliminary but inconclusive evidence for positive outcomes (Hong, Pena-Purcell, & Ory, 2012).

Patients should bring information they obtained online or elsewhere to their appointments and ask their healthcare providers to clarify the information and confirm how it applies to them. When patients get information from the Internet, clinicians need to take the time to review the materials and answer patients' and family members' questions. Healthcare providers need to become familiar with and refer appropriate patients to reputable Internet-based information, even if not prompted by patients (Emond, de Groot, Wetzels, & van Osch, 2013).

If patients use the Internet, clinicians can recommend they review the National Cancer Institute (NCI) fact sheet "Evaluating Online Sources of Health Information" (NCI, 2012). It provides questions to ask as well as a video titled "Anatomy of a Cancer Treatment Scam" that can help people to decide whether the health information they find online is likely to be reliable. Some cancer websites offer accurate, detailed, and up-to-date information on multiple myeloma. For example, the site for Cancer*Care* (www.cancercare.org), a national nonprofit organization, provides general information about cancer and also has current, detailed information on multiple myeloma, its sequelae, and treatments; podcasts, medical updates, and workshop information also are provided. The American Cancer Society (ACS) is a nationwide nonprofit organization that provides cancer resources online as well as services within many communities. Its website (www.cancer.org) has information on complementary and alternative medicine (CAM) therapies, radiation, multiple myeloma treatment, drug details including bisphosphonates, and plasmapheresis. It also offers planning and survivorship information. Other websites also offer survivorship information and blogs, particularly the Livestrong Foundation (www.livestrong.org), which features the Cancer Guide and Tracker iPad® app, the National Coalition for Cancer Survivorship (www.canceradvocacy.org), and OncoLink (www.oncolink.com), a service of the University of Pennsylvania Medical Center. These sites address practical aspects of living with cancer, such as finances, legal planning, and employment, so that patients can then navigate through hospital-based and local services. The National Coalition for Cancer Survivorship site features the free Cancer Survival Toolbox® (www.canceradvocacy.org/resources/cancer-survival-toolbox), which contains a set of basic skills to help patients with cancer to navigate a diagnosis and special topics on key issues. It is available in both written and audio versions. The International Myeloma Foundation (IMF) (www.myeloma.org) provides information online as well as free brochures on all aspects of the disease, diagnostic tests, treatments, and treatment side effects. This organization also offers free patient and family seminars and webcasts as well as a 24-hour hotline staffed by trained information specialists. IMF publishes a quarterly newsletter, *Myeloma Today*, and two disease- and treatment-related handbooks (one is a more concise review of disease and treatment, and the other is a simpler patient handbook providing a myeloma overview). While other organizations provide websites and written materials in English and Spanish, IMF provides information in several languages (English, Spanish, French, German, Italian, Chinese, Portuguese, Polish, Hebrew, Russian, and Arabic), which visitors can select from the home page. Even Wikipedia (http://en.wikipedia.org/wiki/Multiple_myeloma) contains multiple myeloma disease and treatment information that is referenced but may not be current. It does, however, have information in many languages as well as links to IMF and other reputable sources. If patients are consulting these resources, nurses should ensure that the healthcare team explains their situation in reference to the general treatment guidelines and why decisions in their particular case were recommended.

The Multiple Myeloma Research Foundation (MMRF) (www.themmrf.org) has information on multiple myeloma as well as a particular focus on helping patients and healthcare workers find clinical trials. The Leukemia and Lymphoma Society (LLS) (www.lls.org) also has information on the disease and its treatments. LLS will ship written materials free; it also offers education programs that patients can listen to online and an information resource center.

Livestrong Fertility (www.livestrong.org/we-can-help/fertility-services) provides reproductive information, support, and hope to patients with cancer and cancer survivors whose medical treatments present the risk of infertility. Nurses should not assume that fertility is not an issue with patients with multiple myeloma. In addition to the aforementioned information and local support resources, nurses could refer younger patients to a resource such as Stupid Cancer (www.stupidcancer.org), a national, survivor-led advocacy, support, and research organization working exclusively on behalf of survivors and care providers younger than age 40. It has links for support activities, chat rooms, local events, excursions, and retreats, as well as a local chapter finder.

To assist patients and caregivers in navigating the Internet, a handout on reputable websites could be made available and displayed in the clinic. In this way, the healthcare team could be assured that information provided is prudent and consistent. Many institutions have systems in place that require approval of materials provided to patients because of the potential legal impact. Figure 11-3 lists reputable websites for multiple myeloma and related information. Specific brochures could be displayed in the cancer clinic or unit or be in a storage area for clinicians to access.

The Internet may be helpful in providing information on CAM. As patients search the Internet and speak to friends and family members, it is likely they will inquire about CAM therapies they encounter. In listening openly to patients regarding CAM, a good rule of thumb is to offer that credible websites include those ending with ".gov" (indicating a governmental

> **Figure 11-3. Websites for Information and Support for Patients With Multiple Myeloma and Their Caregivers***
>
> - **American Cancer Society**: www.cancer.org
> - **Be the Match: National Marrow Donor Program**: http://bethematch.org
> - **Blood and Marrow Transplant Information Network**: www.BMTInfoNet.org
> - **Bone Marrow Foundation**: www.bonemarrow.org
> - **Cancer*Care***: www.cancercare.org
> - **Cancer Legal Resource Center**: www.disabilityrightslegalcenter.org
> - **Cancer.Net** (patient information from the American Society of Clinical Oncology): www.cancer.net
> - **Caregiver Action Network**: www.caregiveraction.org
> - **Caring Bridge**: www.caringbridge.org
> - **Coalition of Cancer Cooperative Groups**: www.CancerTrialsHelp.org
> - **Family Caregiver Alliance**: http://caregiver.org
> - **International Association for Hospice and Palliative Care**: www.hospicecare.com
> - **International Myeloma Foundation**: www.myeloma.org
> - **Leukemia and Lymphoma Society**: www.lls.org
> - **Livestrong Fertility**: www.livestrong.org/we-can-help/fertility-services
> - **Livestrong Foundation**: www.livestrong.org
> - **MedlinePlus U.S. National Library of Medicine, National Institutes of Health**: www.nlm.nih.gov/medlineplus
> - **MetaCancer Foundation**: www.metacancermosaic.org
> - **Multiple Myeloma Library**: www.navigatingcancer.com/library/multiple-myeloma
> - **Multiple Myeloma Research Foundation**: www.themmrf.org
> - **National Alliance for Caregiving**: www.caregiving.org
> - **National Bone Marrow Transplant Link**: www.nbmtlink.org
> - **National Cancer Institute**: www.cancer.gov
> - **National Coalition for Cancer Survivorship**: www.canceradvocacy.org
> - **National Comprehensive Cancer Network**: www.nccn.org/patients/guidelinesmyeloma
> - **OncoLink OncoLife Survivorship Care Plan**: www.oncolink.com/oncolife
> - **Stupid Cancer**: www.stupidcancer.org
>
> * Not all-inclusive
>
> *Note.* Based on information from Economou et al., 2012; Hanson et al., 2013; Miceli et al., 2013.

agency), ".org" (indicating a professional and/or nonprofit organization), or ".edu" (indicating an educational institution); URLs ending in ".com" indicate a for-profit commercial site (Williams, 2013). Figure 11-4 offers a list of reliable CAM websites.

Commercial materials, such as those produced by pharmaceutical companies, may be appropriate, particularly with new treatments, as long as they are not promotional in nature. Guidelines exist to assist nurses in developing written materials for an institution. A nurse who is in a position to develop written materials may want to form a team of healthcare professionals such as a physician, social worker, registered dietitian, and physical therapist. Recommendations include incorporating pictures; focusing on a central message; emphasizing key points by highlighting, coloring, or underlining text;

Figure 11-4. Websites for Information on Complementary and Alternative Medicine
• **American Cancer Society**: www.cancer.org • **Bandolier**: www.medicine.ox.ac.uk/bandolier/index.html • **Cochrane Review Organization**: www.cochrane.org • **Memorial Sloan Kettering Cancer Center**: www.mskcc.org/aboutherbs • **National Cancer Institute Office of Cancer Complementary and Alternative Medicine**: www.cancer.gov/cam • **National Center for Complementary and Integrative Health**: https://nccih.nih.gov • **Natural Medicines**: http://naturalmedicines.therapeuticresearch.com • **University of Texas MD Anderson Cancer Center**: www.mdanderson.org/cimer
Note. Based on information from Williams, 2013.

leaving plenty of white space; and using fonts sized 12 or larger (Ferguson & Pawlak, 2011). MedlinePlus, a service of the National Library of Medicine, provides helpful tips for creating easy-to-read health information (www.nlm.nih.gov/medlineplus/etr.html).

Multimedia methods for educating patients with multiple myeloma are not as numerous as written methods. However, they could be utilized in specific settings, such as in waiting areas. In a pilot study with patients undergoing radiation therapy, Matsuyama, Lyckholm, Molisani, and Moghanaki (2013) demonstrated the utility of a brief video presented before the initial radiation oncology consultation, which significantly improved health literacy across all socioeconomic subgroups. Several websites shown in Figure 11-3, such as IMF and MMRF, provide webcasts and teleconferences that may be helpful in augmenting and reinforcing verbal and written methods of patient education.

Social Support and Caregivers

The Internet provides a gateway to an inexhaustible volume of virtual communities, networks, and support groups. Many websites for patients with multiple myeloma also have caregiver information (Hanson, Ferrell, & Grant, 2013). A few are listed in Figure 11-3 and include the Family Caregiver Alliance, the Caregiver Action Network, and the National Alliance for Caregiving.

Even in the age of readily accessible information, simply referring patients to one of these sites should not replace therapeutic communication and teaching. Some patients are not comfortable in a group setting or may feel overwhelmed by too much information. Busy clinics and inpatient settings do not always establish an environment in which nurses have time to explore all of the emotional and social support needs of patients and families. A social worker may help with psychosocial issues and provide referrals to support groups and resources. Advanced practice nurses, psychologists, social workers, pharmacists, clergy members, dietitians, physical therapists, and pain management or palliative care specialists can augment a nurse's teaching and enhance patient and family education and support. As part of education, the importance of caregivers should be addressed and their learning needs included (Aizer et al., 2013).

What to Teach

The Disease

The concepts surrounding the disease of multiple myeloma most likely will be foreign to patients and their family, even if a family member is in the healthcare field. An LLS (2013) survey found that 82% of individuals were surprised to learn that more than one million U.S. adults currently are living with a hematologic malignancy. Only 46% knew that blood cancers are the third leading cause of cancer death in the United States. As previously mentioned, multiple myeloma accounts for just 1% of all malignancies; the 5- and 10-year survival rates have improved with the availability of newer treatment options (Pulte et al., 2011; Siegel et al., 2015). Although long-term cure statistics cannot be given, nurses still can offer hope for long-term quality of life. Hope can be instilled realistically in the setting of newer, targeted therapies. This may not be sufficient for younger individuals to be hopeful; thus, nurses must address emotional needs and concerns when educating patients about the disease.

The most common presenting symptoms of myeloma are fatigue and bone pain (Rajkumar & Dispenzieri, 2013). Some patients may be asymptomatic. Other signs and symptoms include malaise, weakness, anorexia, nausea, weight loss, polydipsia, neuropathy, anemia, renal insufficiency, paraproteinemia, and hypercalcemia (Palumbo & Anderson, 2011). As with many serious illnesses, general symptoms may at first mimic a common symptom, such as a backache (e.g., pulled back muscle while gardening) or bone pain, thus delaying diagnosis. Helping patients to sort through the diagnostic process often is helpful in correcting misconceptions regarding "missed" diagnoses. Helping them to then understand the appropriate workup and staging, such as laboratory tests, bone marrow biopsy, skeletal radiographs, and magnetic resonance imaging, can help them to understand the extent of their disease, what questions to ask, and why physicians may be prescribing particular treatments. The primary healthcare provider should explain the International Staging System for multiple myeloma and its significance to the patient's particular case (National Comprehensive Cancer Network®

[NCCN®], 2015). The nurse can then explore the patient's and family's understanding, clarify misconceptions, and make sure they are readdressed as needed.

The concepts of the immune system, plasma cells, bone marrow function, lytic lesions, and diagnostic laboratory tests may be difficult for patients to understand and should be reviewed both in concept and as they relate to the particular case. A basic handout on multiple myeloma may be helpful (see Figure 11-5 for an example). Visual aids of the bone marrow, immunoglobulins versus light chains, and other concepts may be needed, not just the written word. The Internet resources in Figure 11-3 can help clarify these advanced concepts, as many of them provide varying written levels, from basic to advanced, and often include simple diagrams, pictures, and glossaries.

When providing education about myeloma, nurses should inform patients that each case is slightly different and that the written information may not pertain to their case. This is particularly true in cases in which the patient presents with a variant of multiple myeloma, such as those with a solitary plasmacytoma, nonsecretory multiple myeloma, or plasma cell leukemia.

Important concepts related to multiple myeloma include the effect of the disease on the bones, the immune system, and renal function. Failure to monitor and treat these organs can result in often preventable patient morbidity. As it is clinically apparent in most cases, it is important to inform patients that plasma cells proliferate and overproduce an abnormal immunoglobulin (Ig) or "M" protein (IgG, IgA, or rarely IgM, IgE, or IgD), as well as abnormal smaller or light-chain proteins (kappa or lambda light chain), cytokines (proteins) that stimulate osteoclasts and suppress osteoblasts, and angiogenesis. Therefore, uncontrolled disease leads to excessive proteins, hyperviscosity, osteoporosis, hypercalcemia, bone pain, and end-organ damage, especially in the kidneys, bones, and peripheral nerves, as well as anemia and infections (NCCN, 2015; Wood & Payne, 2011).

Medical advances in the past decade have made myeloma a chronic disease with hope for cure. Because it can be considered a chronic condition, teaching about the disease, the manifestations, and sequelae related to the manifestations needs to be ongoing, with respect given to patients' and families' ability and willingness to learn. For example, a patient may be initially diagnosed after presenting with malaise and change in urine output, and the typical bone pain may not have been present. However, the risk of future bone manifestations and serious fractures, including cord compression, needs to be discussed in a way that informs the patient and caregivers of the potential but without initiating undue anxiety. Therefore, the patient and family will know the importance of reporting any new pain or changes in physical function. Another example of specific teaching is that fever and infection may not be the presenting symptoms (Palumbo & Anderson, 2011). However, because of the impact of the disease and treatments

Figure 11-5. What Is Multiple Myeloma?

Multiple myeloma is a cancer of plasma cells. Multiple myeloma cells are abnormal *plasma cells*. Some normal plasma cells are found in the bone marrow (the middle of the bones), and some are in the blood. Normal plasma cells are part of our *immune system*.

The immune system helps our body prevent and fight infection. The immune system has several types of cells that work together to prevent and fight infection. *Lymphocytes* are one type of immune system cells. Two types of lymphocytes exist: T cells and B cells.

B cells change into plasma cells when they react to an infection in our body. The plasma cells make proteins called *antibodies* that attack and kill the germs causing the infection.

When plasma cells grow out of control, they can form a tumor. If only one tumor is formed, it is called a *solitary plasmacytoma*. In most cases, this single tumor will become many tumors. This is called *multiple myeloma*.

Other cells are made in the bone marrow, such as the lymphocytes. They then go into the blood to do their job. These include red blood cells, white blood cells, and platelets. Thus, when abnormal plasma cells grow in the bone marrow, the bone marrow is unable to make enough of these normal cells. The following problems can occur from the growth of myeloma cells in the bone marrow:
- Anemia: A shortage of red blood cells, which can cause you to be weak, tired, and pale
- Bleeding: A shortage of platelets, which can lead to a lot of bruising or bleeding
- Neutropenia: A shortage of a specific white blood cell (the neutrophil), which can increase your risk for infection

Myeloma cells do not act like normal plasma cells. They make antibodies, but these antibodies do not work to kill germs and fight infection. These antibodies may hurt your kidneys and thicken your blood.

Myeloma cells also affect the cells that help keep bones strong. Myeloma cells cause the bones to soften. The body is not able to replace the bone that is thinned and softened. This makes the bones weak, and they may break more easily.

Talk with your nurses and doctors regarding your specific case of multiple myeloma. Ask
- How has the myeloma affected my body?
- What is the treatment plan?
- What are the side effects of the treatment?
- How is the healthcare team going to reduce or prevent side effects of the treatment?
- What can I do to help with the treatment plan?

Make sure you share all of your concerns with your healthcare team.

Note. Based on information from American Cancer Society, 2014; Navigating Cancer, Inc., 2013; Pluta et al., 2010.

on the bone marrow and immune system, the patient and family need to be informed on what to report, hygiene practices, and the importance of immunizations when appropriate.

Nurses need to be aware of their scope of practice when providing patient and family education. Ideally, the nurse should be with the patient when the primary healthcare provider reviews the disease, staging, prognosis, diagnostic tests, and treatment plan so that he or she can augment and document the additional teaching appropriately.

Renal Problems

Even if patients do not present with renal problems, patient teaching should include the potential complications of renal dysfunction (Faiman, Mangan, Spong, Tariman, & the IMF Nurse Leadership Board, 2011). Instructing patients to be observant for any changes in urine output or characteristics (e.g., decreased amount, decreased frequency, cloudy, bloody) is important. Often, it is appropriate to instruct the patient to drink up to three liters of fluids a day to maintain kidney health; this instruction needs to include showing what a liter is and may be done by using a specific water bottle or canister as a visual example of the volume discussed. However, some patients may already have renal disease or comorbid conditions such as congestive heart failure, warranting education on fluid restrictions and special dietary modifications as specified in the primary care provider's plan. Patients should be instructed not to take any over-the-counter medications without letting the doctor know, as they may contribute to renal problems. Patients also need to know that other prescription medications can affect the kidneys and need to make sure that the doctor is aware of all medications the patient has taken (Faiman et al., 2011).

Bone Disease

Bone disease occurs in approximately 80% of patients with multiple myeloma and is associated with bone pain, fractures, and hypercalcemia (NCCN, 2015; Palumbo & Anderson, 2011). In addition to the vertebral column, the long bones, ribs, skull, hip, humerus, and pelvis are commonly involved. More than half of patients with multiple myeloma will experience at least one new fracture, and bone disease has a major impact on quality of life and potentially on patient outcome (Roodman, 2011). For this reason, it is important to educate patients and families regarding the ongoing risk of bone disease and the importance of strict adherence to receiving scheduled bisphosphonates to reduce and delay skeletal-related events (Terpos et al., 2013). Patients and caregivers need to be instructed to promptly report any new pain or ache and to make sure to obtain diagnostic tests. Computed tomography scans may be used in lieu of conventional x-ray imaging. Magnetic resonance imaging can be helpful in distinguishing between benign and malignant compression fractures and particularly for suspected cord compression (Miceli et al., 2011). Education regarding these diagnostic tests, as always, should be provided. Several of the websites in Figure 11-3 offer excellent information on diagnostic tests, such as NCI and ACS.

Treatments

Bisphosphonates

As part of ongoing care for multiple myeloma, patients will receive bisphosphonates regardless of the presence of bone lesions, and the physician may or may not continue this treatment after two years (Terpos, Morgan, et al., 2013; Terpos, Roodman, & Dimopoulos, 2013). It is recommended that bisphosphonates be given to all patients with myeloma-related bone disease. Patients should be treated with either pamidronate 90 mg IV piggyback or zoledronic acid 4 mg IV piggyback every three to four weeks for up to two years (NCCN, 2015; Terpos, Morgan, et al., 2013). The doses will be adjusted for patients with renal problems. There is no clear consensus on the duration of bisphosphonate therapy, but patients with active myeloma may benefit from remaining on treatment longer than two years (Terpos, Roodman, et al., 2013).

Nurses should provide patients with a basic explanation of why this medication is indicated in patients with myeloma-related bone disease (the aim is to reduce bone-related events such as fractures and pain), along with the potential side effects. Patients should be instructed that they will receive an IV infusion in the office or clinic once every three to four weeks. Laboratory work also will be performed to monitor side effects, such as calcium levels and potential effects on the kidneys.

In general, these infusions are well tolerated. Although some patients may have flulike symptoms the day after the infusion, these often subside with subsequent infusions. Osteonecrosis of the jaw (ONJ), a rare and potentially serious complication of IV bisphosphonates, is characterized by the presence of exposed bone in the mouth. It typically occurs after dental extraction, implant placement, and periodontal surgery (Faiman, Pillai, & Benghiac, 2013). Although the risk of ONJ in patients with cancer ranges from 0.7%–40%, the incidence is higher in patients with breast cancer and multiple myeloma and the risk increases over time (Faiman, Pillai, et al., 2013). Thus, all patients should be informed of this risk up front and be reminded throughout their treatment. Initially, patients need to receive a comprehensive dental examination and appropriate preventive dental work before starting bisphosphonate therapy. Active oral infections should be treated, and sites that are at high risk for infection should be eliminated (Faiman, Pillai, et al., 2013). The potential for ONJ, how to reduce one's risk, and signs and symptoms should be reviewed with the patient. The use of alcohol and tobacco appear to increase the risk, so patients should be counseled on healthy lifestyle behaviors. While on therapy, patients should avoid undergoing invasive dental procedures, if possible. If they are necessary, patients should make sure to inform the oncology physician. Nurses can assist in assessing patients' oral health and oral hygiene regimen. Simply instructing patients to "maintain excellent oral hygiene" is not specific enough. General excellent and consistent oral hygiene, which includes brushing with a soft toothbrush, using dental floss once daily, and using an alcohol-free rinse, has been shown to improve oral health outcomes in patients with cancer (Epstein et al., 2012; Lalla et al., 2014). Most studies have shown that it is primarily the frequency and consistency of mouth care that maximizes oral health (Epstein et al., 2012). Patients should be informed of the early signs and symptoms of any oral or tooth pain, any change in the oral mucosa or gums, and any swelling in the jaw or gumlines. Patients also should be counseled on the importance of adequate hydration, the need for calcium and vitamin D supplements, as appropriate, and how to best manage potential side effects (Miceli et al., 2011). For patients with dentures, nurses should check that the dentures are well-fitting and confirm that they are cleaned regularly. Poor-fitting dentures may increase the risk of ONJ (Miceli et al., 2011). Patients should remove them, if possible, when not eating and certainly for sleep. If ONJ develops, nurses should ensure that patients understand and adhere to the antibiotic therapy and oral care directed by the physician or dentist.

Balloon Kyphoplasty and Vertebroplasty

Information on potentially recommended percutaneous balloon kyphoplasty or vertebroplasty can be provided as needed. Nurses can inform patients that percutaneous vertebroplasty is performed under fluoroscopy or computed tomography with the patient under sedation in either the prone or lateral lying position. The vertebroplasty needle is fluoroscopically guided into the diseased bone, and cement is injected into the malignant bone cavity, leading to strengthening of the vertebra and stabilizing against vertebral collapse (National Library of Medicine, 2013). The procedure has a low rate of complications, which should be explained by the physician via informed consent before the procedure, and most patients will experience significant immediate and long-term pain relief (Khan, Brinjikji, & Kallmes, 2013). In contrast to vertebroplasty, during a balloon kyphoplasty, a small incision is made where a working cannula is placed through the pedicle, and an orthopedic balloon is guided into the fractured vertebral body. The balloon is then inflated, reducing the fracture and elevating the superior end plate. The approach is bilateral, using two balloons, to achieve en masse reduction. After reduction of the fracture has taken place, the balloons are deflated and removed. Inflation and deflation of the balloons creates a void that serves as a repository for the bone cement. The void is filled with bone cement under low manual pressure. The procedure usually takes at least one hour for each fracture treated and may necessitate a short stay in the hospital (Anselmetti, Muto, Guglielmi, & Masala, 2010). Many of the websites listed in Figure 11-3 provide written and visual information on this procedure, as well as information on bone health and bone pain; MedlinePlus® has a useful one-page handout.

Patients may potentially need education and support regarding surgery to stabilize long bone fractures. Prevention is an important teaching point. Nurses, as part of the interdisciplinary team, can ensure that patients with multiple myeloma receive a comprehensive screening to minimize bone complications and include optimal functioning in the plan of care. Before addressing potential activity or referral to an exercise regimen, nurses should be aware of the presence of any activity restrictions associated with lytic lesions, especially potential cord compression. Comorbid conditions that are myeloma related (e.g., amyloid cardiac deposition, severe neuropathies) and those that are not myeloma related (e.g., vitamin D deficiency, age-related osteoporosis, arthritis) need to be considered in the teaching plan for bone health.

Radiation

Radiation may be effective in relieving metastatic bone disease and related pain. Spinal cord compression often is treated with external beam radiation therapy, but surgical decompression also may be needed for spinal instability (Palumbo & Anderson, 2011). By first assessing patients' understanding of the treatment, nurses can tailor teaching accordingly. As with education about radiation treatment for other malignancies, it is helpful to explain the treatment room equipment and personnel to relieve patients' concerns, making sure that they understand the information. Patients may not understand that external beam radiation does not pose a risk of radiation exposure to loved ones. Although a small study, Wilson, Mood, and Nordstrom (2010) demonstrated that the reading skill level of patients undergoing radiation therapy may be lower than self-reported. Thus, printed health information on radiation therapy self-care management strategies could be difficult to understand for some patients. Additionally, aside from constitutional symptoms, patients should understand that the side effects are related to the area that will be irradiated and the surrounding area. Patients should be instructed to call their oncologist or radiation oncologist if they have any problems related to the radiation therapy. The side effects most likely will start a week or two after treatment begins and can include skin reactions, urinary problems, and diarrhea, depending on the area irradiated. NCI (2007) has a comprehensive booklet on radiation therapy titled *Radiation Therapy and You: Support for People With Cancer* that can be downloaded or ordered in print format. The American Society for Radiation Oncology (2014) also has a website for patient information, although content specific to patients with multiple myeloma can be difficult to find.

Pharmacologic Treatments

Specific patient education on all of the medical treatments, such as traditional chemotherapy and immunomodulatory agents, is beyond the scope of this writing. Thus, the following information focuses on treatments most specific to multiple myeloma. Some patients may receive treatment with chemotherapeutic drugs, such as liposomal doxorubicin, cyclophosphamide, or vincristine, but this chapter will not cover those, as information is widely available elsewhere. A good website to recommend to patients or to print off for reading material is MedlinePlus. An important point to keep in mind when providing patients with informational materials on treatments is that while side effects from standard chemotherapy may apply, others, such as deep vein thrombosis and neuropathy, may not be addressed. ACS (n.d.) has a Chemotherapy Side Effects Worksheet that could work as a weekly diary for patients to monitor their side effects as well as directives on when to call their healthcare provider. Figure 11-6 provides information that can

---

Figure 11-6. How to Take Your Medications Safely

- Find out what drug you are taking and what it's for. Make sure that is part of the prescription on the order. When in the hospital, make sure you ask what drugs are being given to you and why.
- Find out how to take the drugs, and make sure you understand the directions. If you are told to take a drug three times a day, does that mean eight hours apart exactly or at mealtimes? If you have to take it in the clinic or hospital, how will it be given and how long will the treatment take each time?
- What is the goal of this treatment? How long will this treatment last?
- Where should the medicines be stored and disposed of?
- Are there drugs, beverages, or foods you should avoid?
- What are the side effects (short-term and long-term), and are there things you can do to reduce them? What symptoms should trigger a call to the healthcare provider?
- What should you do if you miss a dose?
- Are there fertility and/or major safety issues?
- Read the bottle's label every time you take the drug to avoid mistakes. If you have difficulty with reading the label or opening the package, speak to your pharmacist for alternatives.
- If you take multiple medications, ask your doctor or pharmacist about compliance aids.
- Who do you call if you have questions, and when can they be reached? In what situations should you go to clinic or emergency department?
- What is the plan to monitor for side effects? How often will the follow-up be? Are there laboratory tests or others that will be done, and how often?
- Keep a list of all medications, including over-the-counter drugs, dietary supplements, medicinal herbs, and other substances you take, with you and report it to your healthcare provider.
- Usually, it is best to bring your medications to each physician or clinic visit and review them with the nurse or other healthcare provider.
- Make sure all of your healthcare providers are aware of medication allergies or other unpleasant drug reactions you may have experienced.
- If in doubt, ask! Be on the lookout for clues of a problem, such as your pills look different than normal, or you notice a different drug name or directions than what you thought.

Note. Based on information from Neuss et al., 2013; U.S. Food and Drug Administration, 2013.

be imparted to patients and caregivers on how to take medications safely (Neuss et al., 2013; U.S. Food and Drug Administration, 2013).

Education is only one aspect that affects medication safety and adherence to taking oral medications. Other factors include medication side effects, costs and access to medications, and patient behaviors and beliefs (Accordino & Hershman, 2013). In a review of oncolytic studies on underadherence, Spoelstra and Given (2011) found that adherence rates ranged from 20% to 80%. In an interventional study, an automated voice response system (AVR) alone was as effective as the AVR plus a nurse intervention at promoting patient adherence to oral regimens and managing side effects (Spoelstra et al., 2013a). In a subset analysis of the same study, the researchers further found that out of 100 patients, 20 were overadherent (leading to potential life-threatening toxicity), and 13 were underadherent (Spoelstra et al., 2013b). Their recommendations for nursing are

- Be vigilant about overadherence to oral oncolytic agents, as vigilance will most likely help to prevent it, particularly in the outpatient setting.
- Encourage patients to keep a calendar or journal of the prescribed oral oncolytic regimen and when pills were taken.
- Bring attention to drug start dates, particularly if cycling, to prevent overadherence.

In a small focus group study by Simchowitz et al. (2010), some patients reported not adhering to treatment because of a lack of understanding or inadequate preparation. Patients wanted more comprehensive education at the initiation of treatment and more frequent follow-up from providers. Additional findings were that retail pharmacists may not always be familiar with oral cancer medications and may not have the background to provide adequate patient education. Complex treatment schedules also make it difficult. Follow-up phone calls by an RN or another licensed healthcare provider may be helpful (Polovich et al., 2014). Behavioral interventions such as electronic reminders and daily text messaging also can be effective (Moon et al., 2012).

Steroids: Steroids are a cornerstone of multiple myeloma treatment, but they can cause mild to life-threatening side effects that can affect almost every body system, such weight gain, edema, headache, flushing, sweating, insomnia, skin rash, thinning skin or acne, hirsutism, endocrine imbalances (hyperglycemia), gastrointestinal disturbances (ulcers), infection, myopathy, osteoporosis, muscle cramping, cataracts, glaucoma, cardiovascular problems (dysrhythmias, hypertension, thromboembolism), and mood alterations (mania, schizophrenia, delirium) (Faiman, Bilotti, Mangan, Rogers, & the IMF Nurse Leadership Board, 2008; Truven Health Analytics, 2013). Patients and family members need to be informed on how to help to prevent and manage them. General information on steroids, such as a patient information sheet from the pharmacy or a general web page, may not be specific enough in describing the rationale for this treatment, nor on specific things to report to the healthcare provider (e.g., symptoms of hyperglycemia). A more specific fact sheet may be helpful (see Figure 11-7). Information available on the IMF's website (see Figure 11-3) is also specific for steroids used to treat multiple myeloma.

Thalidomide: Patient teaching regarding thalidomide should focus on safety without imposing unwarranted fear. Patients may or may not be aware of the birth defects that arose from its use as an antiemetic and sleeping aid for pregnant women (Latif, Chauhan, Khan, Moran, & Usmani, 2012). This drug can only be prescribed and distributed through Celgene Corporation's Thalomid REMS® program to ensure that proper patient instruction is provided regarding the severe, life-threatening birth defects and contraindication in pregnant women (Celgene Corporation, 2013c). The main points of education should include the importance of birth control as well as the risk and prevention of deep venous thrombosis and the potential for neuropathies and somnolence, increasing the risk of injuries and falls. Additionally, although rare, serious Stevens-Johnson syndrome and toxic epider-

---

Figure 11-7. Patient and Family Instructions for Steroids

This medication is used to treat multiple myeloma and may be used in combination with other medications. You will need to follow these precautions while you are taking this medication.
- Swallow the capsule whole; do not crush, break, or chew it. Drink a full glass of water (about 8 ounces) when you take this medication. You may take it with or without food. Take it early in the morning, if possible.
- Tell your doctor if you have any flushing, sweating, difficulty sleeping or hyperactivity, personality or mood changes, difficulty concentrating, muscle weakness, joint or bone pain, muscle cramps, blurred vision, heartburn, changes in appetite, hiccups that do not go away, or skin rashes.
- This medication may cause temporary diabetes. Signs and symptoms of high and low blood sugar include aggressiveness, confusion, difficulty waking, increased thirst, and frequent urination. Call your doctor right away if you have any of these.
- Keep this medication in a secure location so that other people in your home do not accidentally take it.
- Avoid getting an infection by washing your hands frequently and avoiding people who are ill. Stay away from activities where you could be bruised, cut, or injured. Brush and floss your teeth regularly and gently. Be careful when using sharp objects, such as razors and fingernail clippers.
- Make sure to keep all appointments with your doctor as instructed. This medication may affect your blood glucose level.
- Call your doctor right away if you notice any of the following: fever or signs of infection anywhere on or in the body (redness, swelling, pain); swelling of your hands, feet, or ankles; increased or decreased urination; small blisters anywhere on the body; a white coating on the tongue; or aggressiveness, increased thirst, confusion, or difficulty waking.

Note. Based on information from Truven Health Analytics, 2013.

mal necrolysis have occurred (Celgene Corporation, 2013c). Patients need to be watchful for possible skin reactions and report them immediately. For mild skin reactions that are more common, prescribers can recommend topical steroids and antipruritics, and nurses can provide education regarding the application or administration of these, as well as recommend oatmeal baths. General good skin care and hygiene can be reinforced by teaching patients that the skin is the largest part of the immune system and keeping it healthy and intact is an important aspect of infection prevention. Although less likely, neutropenia can occur, so patients should be instructed to keep all blood count appointments and to call the physician if any signs or symptoms of infection develop. A patient handout on thalidomide is provided in Figure 11-8.

Lenalidomide: As with thalidomide, patient teaching regarding lenalidomide should focus on safety. As this medication is only available under Celgene Corporation's restricted distribution program called Revlimid REMS®, prescribers as well as pharmacists must review with patients the high potential for birth defects. The U.S. Food and Drug Administration black box warning reflects this important information, along with the risk of myelosuppression and thromboembolism (Celgene Corporation, 2013b). Instructions on how to take the medication should be reviewed: the patient should be told not to break, chew, or open the capsules; to take them with water; and to make sure that they are stored in a very secure place, away from children. As with all medications, written instructions should outline when side effects warrant going to the emergency department versus simply calling the physician (see Figure 11-9).

Pomalidomide: Pomalidomide is the newest immunomodulatory agent indicated for patients who have received at least two prior therapies and have demonstrated disease progression; it appears to remain effective even in patients resistant to lenalidomide (Lacy & McCurdy, 2013). It often is given with low-dose dexamethasone. As with thalidomide and lenalidomide, this medication is only available under Celgene Corporation's restricted distribution program, Pomalyst REMS™ (Celgene Corporation, 2013a). The side effect profile is similar to the other immunomodulatory agents and, thus, the instructions on how to take the medication are similar to those. Although the risk of thromboembolic events appears to be lower than with other agents, it is because patients in the phase II studies received thromboprophylaxis (Richardson, Mark, & Lacy, 2013). Thus, patients should still be informed as to the importance of adhering to their thromboprophylaxis regimen when taking pomalidomide. Additionally, this medication should be taken on an empty stomach. One major toxicity is myelosuppression, including anemia, thrombocytopenia, and neutropenia, primarily manifested as pneumonia (Lacy & McCurdy, 2013; Richardson et al., 2013). The follow-up and written instructions should outline when side effects warrant going to the emergency department versus simply calling the physician. Fatigue

> **Figure 11-8. Patient and Family Instructions for Thalidomide**
>
> This medication is used to treat multiple myeloma and may be used in combination with dexamethasone. You will need to follow these precautions while you are taking this medication.
> - Use two forms of birth control to prevent pregnancy in yourself and your partner for four weeks before you start using thalidomide, during treatment, and for at least four weeks after your treatment ends. This medication can harm an unborn child and cause serious birth defects. If you are a woman who is able to get pregnant, your doctor will do tests to make sure you are not pregnant before starting thalidomide therapy. Talk to your doctor right away if you have unprotected sex or if you think your birth control has failed.
> - Tell your doctor if you have any shortness of breath, chest pain, arm or leg swelling, or any new skin rash. Thalidomide may increase your risk of having blood clotting problems, so he or she may prescribe a blood thinning medication.
> - Call your doctor right away if you have numbness, tingling, burning, or pain in your hands or feet. Protect your hands and feet from extreme temperature changes. Create a safe environment at home to prevent falls.
> - Avoid driving, using machines, or doing anything that could be dangerous if you are not alert. This medication may make you dizzy, drowsy, or light-headed when standing up, so stand up slowly. It may be helpful to take this medication in the evening. Avoid alcohol and other medications that may cause sedation.
> - Keep this medication in a secure location so that other people in your home do not accidentally take it.
> - Avoid getting an infection by washing your hands frequently and avoiding people who are ill. Stay away from activities where you could be bruised, cut, or injured. Brush and floss your teeth regularly and gently. Be careful when using sharp objects, such as razors and fingernail clippers.
> - Make sure to keep all appointments with your doctor as instructed. This medication may affect your blood counts.
> - Make sure your doctor knows about all other medications you use.
> - Call your doctor right away if you notice any of the following: fever, itching, hives, or swelling in your face, hands, feet, or ankles; rash; swelling or tingling in your mouth or throat; chest tightness, trouble breathing, coughing up blood, blistering or peeling skin, or change in how much or how often you urinate; absence of menstruation or late or missed menstrual periods; confusion, seizures, or tremors; constipation or diarrhea; yellowing of skin or eyes; dry mouth or increased thirst or hunger; or sudden or severe stomach pain, muscle cramps, nausea, or vomiting.
>
> *Note.* Based on information from Celgene Corporation, 2013c; Kurtin & Bilotti, 2013; Truven Health Analytics, 2013.

also seems a frequently reported side effect; thus, patient teaching regarding activity and safety is important (see Figure 11-10).

Bortezomib: Bortezomib is a proteasome inhibitor that is commonly used for myeloma. Patient education on treatment-related peripheral neuropathy associated with bortezomib is crucial to optimize clinical outcomes. Patients should be instructed to report signs and symptoms of progressive neuropathy to clinicians so that bortezomib dose delay or modification can be initiated.

Figure 11-9. Patient and Family Instructions for Lenalidomide

This medication is used to treat multiple myeloma and may be used in combination with dexamethasone. You will need to follow these precautions while you are taking this medication.
- Use two forms of birth control to prevent pregnancy in yourself and your partner for four weeks before you start using lenalidomide, during treatment, and for at least four weeks after your treatment ends. This medication can harm an unborn child and cause serious birth defects. If you are a woman who is able to get pregnant, your doctor will do tests to make sure you are not pregnant before starting lenalidomide therapy. Talk to your doctor right away if you have unprotected sex or if you think your birth control has failed.
- Swallow the capsule whole; do not crush, break, or chew it. Drink a full glass of water (about 8 ounces) when you take this medication. You may take it with or without food.
- Do not take this medication with green tea. Check with your doctor before taking any over-the-counter medications or herbs while taking lenalidomide.
- Tell your doctor if you have any shortness of breath, chest pain, arm or leg swelling, or any new skin rash. Lenalidomide may increase your risk of blood clotting problems, so your doctor may prescribe a blood thinning medication.
- Call your doctor right away if you have numbness, tingling, burning, or pain in your hands or feet. Protect your hands and feet from extreme temperature changes. Create a safe environment at home to prevent falls.
- Avoid driving, using machines, or doing anything that could be dangerous if you are not alert. This medication may make you dizzy, drowsy, or light-headed when standing up, so stand up slowly. It may be helpful to take this medication in the evening. Avoid alcohol and other medications that may cause sedation.
- Keep this medication in a secure location so that other people in your home do not accidentally take it.
- Avoid getting an infection by washing your hands frequently and avoiding people who are ill. Stay away from activities where you could be bruised, cut, or injured. Brush and floss your teeth regularly and gently. Be careful when using sharp objects, such as razors and fingernail clippers.
- Make sure to keep all appointments with your doctor as instructed. This medication may affect your blood counts.
- Make sure your doctor knows about all other medications you use.
- Call your doctor right away if you notice any of the following: fever, itching, hives, or swelling in your face, hands, feet, or ankles; rash; swelling or tingling in your mouth or throat; chest tightness, trouble breathing, coughing up blood, blistering or peeling skin, or change in how much or how often you urinate; absence of menstruation or late or missed menstrual periods; confusion, seizures, or tremors; constipation or diarrhea; yellowing of skin or eyes; dry mouth or increased thirst or hunger; or sudden or severe stomach pain, muscle cramps, nausea, or vomiting.

Note. Based on information from Celgene Corporation, 2013b; Kurtin & Bilotti, 2013; Truven Health Analytics, 2013.

Figure 11-10. Patient and Family Instructions for Pomalidomide

This medication is used to treat multiple myeloma and may be used in combination with dexamethasone. You will need to follow these precautions while you are taking this medication.
- Use two forms of birth control to prevent pregnancy in yourself and your partner for four weeks before you start using pomalidomide, during treatment, and for at least four weeks after your treatment ends. This medication can harm an unborn child and cause serious birth defects. If you are a woman who is able to get pregnant, your doctor will do tests to make sure you are not pregnant before starting pomalidomide therapy. Talk to your doctor right away if you have unprotected sex or if you think your birth control has failed.
- Swallow the capsule whole; do not crush, break, or chew it. Drink a full glass of water (about 8 ounces) when you take this medication. Take this medication on an empty stomach, at least two hours before or two hours after a meal.
- Check with your doctor before taking any over-the-counter medications or herbs while taking pomalidomide.
- Tell your doctor if you have any shortness of breath, chest pain, arm or leg swelling, or any new skin rash. Pomalidomide may increase your risk of blood clotting problems, so your doctor may prescribe a blood thinning medication.
- Call your doctor right away if you have numbness, tingling, burning, or pain in your hands or feet. Protect your hands and feet from extreme temperature changes. Create a safe environment at home to prevent falls.
- Avoid driving, using machines, or doing anything that could be dangerous if you are not alert. This medication may make you dizzy, drowsy, or light-headed when standing up, so stand up slowly. It may be helpful to take this medication in the evening. Avoid alcohol and other medications that may cause sedation.
- Keep this medication in a secure location so that other people in your home do not accidentally take it.
- Avoid getting an infection by washing your hands frequently and avoiding people who are ill. Stay away from activities where you could be bruised, cut, or injured. Brush and floss your teeth regularly and gently. Be careful when using sharp objects, such as razors and fingernail clippers.
- Make sure to keep all appointments with your doctor as instructed. This medication may affect your blood counts.
- Make sure your doctor knows about all other medications you use.
- Call your doctor right away if you notice any of the following: fever, itching, hives, or swelling in your face, hands, feet, or ankles; rash; swelling or tingling in your mouth or throat; chest tightness, trouble breathing, coughing, bleeding, blistering or peeling skin, or change in how much or how often you urinate; absence of menstruation or late or missed menstrual periods; confusion or tremors; constipation or diarrhea; yellowing of skin or eyes; dry mouth or increased thirst or hunger; or sudden or severe stomach pain, muscle cramps, nausea, or vomiting.

Note. Based on information from Celgene Corporation, 2013a; Kurtin & Bilotti, 2013; Truven Health Analytics, 2013.

Safety information to emphasize during patient and family instruction should include calling the physician or 911 right away if the patient experiences seizure, chest pain or discomfort, shortness of breath, cough, confusion, or irregular heartbeat. The physician should be called if the patient has swelling of the feet, ankles, or legs or numbness, tingling, burning, or pain in the hands or feet (Millennium Pharmaceuticals, 2014; Polovich et al., 2014). Nurses should provide patients with physicians' preferred or emergency numbers in writing.

Other safety points of teaching include instructing patients to avoid driving, using machines, or doing anything that could be dangerous if they are not alert. Although rare, a specific cautionary point is that bortezomib can cause extreme drowsiness, confusion, or problems with vision caused by the start of a serious brain condition called *reversible posterior leukoencephalopathy* (Terwiel, Hanrahan, Lueck, & D'Rozario, 2010). Thus, patients who live on their own should have a family member or friend check on them regularly. Because bortezomib may cause myelosuppression, particularly low platelets, patients should be counseled on the importance of follow-up laboratory visits, infection prevention, neutropenia, and potentially thrombocytopenia and bleeding precautions. Recent literature indicates that ingestion of green tea may block the anticancer activity of bortezomib, so patients should be specifically instructed to avoid this drink or any foods, such as ice cream, containing green tea (Jia & Liu, 2013). Because herpes zoster reactivation can occur, patients may be instructed to take a prophylactic antiviral medication as well (NCCN, 2015). If not, they should be informed of the signs and symptoms of herpes zoster. Figure 11-11 provides an example of a patient education handout specific to bortezomib.

Carfilzomib: Carfilzomib is a newer proteasome inhibitor approved for patients who have received at least two prior therapies, including bortezomib and an immunomodulatory agent, and have demonstrated relapsed or refractory disease (Onyx Pharmaceuticals, 2012). It is administered intravenously two consecutive days a week for 28-day cycles. Symptoms of infusion reactions have occurred up to 24 hours after administration: fever, chills, joint or muscle pain, facial flushing or swelling, vomiting, weakness, shortness of breath, low blood pressure, dizziness, and chest tightness or pain. Patients should be instructed on whom to call or what to do if they occur. Premedication with dexamethasone can reduce these reactions (Bilotti, 2013). Because patients may be hydrated to reduce the risk of renal toxicity and tumor lysis syndrome, congestive heart failure and pulmonary hypertension also have been reported (Onyx Pharmaceuticals, 2012). Thus, it is important that patients keep track of their weight daily and report shortness of breath, weight gain, and swelling of the feet or legs. Patients need to make sure they follow up with monitoring of their blood counts and liver and renal function; transient neutropenia, thrombocytopenia, and anemia can occur. Prophylactic antiviral or antibacterial drugs may be prescribed (McBride &

Figure 11-11. Patient and Family Instructions for Bortezomib

This medication is used to treat multiple myeloma. You will receive this medication as a skin injection or by an IV infusion in a cancer clinic or in the hospital. You will need to follow these precautions while you are taking this medication.
- Tell your doctor or nurse right away if you have any nausea or vomiting. You will receive medication to prevent this and should have medications at home in case you have nausea or vomiting. Call your doctor if you are unable to drink enough fluids (eight 8-oz glasses a day or as instructed by your doctor).
- Call 911 right away if you have chest pain or discomfort, shortness of breath, irregular heartbeat, or seizures. Call your doctor if you have swelling of the feet, ankles, or legs while you are taking this medication. It can cause serious heart problems.
- Call your doctor right away if you have numbness, tingling, burning, or pain in your hands or feet. Protect your hands and feet from extreme temperature changes. Create a safe environment at home to prevent falls.
- Avoid driving, using machines, or doing anything that could be dangerous if you are not alert. This medication may make you dizzy, drowsy, or light-headed when standing up, so stand up slowly. It may be helpful to take this medication in the evening. Avoid alcohol and other medications that may cause sedation.
- Dangle your feet before standing, and stand up slowly.
- Call your doctor right away if you start having headaches, extreme drowsiness, confusion, or problems with vision while you are taking this medication. This may be the start of a serious, treatable brain condition called *reversible posterior leukoencephalopathy*.
- Make sure to report any signs of infection or bleeding to your doctor right away. Herpes zoster or "shingles" can occur; report any rash or lesions to your doctor. This medication may affect your blood counts. Because of this, you may get an infection or bleed more easily.
- Avoid getting an infection by washing your hands frequently and avoiding people who are ill. Stay away from activities where you could be bruised, cut, or injured. Brush and floss your teeth regularly and gently. Be careful when using sharp objects, such as razors and fingernail clippers.
- Make sure to tell your doctor about any medications and herbal products you are taking. This medication may interact with some of them.
- This medication should not be taken while you are pregnant. Use an effective form of birth control while using this medicine. Do not breast-feed while you are taking this medication.
- Make sure to keep all appointments with your doctor as instructed. This medication may affect your blood counts.
- Call your doctor right away if you notice any of the following: fever, itching, hives, or swelling in your face, hands, feet, or ankles; rash; swelling or tingling in your mouth or throat; chest tightness, trouble breathing, coughing up blood, blistering or peeling skin, or change in how much or how often you urinate; absence of menstruation or late or missed menstrual periods; confusion or tremors; constipation or diarrhea; yellowing of skin or eyes; dry mouth or increased thirst or hunger; or sudden or severe stomach pain, muscle cramps, nausea, or vomiting.

Note. Based on information from Kurtin & Bilotti, 2013; Millennium Pharmaceuticals, 2013; Truven Health Analytics, 2013.

Samuel, 2013). Peripheral neuropathy occurred in up to 14% of patients in clinical trials, so patients should monitor for new onset and progression of existing neuropathy. Carfilzomib also can cause fatigue, dizziness, fainting, or a drop in blood pressure, so instruction for safety is another intervention (Bilotti, 2013; Onyx Pharmaceuticals, 2012). A patient handout is provided in Figure 11-12.

Panobinostat: Panobinostat is an oral agent that is approved by the U.S. Food and Drug Administration for treatment of relapsed and refractory multiple myeloma. The drug is approved to be given in combination with bortezomib and dexamethasone and belongs to a new class of drugs to treat multiple myeloma, histone deacetylase inhibitors. Patients who take panobinostat in combination with bortezomib and dexamethasone will likely experience side effects such as diarrhea, fatigue, anorexia, fever, vomiting, and weakness. Patients also can experience prolongation of QTc interval. Therefore, drugs such as levofloxacin, ondansetron, and others should be avoided, as these drugs also can prolong the QT interval. Baseline electrocardiogram and echocardiogram monitoring should be considered. Other patient education should be focused on infection prevention, fatigue, dosing, and the use of antidiarrheal agents (Novartis Pharmaceuticals Corporation, 2015).

Hematopoietic Stem Cell Transplantation

High-dose chemotherapy supported by hematopoietic stem cell transplantation (HSCT) is an effective therapy for eligible patients with multiple myeloma (Kurtin & Faiman, 2013; NCCN, 2015). Autologous transplant is the most common type for multiple myeloma; allogeneic transplant is recommended for select patients as part of a clinical trial (Faiman, Miceli, Noonan, & Lilleby, 2013; NCCN, 2015). Because several transplantation-related strategies exist (e.g., tandem autologous HSCT, autologous followed by allogeneic HSCT, nonmyeloablative allogeneic stem cell transplantation [SCT], related versus unrelated), as well as different types of infusions (e.g., peripheral stem cells, bone marrow, cord blood), patients will need to understand that not all transplants are alike (NCCN, 2015; Niess, 2013). The word *transplant* implies the transference from one person to another. Thus, the concept of *rescue*, or reconstituting patients' healthy marrow with their own frozen and thawed marrow, should be made clear. Cohen, Jenkins, Holston, and Carlson (2013) performed in-depth interviews of 60 individuals who underwent HSCT. Their findings demonstrated that health literacy was not a simple function of age, ethnicity, race, or education. Although information was provided, it was not in a way that led to understanding. They concluded that "health literacy and communication concerns require a more nuanced approach to provide optimal patient-centered outcomes" (p. 508).

Pretransplant education usually begins when patients are first considered to be candidates for transplantation. Nursing transplant or research

Figure 11-12. Patient and Family Instructions for Carfilzomib

This medication is used to treat multiple myeloma. You will receive this medication as an IV infusion in a cancer clinic or in the hospital. You will need to follow these precautions while you are taking this medication.
- Infusion reactions may occur up to 24 hours after receiving carfilzomib. These include fever, chills, joint or muscle pain, facial flushing or swelling, vomiting, weakness, shortness of breath, low blood pressure, dizziness, and chest tightness or pain. Notify your nurse or physician immediately if these happen. You may receive a steroid before your treatment to reduce these reactions.
- Tell your doctor or nurse right away if you have any nausea or vomiting. You will receive medication to prevent this and should have medications at home in case you have nausea or vomiting. Call your doctor if you are unable to drink enough fluids (eight 8-oz glasses a day or as instructed by your doctor).
- Call 911 right away if you have chest pain or discomfort, shortness of breath, irregular heartbeat, or seizures. Call your doctor if you have swelling of the feet, ankles, or legs while you are taking this medication. It can cause serious heart problems.
- Call your doctor right away if you have numbness, tingling, burning, or pain in your hands or feet. Protect your hands and feet from extreme temperature changes. Create a safe environment at home to prevent falls.
- Avoid driving, using machines, or doing anything that could be dangerous if you are not alert. This medication may make you dizzy, drowsy, or light-headed when standing up, so stand up slowly. It may be helpful to take this medication in the evening. Avoid alcohol and other medications that may cause sedation.
- Dangle your feet before standing, and stand up slowly.
- Make sure to report any signs of infection or bleeding to your doctor right away. This medication may affect your blood counts. Because of this, you may get an infection or bleed more easily.
- Avoid getting an infection by washing your hands frequently and avoiding people who are ill. Stay away from activities where you could be bruised, cut, or injured. Brush and floss your teeth regularly and gently. Be careful when using sharp objects, such as razors and fingernail clippers.
- Make sure to tell your doctor about any medications and herbal products you are taking. This medication may interact with some of them.
- This medication should not be taken while you are pregnant. Use an effective form of birth control while using this medicine. Do not breast-feed while you are taking this medication.
- Make sure to keep all appointments with your doctor as instructed. This medication may affect your blood counts.
- Call your doctor right away if you notice any of the following: fever, chills, itching, hives, or swelling in your face, hands, feet, or ankles; rash; swelling or tingling in your mouth or throat; chest tightness, trouble breathing, coughing, or change in how much or how often you urinate; absence of menstruation or late or missed menstrual periods; constipation or diarrhea; yellowing of skin or eyes; dry mouth or increased thirst or hunger; or sudden or severe stomach pain, muscle cramps, nausea, or vomiting.

Note. Based on information from Kurtin & Bilotti, 2013; Onyx Pharmaceuticals, 2012; Truven Health Analytics, 2013.

coordinators often perform this function, providing patients with general information on the expected trajectory of the treatment (Clifford, Acheson, & Hall, 2013). Because some of the pre- and post-transplant care may be provided in outpatient settings, nurses in all settings providing care to patients with myeloma should be able to explain these basic concepts as well. Education begins prior to transplant, and different stages of patient and caregiver interaction provide opportunities for education. These include pretransplant, mobilization, central venous line placement, apheresis, transplant and admission to the hospital (or outpatient), post-transplant discharge, and follow-up care (Clifford et al., 2013). Coordinators will provide detailed information on concepts including stem cells, bone marrow, cord blood, autologous transplant, matched related allogeneic transplant, and matched unrelated allogeneic transplant to patients and caregivers as appropriate. Once the transplant treatment is confirmed, topics should be individualized according to the specific type of transplant, such as mobilizing stem cells, harvesting stem cells, the conditioning regimen, the infusion, and the expected side effects and management (Miceli et al., 2013). High-dose melphalan 200 mg/m^2 supported by previously collected peripheral stem cells is a well-established conditioning regimen; gastrointestinal side effects (e.g., diarrhea) are common (Palumbo & Cavallo, 2012). Prior to transplant and as part of the informed consent process, serious side effects such as fever, bleeding, uncontrolled diarrhea, nausea, vomiting, and unusual toxicities of high-dose therapy should be reviewed. Adjunctive teaching by nurses should include the supportive care measures that will be initiated to prevent or minimize these sequelae. Nurses, along with the rest of the healthcare team, can reassure patients that care will be taken to prevent and minimize side effects as well as toxicities.

Patients often have many questions even before meeting with the transplant physician or transplant coordinator. Miceli et al. (2013) provided an overview on autologous HSCT for nurses in community practice that could be helpful to nontransplant nurses. Several organizations, including ACS (www.cancer.org) and NCI (www.cancer.gov), provide good general information that nurses can share with patients. The National Bone Marrow Transplant Link (www.nbmtlink.org) has detailed information about stem cell and bone marrow transplantation online; printed brochures are available for a fee, but free PDF versions are available for download (see www.nbmtlink.org/resources_support/resources.htm). Although they do not include specific information about indications for transplantation in patients with multiple myeloma, they do provide a comprehensive explanation of the variety of HSCTs, as well as the role of the caregiver, insurance information, and an extensive glossary.

Aside from the clinical process of the pretransplant harvesting of stem cells, patients and caregivers will need education and assistance regarding the diagnostic tests required to ensure patient suitability for transplant and the potential need for financial assistance, time away from work, and other factors (Miceli et al., 2013).

Patients receive a calendar plan, and each aspect of the treatment and recovery trajectory is reviewed in a global nature; each part prior to that particular event within the HSCT plan then is reviewed again. Providing an overview, and then tailoring education to a small session focused on the upcoming and current events, may be helpful in minimizing the potentially overwhelming amount of information. Table 11-2 provides a list of potential adverse effects of HSCT and a few simple patient education goals related to each. This could provide a framework for helping clinicians to focus on important aspects of this overwhelming topic.

During the transplant, transplant nurses should provide guidance and ongoing education in daily activities and the plan of care, including activity, hygiene,

Table 11-2. Potential Adverse Effects of Autologous and Allogeneic Stem Cell Transplant and Education Goal Considerations for Patients and Families

Concept/Potential Problem	Patient/Family Education Goals
	The patient and family will be able to verbalize understanding of the following.
Nausea and vomiting	Medication will be given to prevent nausea and vomiting and also as needed. Inform the nurse when even mild nausea occurs. Prevention of nausea and vomiting, particularly when platelets are low, is critical to prevent bleeding.
Mucositis (mouth and throat soreness)	Oral sores may not be 100% preventable. Sucking on ice before, during, and after melphalan administration can minimize them. Inflammation of the entire gastrointestinal tract is common, leading to diarrhea.
Diarrhea	Any change in bowel pattern must be reported to the nurse as soon as it occurs. Stool samples must be sent to make sure it is related to the chemotherapy, not an infection. Medications can be given to minimize diarrhea. Inform the nurse or doctor if you have abdominal pain or if the perirectal area becomes sore or irritated.
Malnutrition/dehydration	Loss of appetite is common. Few patients need high-calorie IV infusions, but blood tests will be done to monitor your nutrition and fluid balance. You can help the healthcare team by letting them know how much you eat and drink and by saving urine and stool as instructed.

(Continued on next page)

Table 11-2. Potential Adverse Effects of Autologous and Allogeneic Stem Cell Transplant and Education Goal Considerations for Patients and Families *(Continued)*	
Concept/Potential Problem	**Patient/Family Education Goals**
Infection	Fever is common and may be the result of an infection. Blood tests will be done to check for infection. IV antibiotics will be given to you even if an infection is not found. Notify the nurse or doctor if you have any chills, redness, swelling, or pain in or on any part of your body.
Bleeding	Minor bleeding may occur because of low platelet counts. You will be given platelet transfusions as needed to prevent this. Tell your nurse or doctor immediately if you notice any bruising, red spots on your skin, or bleeding.
Anemia and fatigue	A low red cell count can cause anemia and contribute to weakness. You will be given red cell transfusions as needed. Tell your nurse or doctor immediately if you feel short of breath or dizzy, or if your heart is pounding or beating very fast.
Graft-versus-host disease	This is a side effect associated with receiving a stem cell transplant using cells from someone else. Immune suppression medications must be taken as directed. You must report any signs or symptoms of skin or gastrointestinal problems such as diarrhea, or weight gain.
Liver problems	Some chemotherapy and other medications can affect the liver. You will have blood tests done to monitor this, and the doctors will adjust medications if needed.
Skin problems	The skin is the largest organ of the immune system. You and your family need to inform the healthcare team if you have any skin discomfort or notice any skin changes, lesions, etc., and participate as directed in skin care.
Emotional problems	Fatigue, difficulty sleeping or concentrating, irritability, and other emotions can be a result of this treatment and its side effects. Tell your healthcare team all of your concerns so they can provide support and additional services, such as social workers, therapy, rest periods, or whatever is needed.

Note. Based on information from Clifford et al., 2013; Ezzone, 2013; Kiviat, 2013; McAdams & Burgunder, 2013; Miceli et al., 2013; Neumann, 2013; Rosselet, 2013.

laboratory results, and plan for each day, such as the need for electrolyte replacement and blood products. Nurses should reassure patients and caregivers as side effects occur by giving supportive and educational statements. Nurses should explain that neutropenic fever, "stat" cultures, and the administration of broad-spectrum antibiotics are common and that the team is qualified and prepared to help patients through the experience (Miceli et al., 2013).

At discharge, patients should be instructed on the importance of taking the prescribed medications, as well as making sure to come to follow-up appointments at the transplant center. Because patients with multiple myeloma may have immune deficits for some time even though they have recovered from their neutropenia, they may need to be on acyclovir and fluconazole (Miceli et al., 2013). Nurses must provide instructions to call the physician or another healthcare provider for any signs or symptoms of infection. Additionally, engraftment of platelets may lag behind. Patients may be discharged before full platelet engraftment is achieved, depending on the preference of the primary care provider, and they may need to adhere to activity restrictions until platelet counts reach $100,000/mm^3$ or per institutional guidelines.

Infection

Patients may still be at risk for infection after transplant whether or not they are neutropenic. They are always at risk for infection, even if they have not undergone HSCT. Infection is the leading cause of death in patients with multiple myeloma (Nucci & Anaissie, 2009). These patients often are functionally hypogammaglobulinemic with restricted production of effective antibodies. Patients with multiple myeloma often are receiving steroids as part of their treatment, which also blunts fever and local signs of infection, so patients should be educated that any new symptom (e.g., chills, generalized pain) could in fact be the first sign of an infection. Intravascular catheters also may be a source of infection, and patients should be thoroughly educated as to their care. The number of patients developing *Clostridium difficile*–associated enterocolitis has risen dramatically, and patients need to be prudent in notifying healthcare providers if they experience any diarrhea (Wood & Payne, 2011).

Patients need to be informed not only of the risk of infection but also of the importance of specific hygiene practices (e.g., hand washing, oral care, central line care). Patients need to immediately report to their healthcare provider any signs and symptoms of infection, even subtle ones, such as a low-grade fever or thrush caused by being on steroids alone. Patients need to know what to do, as well as the importance of taking any prescribed antimicrobial agents.

Thrombosis Versus Bleeding

Patients with multiple myeloma should be instructed regarding the potential risk of venous thromboembolic disease. Many patients are at risk for venous thromboembolism because of their own risk factors (e.g., immobility, obesity), as well as treatment factors (e.g., thalidomide, lenalidomide, steroids) (NCCN, 2014). However, at different times, they may be at risk for bleeding as a result of thrombocytopenia, such as after HSCT or associated with bortezomib or carfilzomib (Kurtin & Bilotti, 2013). Thus, measures to reduce risk and prevent these events are important in ongoing assessment and patient education.

Pain Management

Pain control should be assessed at every encounter, as it likely will be an important aspect in patients' functioning (Boland et al., 2013). Patients' and families' understanding of pain and the plan to treat the pain should be assessed. Patients with advanced cancer can even benefit from education to help modify their potentially negative attitudes or beliefs toward pain. They should be involved in appropriate pain monitoring and treatment modification; this will establish better pain control. Careful patient interviews should probe not only the degree of patient distress from pain but also psychological and social factors; thus, these aspects of the pain experience should be included in the teaching as well (Paice & Ferrell, 2011).

Patients should understand that they may have different types of pain and may need several different methods to control each type. Education should include what specific over-the-counter drugs can be taken and how much per day they can take safely, as some patients should not take them at all because of adverse renal effects (Paice & Ferrell, 2011). For example, patients should be informed when it is acceptable to use nonsteroidal anti-inflammatory drugs (NSAIDs); these drugs usually are contraindicated in patients with multiple myeloma because of their adverse effects on the kidneys (Faiman et al., 2011). Nurses should explain that if NSAIDs are recommended, they may augment a reduction in inflammation caused by tumors and aid with other pain relief measures, such as radiation and opioids. Opioids are the preferred medication for cancer pain control; thus, nurses should explain the importance of taking opioids preventively, as well as the potential side effects. Other modalities that may be part of the pain management regimen in patients with multiple myeloma include interventional procedures such as nerve blocks and kyphoplasty. Steroids may help with reducing pain caused by inflammation as well as treating the myeloma (Faiman et al., 2008). Prevention of bone-related problems through administration of bisphosphonates also helps to reduce pain problems because they decrease vertebral fractures (Miceli et al., 2011). Inform patients of the high potential for peripheral neuropathic pain, which may occur from myeloma, comorbid conditions such as diabetes, or treatments (Tariman, Love, McCullagh, Sandifer, & the IMF Nurse Leadership Board, 2008). Although most neuropathies are not curable, they can be reduced with treatment. Patients may be hesitant to report treatment-related neuropathic pain for fear that an effective treatment may be stopped or dose-reduced. It is important to explore this possibility, reeducate patients, and offer plausible and hopeful scenarios so that this does not occur.

Partnering with patients and families optimizes pain management. A study by Thomas et al. (2012) demonstrated that patients who received education and coaching (e.g., follow-up telephone sessions with an advanced practice nurse) noted significant improvements in pain-related interference with function, as well as general health, vitality, and mental health.

Pain education should include the following.
- Terminology associated with pain management
- Pain assessment at home (via a diary/log)
- Facts about opioids and the rarity of addiction when used for pain management
- Adjuvant therapies for pain management
- Alternative and complementary therapies for pain management
- Importance of communication with the interdisciplinary team, especially related to the pain experience, effectiveness of medications and other interventions, and any side effects. The team may consist of physicians, nurses (including pain specialists), psychologists, social workers, physical therapists, and others.

General handouts on pain are available through many of the websites already mentioned. Examples of two simple patient education materials from NCI cover the chemotherapy side effects of pain (www.cancer.gov/cancertopics/chemo-side-effects/pain.pdf) and nerve changes (www.cancer.gov/cancertopics/chemo-side-effects/nerve.pdf). NCI also provides information about cancer-related pain (www.cancer.gov/cancertopics/pdq/supportivecare/pain/patient). This information reviews the important aspects of patient self-reporting, which is helpful during clinical assessment of patients' pain. It delineates the aspects of pain that patients must describe, including the pain itself (e.g., when it started, how long it lasts, if it is worse at certain times), location, pattern, intensity or severity, aggravating and relieving factors, and personal response. It includes an excellent glossary of terms, including clarification of drug abuse, drug addiction, and drug tolerance.

ACS provides many pain-related resources (see www.cancer.org/treatment/treatmentsandsideeffects/physicalsideeffects/pain/index), including an online "I Can Cope" educational program on relieving cancer pain and a detailed monograph, *Guide to Controlling Cancer Pain*. It includes specific medications and their actions and side effects. For example, the monograph specifically explains that NSAIDs can irritate the stomach, cause bleeding, reduce fever, and cause kidney problems. Opioid side effects, such as drowsiness, constipation, and nausea and vomiting, also are discussed. A printable pain diary for patients is included. A pain management video also is available on the ACS website.

The Livestrong Guidebook (see http://store.livestrong.org/guidebook.html) provides a simple health diary format for recording the date, time, and any changes in physical or emotional health that can be used for patient self-report and recording of health status in any setting.

Exercise and Safety

Myeloma treatments can affect bone health and physical functioning. For example, fatigue and weakness, either generalized or caused by treatment (e.g., steroid-induced proximal muscle weakness), can occur. Gastrointestinal problems, such as nausea and vomiting, can lead to electrolyte imbalances; other myeloma and treatment effects, such as anemia, can affect patients' ability to adhere to recommendations regarding maximizing bone health and functioning (Rome et al., 2011).

Craike, Hose, and Livingston (2013) surveyed 229 patients with multiple myeloma regarding perceived benefits and barriers to exercise. The strongest barriers to participation were fatigue, injuries, and pain. Forty-one percent reported they were likely to attend an exercise program if offered. Patients who were active before diagnosis were 4.79 times more likely to be active after treatment. Patients with multiple myeloma reported low levels of physical activity across all levels of intensity, but they were interested in attending a physical activity program. The authors recommended that interventions should target perceived barriers with particular focus on those who were not physically active prior to diagnosis (Craike et al., 2013). Larger cancer centers offer a variety of physical activity programs, including yoga, Pilates, and Tai Chi. Yoga, walking, biking, and swimming provide health benefits for patients with cancer. Even patients with advanced-stage cancer may benefit from exercise, which can help to reduce anxiety, stress, and depression and decrease pain, fatigue, shortness of breath, constipation, and insomnia (Albrecht & Taylor, 2012). Moderate exercise such as walking is safe even in patients undergoing HSCT and may reduce fatigue (Chiffelle & Kenny, 2013).

The ACS website (www.cancer.org/healthy/eathealthygetactive/index) provides general physical activity guidance for cancer survivors. The American College of Sports Medicine guidelines recommend that cancer survivors engage in at least 150 minutes of moderate-intensity aerobic physical activity per week or at least 75 minutes of vigorous-intensity activity per week, two to three sessions of resistance training, as well as flexibility training on all days that include physical activity (Schmitz et al., 2010). Nurses and other clinicians frequently provide physical activity counseling and referral (Karvinen, Carr, & Stevinson, 2013). It is important that nurses routinely inquire about patients' activity patterns and offer advice, counseling, and encouragement. They should educate patients about the benefits and advise them to discuss with their healthcare provider to identify safe and easy ways they can incorporate exercise into their daily lives. Patient preferences also should be considered (Albrecht & Taylor, 2012).

Clinical Trials

Ongoing education regarding the availability of clinical trials, as appropriate, should be discussed with patients. Patients should be directed to appropriate websites if needed. NCI (www.cancer.gov/about-cancer/treatment/clinical-trials), a myeloma-specific clinical trial search engine (http://sparkcures.com), and the Coalition of Cancer Cooperative Groups (www.cancertrialshelp.org) provide information about ongoing clinical trials.

Long-Term and Late Side Effects and Survivorship

Long-term and late side effects of chemotherapy may include fatigue, pain (including neuropathic pain), sexual dysfunction, cardiac problems, psychological distress, and other conditions (Greer, Jackson, Meier, & Temel, 2013). Nurses should make appropriate referrals for psychosocial support and to other previously described resources. Some patients prefer one-on-one counseling, whereas others prefer support groups. The Cancer Survival Toolbox from the National Coalition for Cancer Survivorship, as mentioned previously, includes a basic skill set that covers communicating, finding information, making decisions, solving problems, negotiating, and standing up for one's rights. Patients who are not able or are not interested in using the Internet can be encouraged to keep a notebook or organized file folder. More information on survivorship appears in Chapter 8 of this text.

Palliative Care and Hospice

Patient and family education regarding the right to accept or refuse medical treatments and even supportive care should be done by the physician; the role of nurses and the rest of the healthcare team is to work collaboratively with physicians, patients, and families and to help to ensure understanding of this topic. Educational interventions can increase the likelihood that patients will complete advance directives. The International Association for Hospice and Palliative Care website (www.hospicecare.com) provides resources for healthcare providers, patients, and families.

Evaluation

Communicating effectively is crucial to ensure that patients feel respected and to establish a therapeutic relationship. It promotes greater satisfaction and ensures better adherence to treatment plans and better health outcomes for patients. Patients often are uncomfortable expressing that they do not understand what a clinician is telling them. Evaluation that effective learning has been done is essential. Patients and significant others should be able to verbalize an understanding of the information presented, such as the diagnosis and related problems or potential problems, the proposed treatment, key instructions for self-care, symptoms and side effects to report and whom to call, and return demonstration on items such as temperature monitoring and hand washing. They need to be able to accurately verbalize dates and times of next follow-up visits and to verbalize the names of medications, correct procedures for administration, and safe handling and disposal procedures (Polovich et al., 2014).

Hyde and Kautz (2013) performed an interventional strategy to help their rehabilitation patients in their health promotion. They demonstrated that by information-giving strategies, partnership-building behaviors, and the teach-back method, practitioners could increase the likelihood that patients would lose weight, adopt a regular exercise program, and bring chronic illnesses such as hypertension and diabetes under control. The National Quality Forum identified "teaching back" as one of 50 essential safe practices to improve health care. Although using this method does take time, early adopters found that once practitioners became accustomed to using the technique, it actually took less than a minute (National Center for Ethics in Health Care, 2006).

"Teach back" involves having patients or their surrogates explain, in everyday words, the "diagnosis/health problem for which they need care; name/type/general nature of treatment, service or procedure, including what receiving it will entail; risks, benefits, and alternatives to the treatment, service, or procedure" (National Center for Ethics in Health Care, 2006, p. 1). Clinicians should request "teach back" early in the process and as new information is given. Appropriate questions to ask include (National Center for Ethics in Health Care, 2006, p. 1)

- "I want to be sure I was clear. Can you tell me, in your own words, how you should take this medication?"
- "To be sure I've explained your treatment clearly, please tell me, in your own words, how you'd describe it to your wife/husband."
- "It's important that we're on the same page about your care. Can you tell me, in your own words, what our plan is?"

Questions such as "Do you understand?" or "Do you have questions?" are insufficient to ensure understanding of the information presented.

Although it may be difficult in a busy healthcare environment, it is important that nurses allow patients and caregivers to demonstrate their understanding of what was taught, give them feedback, and reeducate as needed. This will allow clinicians to further tailor education and concepts that need to be clarified. After reading written information, patients should bring it to their next appointment so that the healthcare team can validate patients' understanding and clarify any outlying aspects. Methods to evaluate recall of information should be tailored for each patient.

Conclusion

Multiple myeloma is a complex disease affecting multiple organs of the body, and most patients receive different therapies over time. Thorough and attentive assessment and subsequent tailored education should be done at every patient and family encounter. In a study of 1,197 long-term cancer survivors, Kent et al. (2012) showed that information needs were unmet regarding side effects and symptoms (75.8%), tests and treatment (71.5%), health promotion (64.5%), interpersonal and emotional factors (60.2%), insurance (39%), and sexual functioning and fertility (34%). Moreover, a recent study showed that the top three information needs of patients with myeloma relate to treatment, disease, and self-care (Tariman, Doorenbos, Schepp, Singhal, & Berry, 2015). This illustrated "a need for tailored interventions to equip survivors with comprehensive health information and to bolster skills for obtaining information" (Kent et al., 2012, p. 345). Nurses and other healthcare providers have opportunities to improve patient and caregiver education. Education is part of the nurturing relationship nurses have with their patients and patients' caregivers. Education, and evaluation of its effectiveness as part of the healthcare teams' ongoing support and encouragement, is essential for helping patients to maximize their quality of life as they live with multiple myeloma.

References

Accordino, M., & Hershman, D. (2013). Disparities and challenges in adherence to oral antineoplastic agents. *2013 ASCO Educational Book,* pp. 271–276. doi:10.1200/EdBook_AM.2013.33.271

Aizer, A.A., Chen, M., McCarthy, E.P., Mendu, M.L., Koo, S., Wilhite, T.J., ... Nguyen, P.L. (2013). Marital status and survival in patients with cancer. *Journal of Clinical Oncology, 31,* 3869–3876. doi:10.1200/JCO.2013.49.6489

Albrecht, T.A., & Taylor, A.G. (2012). Physical activity in patients with advanced-stage cancer: A systematic review of the literature. *Clinical Journal of Oncology Nursing, 16,* 293–300. doi:10.1188/12.CJON.293-300

American Cancer Society. (n.d.). Chemotherapy side effects worksheet. Retrieved from http://www.cancer.org/Treatment/chemotherapy-side-effects-worksheet

American Cancer Society. (2014). What is multiple myeloma? Retrieved from http://www.cancer.org/cancer/multiplemyeloma/detailedguide/multiple-myeloma-what-is-multiple-myeloma

American Society for Radiation Oncology. (2014). For your patients. Retrieved from https://www.astro.org/Practice-Management/For-Your-Patients/Index.aspx

Anselmetti, G.C., Muto, M., Guglielmi, G., & Masala, S. (2010). Percutaneous vertebroplasty or kyphoplasty. *Radiologic Clinics of North America, 48,* 641–649. doi:10.1016/j.rcl.2010.02.020

Bartlett, E.E. (1985). Editorial: At last, a definition. *Patient Education and Counseling, 7,* 323–324. doi:10.1016/0738-3991(85)90041-2

Bilotti, E. (2013). Carfilzomib: A next-generation proteasome inhibitor for multiple myeloma treatment [Online exclusive]. *Clinical Journal of Oncology Nursing, 17,* E35–E44. doi:10.1188/13.CJON.E35-E44

Boland, E., Eiser, C., Ezaydi, Y., Greenfield, D.M., Ahmedzai, S.H., & Snowden, J.A. (2013). Living with advanced but stable multiple myeloma: A study of the symptom burden and cumulative effects of disease and intensive (hematopoietic stem cell transplant-based) treatment on health-related quality of life. *Journal of Pain and Symptom Management, 46,* 671–680. doi:10.1016/j.jpainsymman.2012.11.003

Bucher, L., & Kotecki, C.N. (2014). Patient and caregiver teaching. In S. Lewis, S. Dirksen, M. Heitkemper, & L. Bucher (Eds.), *Medical-surgical nursing: Assessment and management of clinical problems* (pp. 47–60). St. Louis, MO: Elsevier.

Celgene Corporation. (2013a). *Pomalyst® (pomalidomide)* [Package insert]. Retrieved from http://www.pomalyst.com/docs/prescribing_information.pdf

Celgene Corporation. (2013b). *Revlimid® (lenalidomide)* [Package insert]. Retrieved from http://www.revlimid.com/pdf/MCL_PI.pdf

Celgene Corporation. (2013c). *Thalomid® (thalidomide)* [Package insert]. Retrieved from http://www.thalomid.com/pdf/Thalomid_PI.pdf

Cheung, Y., Shwe, M., Tan, Y., Fan, G., Ng, R., & Chan, A. (2012). Cognitive changes in multi-ethnic Asian breast cancer patients: A focus group study. *Annals of Oncology, 23,* 2547–2552. doi:10.1093/annonc/mds029

Chiffelle, R., & Kenny, K. (2013). Exercise for fatigue management in hematopoietic stem cell transplant recipients. *Clinical Journal of Oncology Nursing, 17,* 241–244. doi:10.1188/13.CJON.241-244

Clifford, K.N., Acheson, J.B., & Hall, J.J. (2013). Considerations in hematopoietic stem cell transplantation development and sites of care. In S. Ezzone (Ed.), *Hematopoietic stem cell transplantation: A manual for nursing practice* (2nd ed., pp. 67–102). Pittsburgh, PA: Oncology Nursing Society.

Cohen, M.Z., Jenkins, D., Holston, E.C., & Carlson, E.D. (2013). Understanding health literacy in patients receiving hematopoietic stem cell transplantation. *Oncology Nursing Forum, 40,* 508–515. doi:10.1188/13.ONF.508-515

Craike, M., Hose, K., & Livingston, P.M. (2013). Physical activity participation and barriers for people with multiple myeloma. *Supportive Care in Cancer, 21,* 927–934. doi:10.1007/s00520-012-1607-4

Dalby, C.K., Nesbitt, M., Frechette, C.A., Kennerley, K., Lacoursiere, L.H., & Buswell, L. (2013). Standardization of initial chemotherapy teaching to improve care. *Clinical Journal of Oncology Nursing, 17,* 472–475. doi:10.1188/13.CJON.472-475

Economou, D., Grant, M., & McCabe, M. (2012). Cancer survivorship websites and resources. *Journal of the Advanced Practitioner in Oncology, 3,* 170–173.

Elsevier. (n.d.). *Patient Education and Counseling:* Guide for authors. Retrieved from http://www.elsevier.com/journals.patient-education-and-counseling/0738-3991/guide-for-authors

Emond, Y., de Groot, J., Wetzels, W., & van Osch, L. (2013). Internet guidance in oncology practice: Determinants of health professionals' Internet referral behavior. *Psycho-Oncology, 22,* 74–82. doi:10.1002/pon.2056

Epstein, J.B., Thariat, J., Bensadoun, R., Barasch, A., Murphy, B.A., Kolnick, L., ... Maghami, E. (2012). Oral complications of cancer and cancer therapy. *CA: A Cancer Journal for Clinicians, 62,* 401–422. doi:10.3322/caac.21157

Ezzone, S.A. (2013). Gastrointestinal complications. In S. Ezzone (Ed.), *Hematopoietic stem cell transplantation: A manual for nursing practice* (2nd ed., pp. 173–190). Pittsburgh, PA: Oncology Nursing Society.

Faiman, B., Bilotti, E., Mangan, P., Rogers, K., & the IMF Nurse Leadership Board. (2008). Steroid-associated side effects in patients with multiple myeloma: Consensus statement of the IMF Nurse Leadership Board. *Clinical Journal of Oncology Nursing, 12,* 53–62. doi:10.1188/08.CJON.S1.53-62

Faiman, B., Mangan, P., Spong, J.E., Tariman, J.D., & the IMF Nurse Leadership Board. (2011). Renal complications in multiple myeloma and related disorders: Survivorship care plan of the IMF Nurse Leadership Board. *Clinical Journal of Oncology Nursing, 15*(Suppl. 4), 66–76. doi:10.1188/11.CJON.S1.66-76

Faiman, B., Miceli, T., Noonan, K., & Lilleby, K. (2013). Clinical updates in blood and marrow transplantation in multiple myeloma. *Clinical Journal of Oncology Nursing, 17*(Suppl. 6), 33–41. doi:10.1188/13.CJON.S2.33-41

Faiman, B., Pillai, A., & Benghiac, G. (2013). Bisphosphonate-related osteonecrosis of the jaw: Historical, ethical, and legal issues associated with prescribing. *Journal of the Advanced Practitioner in Oncology, 4,* 25–35.

Fee-Schroeder, K., Howell, L., Kokal, J., Bjornsen, S., Christensen, S., Hathaway, J., ... Vickers, K.S. (2013). Empowering individuals to self-manage chemotherapy side effects. *Clinical Journal of Oncology Nursing, 17,* 369–371. doi:10.1188/13.CJON.369-371

Ferguson, L.A., & Pawlak, R. (2011). Health literacy: The road to improved health outcomes. *Journal for Nurse Practitioners, 7,* 123–129. doi:10.1016/j.nurpra.2010.11.020

Gallup, Inc. (2014, December 18). Americans rate nurses highest on honesty, ethical standards. Retrieved from http://www.gallup.com/poll/180260/americans-rate-nurses-highest-honesty-ethical-standards.aspx

Greer, J.A., Jackson, V.A., Meier, D.E., & Temel, J.S. (2013). Early integration of palliative care services with standard oncology care for patients with advanced cancer. *CA: A Cancer Journal for Clinicians, 63,* 349–363. doi:10.3322/caac.21192

Hanson, J., Ferrell, B., & Grant, M. (2013). Websites and resources for cancer family caregivers. *Journal of the Advanced Practitioner in Oncology, 4,* 269–272.

Hong, Y., Pena-Purcell, N.C., & Ory, M.G. (2012). Outcomes of online support and resources for cancer survivors: A systematic literature review. *Patient Education and Counseling, 86,* 288–296. doi:10.1016/j.pec.2011.06.014

Husson, O., Thong, M.S.Y., Mols, F., Oerlemans, S., Kaptein, A.A., & van de Poll-Franse, L.V. (2013). Illness perceptions in cancer survivors: What is the role of information provision? *Psycho-Oncology, 22,* 490–498. doi:10.1002/pon.3042

Hyde, Y.M., & Kautz, D.D. (2013). Enhancing health promotion during rehabilitation through information-giving, partnership-building, and teach-back. *Rehabilitation Nursing, 39,* 178–182. doi:10.1002/rnj.124

Im, E. (2011). Online support of patients and survivors of cancer. *Seminars in Oncology Nursing, 27,* 229–236. doi:10.1016/j.soncn.2011.04.008

Jansen, C.E. (2013). Cognitive changes associated with cancer and cancer therapy: Patient assessment and education. *Seminars in Oncology Nursing, 29,* 270–279. doi:10.1016/j.soncn.2013.08.007

Jia, L., & Liu, F. (2013). Why bortezomib cannot go with 'green'? *Cancer Biology and Medicine, 10,* 206–213. doi:10.7497/j.issn.2095-3941.2013.04.004

Joint Commission. (2015). Speak Up initiatives. Retrieved from http://www.joint commission.org/speakup.aspx

Karvinen, K.H., Carr, L.J., & Stevinson, C. (2013). Resources for physical activity in cancer centers in the United States [Online exclusive]. *Clinical Journal of Oncology Nursing, 17*, E71–E76. doi:10.1188/13.CJON.E71-E76

Kent, E.E., Arora, N.K., Rowland, J.H., Bellizzi, K.M., Forsythe, L.P., Hamilton, A.S., ... Aziz, N.M. (2012). Health information needs and health-related quality of life in a diverse population of long-term cancer survivors. *Patient Education and Counseling, 89*, 345–352. doi:10.1016/j.pec.2012.08.014

Khan, O.A., Brinjikji, W., & Kallmes, D.F. (2013). Vertebral augmentation in patients with multiple myeloma: A pooled analysis of published case series. *American Journal of Neuroradiology, 35*, 207–210. doi:10.3174/ajnr.A3622

Kiviat, J. (2013). Quality-of-life issues. In S. Ezzone (Ed.), *Hematopoietic stem cell transplantation: A manual for nursing practice* (2nd ed., pp. 283–291). Pittsburgh, PA: Oncology Nursing Society.

Kristinsson, S.Y., Anderson, W.F., & Landgren, O. (2014). Improved long-term survival in multiple myeloma up to the age of 80 years. *Leukemia, 28*, 1346–1348. doi:10.1038/leu.2014.23

Kurtin, S.E., & Bilotti, E. (2013). Novel agents for the treatment of multiple myeloma: Proteasome inhibitors and immunomodulatory agents. *Journal of the Advanced Practitioner in Oncology, 4*, 307–321.

Kurtin, S., & Faiman, B. (2013). The changing landscape of multiple myeloma: Implications for oncology nurses. *Clinical Journal of Oncology Nursing, 17*(Suppl. 6), 9–11. doi:10.1188/13.CJON.S2.7-11

Lacy, M.Q., & McCurdy, A.R. (2013). Pomalidomide. *Blood, 122*, 2305–2309. doi:10.1182/blood-2013-05-484782

Lalla, R.V., Bowen, J., Barasch, A., Elting, L., Epstein, J., Keefe, D.M., ... Mucositis Guidelines Leadership Group of the Multinational Association of Supportive Care in Cancer and International Society of Oral Oncology (MASCC/ISOO). (2014). MASCC/ISOO clinical practice guidelines for the management of mucositis secondary to cancer therapy. *Cancer, 120*, 1453–1461. doi:10.1002/cncr.28592

Latif, T., Chauhan, N., Khan, R., Moran, A., & Usmani, S.Z. (2012). Thalidomide and its analogues in the treatment of multiple myeloma. *Experimental Hematology and Oncology, 1*, 27. doi:10.1186/2162-3619-1-27

Lawrentschuk, N., Sasges, D., Tasevski, R., Abouassaly, R., Scott, A.M., & Davis, I.D. (2011). Oncology health information quality on the Internet: A multilingual evaluation. *Annals of Surgical Oncology, 19*, 706–713. doi:10.1245/s10434-011-2137-x

Leukemia and Lymphoma Society. (2013). National consumer survey reveals alarming knowledge gap about blood cancers. Retrieved from http://www.lls.org/?gclid=CIyj9uO6i7wCFc6Tfgody3gAIQ#/aboutlls/news/newsreleases/082913_national_consumer_survey_knowledgegap_bloodcancers

Levensky, E.R., Forcehimes, A., O'Donohue, W.T., & Beitz, K. (2007). Motivational interviewing. *American Journal of Nursing, 107*(10), 50–58. doi:10.1097/01.NAJ.0000292202.06571.24

Matsuyama, R.K., Kuhn, L.A., Mosilani, A., & Wilson-Genderson, M.C. (2012). Cancer patients' information needs the first nine months after diagnosis. *Patient Education and Counseling, 90*, 96–102. doi:10.1016/j.pec.2012.09.009

Matsuyama, R.K., Lyckholm, L.J., Molisani, A., & Moghanaki, D. (2013). The value of an educational video before consultation with a radiation oncologist. *Journal of Cancer Education, 28*, 306–313. doi:10.1007/s13187-013-0473-1

Matsuyama, R., Wilson-Genderson, M., Kuhn, L., Moghanaki, D., Vachhani, H., & Paasche-Orlow, M. (2011). Education level, not health literacy, associated with information needs for patients with cancer. *Patient Education and Counseling, 85*, e229–e236. doi:10.1016/j.pec.2011.03.022

McAdams, F.W., & Burgunder, M.R. (2013). Transplant treatment course and acute complications. In S. Ezzone (Ed.), *Hematopoietic stem cell transplantation: A manual for nursing practice* (2nd ed., pp. 47–66). Pittsburgh, PA: Oncology Nursing Society.

McBride, L., & Samuel, C.O. (2013). The side effect profile of carfilzomib: From clinical trials to clinical practice. *Journal of the Advanced Practitioner in Oncology, 4*(Suppl. 1), 22–30.

Miceli, T.S., Colson, K., Faiman, B.M., Miller, K., Tariman, J.D., & the IMF Nurse Leadership Board. (2011). Maintaining bone health in patients with multiple myeloma. *Clinical Journal of Oncology Nursing, 15*(Suppl. 4), 9–23. doi:10.1188/11.S1.CJON.9-23

Miceli, T., Colson, K., Gavino, M., Lilleby, K., & the IMF Nurse Leadership Board. (2008). Myelosuppression associated with novel therapies in patients with multiple myeloma: Consensus statement of the IMF Nurse Leadership Board. *Clinical Journal of Oncology Nursing, 12,* 13–20. doi:10.1188/08.CJON.S1.13-19

Miceli, T., Lilleby, K., Noonan, K., Kurtin, S., Faiman, B., & Mangan, P.A. (2013). Autologous hematopoietic stem cell transplantation for patients with multiple myeloma: An overview for nurses in community practice. *Clinical Journal of Oncology Nursing, 17*(Suppl. 6), 13–24. doi:10.1188/13.CJON.S2.13-24

Millennium Pharmaceuticals. (2014). *Velcade® (bortezomib)* [Package insert]. Retrieved from http://www.velcade.com/files/PDFs/VELCADE_PRESCRIBING_INFORMATION.pdf

Mollaoglu, M., & Erdogan, G. (2014). Effect on symptom control of structured information given to patients receiving chemotherapy. *European Journal of Oncology Nursing, 18,* 78–84. doi:10.1016/j.ejon.2013.07.006

Moon, J.H., Sohn, S.K., Kim, S.N., Park, S.Y., Yoon, S.S., Kim, I.H., ... Kim, D.H. (2012). Patient counseling program to improve the compliance to imatinib in chronic myeloid leukemia patients. *Medical Oncology, 29,* 1179–1185. doi:10.1007/s12032-011-9926-8

National Cancer Institute. (2007). *Radiation therapy and you: Support for people with cancer.* Retrieved from http://www.cancer.gov/publications/patient-education/radiation-therapy-and-you

National Cancer Institute. (2012). *Evaluating online sources of health information.* Retrieved from http://www.cancer.gov/cancertopics/cancerlibrary/health-info-online

National Center for Ethics in Health Care. (2006, April). "Teach back": A tool for improving provider-patient communication. *IN Focus: Topics in Health Care Ethics,* pp. 1–2. Retrieved from http://www.ethics.va.gov/docs/infocus/InFocus_20060401_teach_Back.pdf

National Comprehensive Cancer Network. (2014). *NCCN Clinical Practice Guidelines in Oncology (NCCN Guidelines®): Cancer-associated venous thromboembolic disease* [v.2.2014]. Retrieved from http://www.nccn.org/professionals/physician_gls/pdf/vte.pdf

National Comprehensive Cancer Network. (2015). *NCCN Clinical Practice Guidelines in Oncology (NCCN Guidelines®): Multiple myeloma* [v.3.2015]. Retrieved from http://www.nccn.org/professionals/physicians_gls/pdf/myeloma.pdf

National Library of Medicine. (2013). *Kyphoplasty.* Retrieved from http://nlm.nih.gov/medlineplus/ency/article/007511.htm

National Patient Safety Foundation. (n.d.). *Health literacy: Statistics at-a-glance.* Retrieved from http://c.ymcdn.com/sites/www.npsf.org/resource/collection/9220B314-9666-40DA-89DA-9F46357530F1/AskMe3_Stats_English.pdf

Navigating Cancer, Inc. (2013). *Multiple myeloma library.* Retrieved from https://www.navigatingcancer.com/library/multiple-myeloma

Neumann, J.L. (2013). Ethical considerations. In S. Ezzone (Ed.), *Hematopoietic stem cell transplantation: A manual for nursing practice* (2nd ed., pp. 269–281). Pittsburgh, PA: Oncology Nursing Society.

Neuss, M.N., Polovich, M., McNiff, K., Esper, P., Gilmore, T.R., LeFebvre, K.B., ... Jacobson, J.O. (2013). 2013 updated American Society of Clinical Oncology/Oncology Nursing Society chemotherapy administration safety standards including standards for the safe administration and management of oral chemotherapy. *Journal of Oncology Practice, 9*(Suppl. 2), 5s–13s. doi:10.1200/JOP.2013.000874

Niess, D. (2013). Basic concepts of transplantation. In S. Ezzone (Ed.), *Hematopoietic stem cell transplantation: A manual for nursing practice* (2nd ed., pp. 13–46). Pittsburgh, PA: Oncology Nursing Society.

Novartis Pharmaceuticals Corporation. (2015). *Farydak® (panobinostat)* [Package insert]. Retrieved from http://www.pharma.us.novartis.com/product/pi/pdf/farydak.pdf

Nucci, M., & Anaissie, E. (2009). Infections in patients with multiple myeloma in the era of high-dose therapy and novel agents. *Clinical Infectious Diseases, 49,* 1211–1225. doi:10.1086/605664

Oncology Nursing Society. (2009). Tools for oral adherence toolkit. Retrieved from https://www.ons.org/sites/default/files/oral%20adherence%20toolkit.pdf

Onyx Pharmaceuticals. (2012). *Kyprolis® (carfilzomib)* [Package insert]. Retrieved from http://kyprolis.com/Content/pdf/PrescribingInformation.pdf

Paice, J.A., & Ferrell, B. (2011). The management of cancer pain. *CA: A Cancer Journal for Clinicians, 61,* 157–182. doi:10.3322/caac.20112

Palumbo, A., & Anderson, K. (2011). Multiple myeloma. *New England Journal of Medicine, 364,* 1046–1060. doi:10.1056/NEJMra1011442

Palumbo, A., & Cavallo, F. (2012). Have drug combinations supplanted stem cell transplantation in myeloma? *Blood, 120,* 4692–4698. doi:10.1182/blood-2012-05-423202

Pew Research Center. (2014, January 15). The social life of health information. Retrieved from http://www.pewresearch.org/fact-tank/2014/01/15/the-social-life-of-health-information

Pluta, R.M., Lynm, C., & Glass, R.M. (2010). Multiple myeloma (*JAMA* patient page). *JAMA, 304,* 2430. doi:10.1001/jama.304.21.2430

Polovich, M., Olsen, M., & LeFebvre, K.B. (Eds.). (2014). *Chemotherapy and biotherapy guidelines and recommendations for practice* (4th ed.). Pittsburgh, PA: Oncology Nursing Society.

Prochaska, J.O., & Velicer, W.F. (1997). The transtheoretical model of health behavior change. *American Journal of Health Promotion, 12,* 38–48. doi:10.4278/0890-1171-12.1.38

Pulte, D., Gondos, A., & Brenner, H. (2011). Improvement in survival of older adults with multiple myeloma: Results of an updated period analysis of SEER data. *Oncologist, 16,* 1600–1603. doi:10.1634/theoncologist.2011-0229

Rajkumar, S.V., & Dispenzieri, A. (2013). Multiple myeloma and related disorders. In J.E. Niederhuber, J.O. Armitage, J.H. Doroshow, M.B. Kastan, & J.E. Tepper (Eds.), *Abeloff's clinical oncology* (5th ed., Chapter 104). Philadelphia, PA: Saunders. Retrieved from http://www.expertconsultbook.com/expertconsult/ob/book.do?method=display&eid=4-u1.0-B978-0-443-06694-8..X5001-5-TOP&isbn=978-0-443-06694-8&selectBook=true&decorator=none&type=aboutPage

Richardson, P.G., Mark, T.M., & Lacy, M.Q. (2013). Pomalidomide: New immunomodulatory agent with potent antiproliferative effects. *Critical Reviews in Oncology/Hematology, 88,* S36–S44. doi:10.1016/j.critrevonc.2013.02.001

Rome, S.I., Jenkins, B.S., Lilleby, K.E., & the International Myeloma Foundation Nurse Leadership Board. (2011). Mobility and safety in the multiple myeloma survivor: Survivorship care plan of the International Myeloma Foundation Nurse Leadership Board. *Clinical Journal of Oncology Nursing, 15*(Suppl. 4), 41–52. doi:10.1188/11.S1.CJON.41-52

Roodman, G.D. (2011). Bone disease and its management in multiple myeloma. Retrieved from http://meetinglibrary.asco.org/content/43400

Rosselet, R.M. (2013). Hematologic effects. In S. Ezzone (Ed.), *Hematopoietic stem cell transplantation: A manual for nursing practice* (2nd ed., pp. 155–172). Pittsburgh, PA: Oncology Nursing Society.

Schmitz, K.H., Courneya, K.S., Matthews, C., Demark-Wahnefried, W., Galvao, D.A., Pinto, B.M., ... Schwartz, A.L. (2010). American College of Sports Medicine roundtable on exercise guidelines for cancer survivors. *Medicine and Science in Sports and Exercise, 42,* 1409–1426. doi:10.1249/MSS.0b013e3181e0c112

Siegel, R.L., Miller, K.D., & Jemal, A. (2015). Cancer statistics, 2015. *CA: A Cancer Journal for Clinicians, 65,* 5–29. doi:10.3322/caac.21254

Simchowitz, B., Shiman, L., Spencer, J., Brouillard, B.A., Gross, A., Connor, M., & Weingart, S.N. (2010). Perceptions and experiences of patients receiving oral chemotherapy. *Clinical Journal of Oncology Nursing, 14,* 447–453. doi:10.1188/10.CJON.447-453

Spinks, T., Albright, H.S., Feeley, T.W., Walters, R., Burke, T.W., Aloia, E., … Shine, K.I. (2012). Ensuring quality cancer care. *Cancer, 118,* 2571–2582. doi:10.1002/cncr.26536

Spoelstra, S., Given, B., Given, C., Grant, M., Sikorskii, A., You, M., & Decker, V. (2013a). An intervention to improve adherence and management of symptoms for patients prescribed oral chemotherapy agents. *Cancer Nursing, 36,* 18–28. doi:10.1097/NCC.0b013e3182551587

Spoelstra, S., Given, B., Given, C., Grant, M., Sikorskii, A., You, M., & Decker, V. (2013b). Issues related to overadherence to oral chemotherapy or targeted agents. *Clinical Journal of Oncology Nursing, 17,* 604–609. doi:10.1188/13.CJON.17-06AP

Spoelstra, S., & Given, C.W. (2011). Assessment and measurement of adherence to oral antineoplastic agents. *Seminars in Oncology Nursing, 27,* 116–132. doi:10.1016/jsonon.2011.02.004

Tariman, J.D., Doorenbos, A., Schepp, K.G., Singhal, S., & Berry, D.L. (2015). Top information need priorities of older adults newly diagnosed with active myeloma. *Journal of the Advanced Practitioner in Oncology, 6,* 14–21.

Tariman, J.D., Love, G., McCullagh, E., Sandifer, S., & the IMF Nurse Leadership Board. (2008). Peripheral neuropathy associated with novel therapies in patients with multiple myeloma: Consensus statement of the IMF Nurse Leadership Board. *Clinical Journal of Oncology Nursing, 12,* 29–35. doi:10.1188/08.CJON.S1.29-35

Terpos, E., Morgan, G., Dimopoulos, M.A., Drake, M.T., Lentzsch, S., Raje, N., … Roodman, G.D. (2013). International Myeloma Working Group recommendations for the treatment of multiple myeloma-related bone disease. *Journal of Clinical Oncology, 31,* 2347–2357. doi:10.1200/JCO.2012.47.7901

Terpos, E., Roodman, G.D., & Dimopoulos, M.A. (2013). Optimal use of bisphosphonates in patients with multiple myeloma. *Blood, 121,* 3325–3328. doi:10.1182/blood-2012-10-435750

Terwiel, E., Hanrahan, R., Lueck, C., & D'Rozario, J. (2010). Reversible posterior encephalopathy syndrome associated with bortezomib. *Internal Medicine Journal, 40,* 69–71. doi:10.1111/j.1445-5994.2009.02097.x

Thomas, M.L., Elliot, J.E., Rao, S.M., Fahey, K.F., Paul, S.M., & Miaskowski, C. (2012). A randomized, clinical trial of education or motivational-interviewing-based coaching compared to usual care to improve cancer pain management. *Oncology Nursing Forum, 39,* 39–49. doi:10.1188/12.ONF.39-49

Thompson, J., Silliman, K., & Clifford, D.E. (2013). Impact of an early education multimedia intervention in managing nutrition-related chemotherapy side-effects: A pilot study. *SpringerPlus, 2,* 179. doi:10.1186/2193-1801-2-179

Truven Health Analytics. (2013). CareNotes patient education. Retrieved from http://www.micromedex.com/products/carenotes

U.S. Food and Drug Administration. (2013). Strategies to reduce medication errors: Working to improve medication safety. Retrieved from http://www.fda.gov/Drugs/ResourcesForYou/consumers/ucm143553.htm

Williams, J.T. (2013). Credible and complementary and alternative medicine websites. *Journal of the Advanced Practitioner in Oncology, 4,* 123–124.

Wilson, F.L., Mood, D., & Nordstrom, C.K. (2010). The influence of easy-to-read pamphlets about self-care management of radiation side effects on patients' knowledge. *Oncology Nursing Forum, 37,* 774–781. doi:10.1188/10.ONF.774-781

Wood, S.K., & Payne, J.K. (2011). Cancer-related infections. *Journal of the Advanced Practitioner in Oncology, 2,* 356–371.

CHAPTER **12**

Clinical Trials

Joseph D. Tariman, PhD, ANP-BC

Introduction

Novel agents have changed the treatment paradigm for patients with multiple myeloma, leading to dramatic improvements in overall response rates and overall survival (Kurtin & Bilotti, 2013; Venner et al., 2011). In the past decade, therapeutic options have increased significantly with six new drugs approved for patients with multiple myeloma, and further insight has been gained into the biology and genetics of myeloma leading to more therapeutic targets (Lawasut et al., 2013; Minami et al., 2014). Since the release of the first edition of this book in 2010, the U.S. Food and Drug Administration (FDA) has approved three new drugs, pomalidomide (approved in 2013), carfilzomib (approved in 2012), and panobinostat (approved in 2015), leading the way for more therapeutic options for patients with multiple myeloma (International Myeloma Foundation, 2014; Traynor, 2013; U.S. FDA, 2015).

The advent of additional novel agents and the optimization of the therapeutic benefits of existing ones can further improve clinical outcomes. Patients' overall survival will continue to improve with new generations of drugs and with more breakthroughs in clinical drug trials. Oncology nurses play a major role in the safe and effective administration of these novel agents. Furthermore, oncology nurses are critical in monitoring adherence, managing side effects, evaluating treatment outcomes, and providing patient education on treatment options. They play a pivotal role in maximizing the therapeutic benefits of these new drugs, whether already FDA approved or still in early stages of clinical drug trials.

Ongoing Research Studies

Several biologically based therapeutic agents currently are under clinical drug investigation for multiple myeloma (see Table 12-1). Increased under-

Table 12-1. Novel Agents Currently Under Clinical Drug Investigation for Multiple Myeloma

Drug Classification	Generic Drug Name/Number and Associated Publications
Akt inhibitor	Afuresertib (Spencer et al., 2014)
Farnesyltransferase inhibitor	Tipifarnib (Alsina et al., 2004)
Heat-shock protein inhibitor	SNX5422 (Reddy et al., 2013) Tanespimycin (Richardson et al., 2010, 2011)
Histone deacetylase inhibitor	Vorinostat (Badros et al., 2009; Dimopoulos et al., 2013; Richardson et al., 2008; Siegel et al., 2014; Weber et al., 2012)
Monoclonal antibody	BT-062 (de la Puente & Azab, 2013) Daratumumab (Kuroda et al., 2013; Laubach et al., 2014) Denosumab (Cicci et al., 2014; Hageman et al., 2013; Henry et al., 2011; Vij et al., 2009) Elotuzumab (de la Puente & Azab, 2013; Jakubowiak et al., 2012; Kuroda et al., 2013; Lonial et al., 2012; Moreau & Touzeau, 2014; van Rhee et al., 2009; Zonder et al., 2012) Siltuximab (Bagcchi, 2014; Kurzrock et al., 2013; San-Miguel et al., 2014; Voorhees et al., 2013)

standing of osteoblast inhibition (Giuliani, Rizzoli, & Roodman, 2006) and improved comprehension of the role of bone marrow microenvironment and multiple myeloma cell survival pathways have led to the development of several effective therapeutics with promising clinical results as well as identification of novel drug targets (Anderson, 2013; Gorgun et al., 2013; Keane, Glavey, Krawczyk, & O'Dwyer, 2014; Minami et al., 2014; Misso et al., 2013; Podar, Chauhan, & Anderson, 2009). The new and emerging science of epigenetics also offers new therapeutic targets and could potentially lead to the development of a new class of therapy that can improve the response rates, duration of response, and overall survival of patients with multiple myeloma (Chesi & Bergsagel, 2010; Dimopoulos, Gimsing, & Gronbaek, 2014; Fuchs, 2013).

Recently Approved Agent: Panobinostat

Panobinostat is a potent pan-histone deacetylase (HDAC) inhibitor with low nanomolar activity against all HDAC enzymes including class I, II, and IV that are implicated as potential targets in cancer, including multiple myeloma (Atadja, 2009; Neri, Bahlis, & Lonial, 2012). Panobinostat increases acetylation of proteins, particularly the aggresome protein degradation pathway known to be involved in multiple cancer cell pathways including multiple myeloma cells (Catley et al., 2006). Promising phase II clinical trial results of this novel drug have been published recently. The investigators of the PANORAMA 2 trial (N = 55) reported patients with multiple myeloma achieving an overall response rate (ORR) of 34.5% (1 with near complete response [nCR] and 18 with partial response [PR]) and a clinical benefit response (CBR) of 52.7% (10 additional patients achieved minimal response). Panobinostat was combined with bortezomib and dexamethasone for the treatment of patients with relapsed and bortezomib-refractory multiple myeloma with two or more prior lines of therapy, including an immunomodulatory drug. Furthermore, patients already had progressive disease on or within 60 days of the last bortezomib-based therapy (Richardson et al., 2013). Several phase I/Ib and II studies combining panobinostat with bortezomib (San-Miguel et al., 2013), melphalan (Berenson et al., 2014), or melphalan, thalidomide, and prednisone (Offidani et al., 2012) or as a single agent (Wolf et al., 2012) also are showing antitumor activities against myeloma.

The results of the phase III trial (N = 768) of panobinostat (PANORAMA 1), a randomized, double-blind study of panobinostat or placebo plus bortezomib and dexamethasone in relapsed and refractory multiple myeloma (RRMM), were reported during the 2014 American Society of Clinical Oncology annual meeting. The results showed median progression-free survival (PFS) of 12 months versus 8.1 months ($p < 0.0001$; hazard ratio = 0.63, 95% confidence interval 0.52–0.76) for patients treated with panobinostat versus the placebo arm. Moreover, the panobinostat arm had an ORR of 61% versus 55% in the placebo arm. The nCR/CR rate was 28% with panobinostat and 16% with placebo arm with duration of response of 13.1 months (panobinostat arm) versus 10.9 months (placebo arm). No overall survival data were available because of the lack of maturity of the trial (Richardson, Hungria, et al., 2014).

Promising Clinical Trials

Elotuzumab

Elotuzumab is an anti-CS1 monoclonal antibody that has been heavily investigated in patients with RRMM. The first phase I trial of elotuzumab had a dosing range from 0.5 to 20 mg/kg every two weeks. Patients who achieved at least stable disease after four treatments received another four treatments. No maximum tolerated dose (MTD) was reported, even in the maximum dose of 20 mg/kg. The most common adverse events reported by investigators included headache, back pain, fever, and chills. These adverse reactions generally were mild to moderate and primarily were infusion-related, according to the study report. The level of CS1 on bone marrow–derived plasma cells was reliably saturated (≥ 95%) at the 10 mg/kg and 20 mg/kg dose levels. The response rates reported on this phase I study were modest but promising with nine patients (26.5%) achieving stable disease. The investigators concluded that elotuzumab generally is well tolerated and requires further exploration of elotuzumab in combination regimens (Zonder et al., 2012).

A follow-up phase I study combined elotuzumab with lenalidomide and dexamethasone for the treatment of patients with relapsed or refractory multiple myeloma. This study had three cohorts: elotuzumab was administered intravenously on days 1, 8, 15, and 22 of a 28-day cycle in the first two cycles at 5, 10, or 20 mg/kg IV and on days 1 and 15 of each subsequent cycle. The additional two drugs were lenalidomide 25 mg orally on days 1 to 21 and dexamethasone 40 mg orally weekly. The investigators reported that 29 patients with relapsed/refractory multiple myeloma were enrolled in this study. Overall, 28 patients were treated. Three patients each were assigned to the 5 mg/kg and 10 mg/kg cohorts and 22 patients were assigned to the 20 mg/kg cohort. Similar to the prior phase I study, no dose-limiting toxicities were reported, even in the cohort with the maximum dose of 20 mg/kg (Lonial et al., 2012).

The most common adverse reactions were grade 3–4 neutropenia (36%) and thrombocytopenia (21%). The investigators reported two study participants having serious infusion reactions: one study participant had a grade 4 anaphylactic reaction and the other experienced a grade 3 drug reaction, reporting stridor. These two serious adverse events occurred during the first cycle of therapy. Impressively, the ORR seen was 82% (n = 23) of treated patients. Interim analysis done at a median follow-up time of 16.4 months showed that the median time to progression was not reached. Patients who were in the 20 mg/kg cohort were treated until they showed evidence of disease progression. The investigators concluded that elotuzumab plus lenalidomide and dexamethasone demonstrated a remarkably high ORR in this phase I study. Additionally, the observed median time to disease progression suggested that the triple combination could be superior to lenalidomide/dexamethasone double combination therapy. The investigators recognized that elotuzumab is associated with a higher incidence of infusion reactions. However, they suggested that this adverse event can be effectively managed with premedication as stated by the treatment protocol (Lonial et al., 2012).

Another phase I trial evaluated the safety and efficacy of elotuzumab in combination with bortezomib in patients with RRMM. Using a 21-day cycle of therapy, study participants were treated with elotuzumab at 2.5, 5, 10, or 20 mg/kg IV and bortezomib at 1.3 mg/m^2 IV on days 1 and 11 and days 1, 4, 8, and 11, respectively. The study also utilized a 3 + 3 dose-escalation

(35%). One grade 3 peripheral neuropathy (PN) was reported, and fewer patients than expected had PN with only 20% grade 1–2 PN. The ORR was 18% (n = 9), which includes patients who achieved a partial response or better. This response rate included 8 patients (27% of 30 patients enrolled) treated at 2.97 mg/m^2. The terminal half-life of ixazomib was long, ranging from 3.6 to 11.3 days, which makes once-weekly dosing ideal (Kumar et al., 2014).

The second phase I study was reported by Richardson, Baz, et al. (2014). In this study, a larger number of patients with RRMM (N = 60) were enrolled. Patients received single-agent ixazomib 0.24–2.23 mg/m^2 on a twice-a-day dosing schedule (days 1, 4, 8, 11) in a 21-day cycle. Rash (grade 3) and thrombocytopenia (grade 4) were reported as the only two dose-limiting toxicities, which occurred in the 2.23 mg/m^2 patient cohort. The investigators established the MTD for the twice-weekly dosing at 2 mg/m^2, which then enrolled another 40 patients in four expansion cohorts. The median number of treatment cycles was 4 (range = 1–39), but a modest percentage (18%) of patients enrolled received 12 or more cycles. Grade 1–2 side effects were reported in 88% of patients enrolled, which included nausea (42%), thrombocytopenia (42%), fatigue (40%), and rash (40%). No grade 3 or higher PN was reported. Mild (grade 1–2) PN was documented in 12% of study patients. Two deaths were reported during the duration of the study, but both were considered unrelated to ixazomib. For this twice-a-week dosing schedule, the half-life of ixazomib was 3.3–7.4 days. The ORR was high when stable disease was included at 76%. Partial response or better was observed in 15% of the entire study cohort (Richardson, Baz, et al., 2014).

Phase III global studies are underway for ixazomib in RRMM (Millennium Pharmaceuticals Inc., 2014). Ixazomib in combination with lenalidomide and dexamethasone is being studied as a potential new standard treatment for RRMM (National Cancer Institute, 2014). At this point, lenalidomide plus dexamethasone is considered standard of care for RRMM with an FDA indication for this specific myeloma patient population with relapsed and/or refractory disease state (National Comprehensive Cancer Network®, 2015).

Daratumumab

The first report of the potential antimyeloma activity of daratumumab was initiated by de Weers et al. (2011). They reported that daratumumab has shown antimyeloma properties by mediating strong lysis of multiple myeloma cells via complement-dependent cytotoxicity (CDC) and antibody-dependent cellular cytotoxicity (ADCC) despite donor dependency of the cytotoxic activity of the autologous ADCC. Additional experiments combining daratumumab with lenalidomide validated the initial findings. This same design. Study participants who had achieved a stable disease or better after four cycles were allowed to continue treatment until disease progression or unexpected toxicity (Jakubowiak et al., 2012).

The investigators reported the response rates of 28 patients who had a median of two prior therapies. In total, 3 patients received 2.5, 5, and 10 mg/kg of IV elotuzumab and 19 received the 20 mg/kg dose. The investigators found no dose-limiting toxicities during cycle 1 of the dose-escalation phase. Moreover, the MTD was not reached even in the 20 mg/kg patient cohort. The most frequent reported side effects included grade 3–4 lymphopenia (25%) and fatigue (14%). Two infusion-related serious adverse events were reported: one patient had chest pain and the other experienced gastroenteritis. Using the European Blood and Marrow Transplant criteria of response, the overall response (partial response or better) was 48% (n = 13) of 27 evaluable patients. These responses included two of the three patients who were already known to be refractory to bortezomib. The median time to progression was adequate at 9.46 months. This study demonstrated that the combination of elotuzumab and bortezomib generally was well tolerated and a promising combination therapy option for patients with RRMM (Jakubowiak et al., 2012).

Ixazomib

Ixazomib (MLNM9708) is the first oral proteasome inhibitor developed in the United States by Millennium Pharmaceuticals, maker of the first-in-class proteasome inhibitor bortezomib (Millennium Pharmaceuticals Inc., 2014). This is another boronic-based proteasome inhibitor that is reversible, just like its parent compound bortezomib. Similar to bortezomib, ixazomib primarily targets the chymotrypsin-like activity of the 20S proteasome. However, there are differences between bortezomib and ixazomib, which are reported in the literature. First, ixazomib has a shorter half-life (the time it takes for its plasma concentration to decline by 50%). Second, ixazomib demonstrated greater tissue penetration when compared with bortezomib in preclinical study (Kupperman et al., 2010; Moreau, 2014).

Two phase I studies on ixazomib for RRMM with different dosing schedules have been published. The first study was reported by Kumar et al. (2014) using a weekly dosing schedule. In this study, 60 patients with RRMM were enrolled to evaluate safety and tolerability as well as to establish the MTD of single-agent oral ixazomib as a weekly proteasome inhibitor for three to four weeks. The study had four different cohorts based on prior history of refractoriness to bortezomib and carfilzomib. The investigator reported the MTD at 2.97 mg/m^2. The dose-limiting adverse effects were grade 3 nausea, vomiting, and diarrhea in two patients and grade 3 skin rash in one patient. The most common side effects related to ixazomib were grade 1–2 thrombocytopenia (43%), diarrhea (38%), nausea (38%), fatigue (37%), and vomiting group of researchers found that lenalidomide can increase the potency of daratumumab-dependent antimyeloma activity by activating the autologous effector cells within the microenvironment of multiple myeloma cells (van der Veer et al., 2011a, 2011b).

At the 2013 American Society of Clinical Oncology annual meeting, Lokhorst et al. (2013) reported on a phase I/II study conducted in Europe and North America. The study enrolled patients aged 18 years or older who required systemic therapy for RRMM and had been treated with at least two types of chemotherapy. Investigators utilized a 3 + 3 dose escalation design. Daratumumab in various doses was administered IV over a nine-week period as two pre- and seven full doses. The MTD was determined at 8 mg/kg and was used in the phase II trial with a weekly dosing schedule for 8 weeks, then followed every 2 weeks dosing for 16 weeks, and a monthly dose until disease progression for a maximum dose of 24 months.

The Lokhorst et al. (2013) study involved 32 evaluable patients. Response rates were based on the International Myeloma Working Group guidelines. In the cohort of patients who received a dose of 4 mg/kg or greater (n = 12), five patients achieved partial response and three achieved minimal response. The median PFS in this patient cohort was not reached during a median follow-up time of 3.8 months (range = 0–9.6 months). No antidrug antibodies were detected in this group of patients. Infusion-related reactions (IRRs) (44%) across all groups were the most common adverse drug reactions, including two patients who had grade 3 reactions. This IRR typically occurred during the first full infusion. Additionally, one anemia, one thrombocytopenia, two bronchospasms, one cytokine release, and one aspartate aminotransferase increase were reported as serious adverse events observed across all study cohorts. The investigators concluded that daratumumab can significantly reduce the M protein of patients with RRMM and is considered an unprecedented result for a single-agent monoclonal antibody (Lokhorst et al., 2013). In 2014, FDA designated a breakthrough drug status for daratumumab in RRMM (Laubach, Tai, Richardson, & Anderson, 2014).

Conclusion

Several advances have taken place in the area of therapeutics for patients with myeloma. The approvals of carfilzomib, pomalidomide, and panobinostat provided additional options for patients with RRMM. An array of promising drugs such as elotuzumab, ixazomib, and daratumumab are discussed in this chapter. These drugs have shown partial response or better in the RRMM setting. Many more new drugs are outlined in Table 12-1. Their applications in myeloma therapeutics in the near future will undoubtedly change the landscape and paradigm of myeloma therapy. Large prospective, randomized trials are needed to establish new standards in therapeutics. Oncology nurses are key members of the healthcare team for the recruitment of patients during clinical trials as well as in the safe monitoring of patients' health status throughout the chemotherapy period.

References

Alsina, M., Fonseca, R., Wilson, E.F., Belle, A.N., Gerbino, E., Price-Troska, T., ... Sebti, S.M. (2004). Farnesyltransferase inhibitor tipifarnib is well tolerated, induces stabilization of disease, and inhibits farnesylation and oncogenic/tumor survival pathways in patients with advanced multiple myeloma. *Blood, 103*, 3271–3277. doi:10.1182/blood-2003-08-2764

Anderson, K.C. (2013). Therapeutic advances in relapsed or refractory multiple myeloma. *Journal of the National Comprehensive Cancer Network, 11*(Suppl. 5), 676–679.

Atadja, P. (2009). Development of the pan-DAC inhibitor panobinostat (LBH589): Successes and challenges. *Cancer Letters, 280*, 233–241. doi:10.1016/j.canlet.2009.02.019

Badros, A., Burger, A.M., Philip, S., Niesvizky, R., Kolla, S.S., Goloubeva, O., ... Grant, S. (2009). Phase I study of vorinostat in combination with bortezomib for relapsed and refractory multiple myeloma. *Clinical Cancer Research, 15*, 5250–5257. doi:10.1158/1078-0432.CCR-08-2850

Bagcchi, S. (2014). Siltuximab in transplant-ineligible patients with myeloma. *Lancet Oncology, 15*, e309. doi:10.1016/S1470-2045(14)70446-2

Berenson, J.R., Hilger, J.D., Yellin, O., Boccia, R.V., Matous, J., Dressler, K., ... Vescio, R. (2014). A phase 1/2 study of oral panobinostat combined with melphalan for patients with relapsed or refractory multiple myeloma. *Annals of Hematology, 93*, 89–98. doi:10.1007/s00277-013-1910-2

Catley, L., Weisberg, E., Kizilitepe, T., Tai, Y.T., Hideshima, T., Neri, P., ... Anderson, K.C. (2006). Aggresome induction by proteasome inhibitor bortezomib and alpha-tubulin hyperacetylation by tubulin deacetylase (TDAC) inhibitor LBH589 are synergistic in myeloma cells. *Blood, 108*, 3441–3449. doi:10.1182/blood-2006-04-016055

Chesi, M., & Bergsagel, P.L. (2010). Epigenetics and microRNAs combine to modulate the MDM2/p53 axis in myeloma. *Cancer Cell, 18*, 299–300. doi:10.1016/j.ccr.2010.10.004

Cicci, J.D., Buie, L., Bates, J., & van Deventer, H. (2014). Denosumab for the management of hypercalcemia of malignancy in patients with multiple myeloma and renal dysfunction. *Clinical Lymphoma, Myeloma and Leukemia, 14*, e207–e211. doi:10.1016/j.clml.2014.07.005

de la Puente, P., & Azab, A.K. (2013). Contemporary drug therapies for multiple myeloma. *Drugs of Today, 49*, 563–573. doi:10.1358/dot.2013.49.09.2020941

de Weers, M., Tai, Y.T., van der Veer, M.S., Bakker, J.M., Vink, T., Jacobs, D.C., ... Parren, P.W. (2011). Daratumumab, a novel therapeutic human CD38 monoclonal antibody, induces killing of multiple myeloma and other hematological tumors. *Journal of Immunology, 186*, 1840–1848. doi:10.4049/jimmunol.1003032

Dimopoulos, M., Siegel, D.S., Lonial, S., Qi, J., Hajek, R., Facon, T., ... Anderson, K.C. (2013). Vorinostat or placebo in combination with bortezomib in patients with multiple myeloma (VANTAGE 088): A multicentre, randomised, double-blind study. *Lancet Oncology, 14*, 1129–1140. doi:10.1016/S1470-2045(13)70398-X

Dimopoulos, K., Gimsing, P., & Gronbaek, K. (2014). The role of epigenetics in the biology of multiple myeloma. *Blood Cancer Journal, 4*, e207. doi:10.1038/bcj.2014.29

Fuchs, O. (2013). Targeting of NF-kappaB signaling pathway, other signaling pathways and epigenetics in therapy of multiple myeloma. *Cardiovascular and Hematological Disorders—Drug Targets, 13*, 16–34. doi:10.2174/1871529X11313010003

Giuliani, N., Rizzoli, V., & Roodman, G.D. (2006). Multiple myeloma bone disease: Pathophysiology of osteoblast inhibition. *Blood, 108,* 3992–3996. doi:10.1182/blood-2006-05-026112

Gorgun, G.T., Whitehill, G., Anderson, J.L., Hideshima, T., Maguire, C., Laubach, J., ... Anderson, K.C. (2013). Tumor-promoting immune-suppressive myeloid-derived suppressor cells in the multiple myeloma microenvironment in humans. *Blood, 121,* 2975–2987. doi:10.1182/blood-2012-08-448548

Hageman, K., Patel, K.C., Mace, K., & Cooper, M.R. (2013). The role of denosumab for prevention of skeletal-related complications in multiple myeloma. *Annals of Pharmacotherapy, 47,* 1069–1074. doi:10.1345/aph.1R776

Henry, D.H., Costa, L., Goldwasser, F., Hirsh, V., Hungria, V., Prausova, J., ... Yeh, H. (2011). Randomized, double-blind study of denosumab versus zoledronic acid in the treatment of bone metastases in patients with advanced cancer (excluding breast and prostate cancer) or multiple myeloma. *Journal of Clinical Oncology, 29,* 1125–1132. doi:10.1200/JCO.2010.31.3304

International Myeloma Foundation. (2014). Myeloma matrix—Drugs in development or recently-approved. Retrieved from http://myeloma.org/ResearchMatrix.action?tabId=4&menuId=206&queryPageID=14

Jakubowiak, A.J., Benson, D.M., Bensinger, W., Siegel, D.S., Zimmerman, T.M., Mohrbacher, A., ... Anderson, K.C. (2012). Phase I trial of anti-CS1 monoclonal antibody elotuzumab in combination with bortezomib in the treatment of relapsed/refractory multiple myeloma. *Journal of Clinical Oncology, 30,* 1960–1965. doi:10.1200/JCO.2011.37.7069

Keane, N.A., Glavey, S.V., Krawczyk, J., & O'Dwyer, M. (2014). AKT as a therapeutic target in multiple myeloma. *Expert Opinion on Therapeutic Targets, 18,* 897–915. doi:10.1517/14728222.2014.924507

Kumar, S.K., Bensinger, W.I., Zimmerman, T.M., Reeder, C.B., Berenson, J.R., Berg, D., ... Niesvizky, R. (2014). Phase 1 study of weekly dosing with the investigational oral proteasome inhibitor ixazomib in relapsed/refractory multiple myeloma. *Blood, 124,* 1047–1055. doi:10.1182/blood-2014-01-548941

Kupperman, E., Lee, E.C., Cao, Y., Bannerman, B., Fitzgerald, M., Berger, A., ... Bolen, J. (2010). Evaluation of the proteasome inhibitor MLN9708 in preclinical models of human cancer. *Cancer Research, 70,* 1970–1980. doi:10.1158/0008-5472.CAN-09-2766

Kuroda, J., Nagoshi, H., Shimura, Y., & Taniwaki, M. (2013). Elotuzumab and daratumumab: Emerging new monoclonal antibodies for multiple myeloma. *Expert Review of Anticancer Therapy, 13,* 1081–1088. doi:10.1586/14737140.2013.829641

Kurtin, S.E., & Bilotti, E. (2013). Novel agents for the treatment of multiple myeloma: Proteasome inhibitors and immunomodulatory agents. *Journal of the Advanced Practitioner in Oncology, 4,* 307–321.

Kurzrock, R., Voorhees, P.M., Casper, C., Furman, R.R., Fayad, L., Lonial, S., ... van Rhee, F. (2013). A phase I, open-label study of siltuximab, an anti-IL-6 monoclonal antibody, in patients with B-cell non-Hodgkin lymphoma, multiple myeloma, or Castleman disease. *Clinical Cancer Research, 19,* 3659–3670. doi:10.1158/1078-0432.CCR-12-3349

Laubach, J.P., Tai, Y.T., Richardson, P.G., & Anderson, K.C. (2014). Daratumumab granted breakthrough drug status. *Expert Opinion on Investigational Drugs, 23,* 445–452. doi:10.1517/13543784.2014.889681

Lawasut, P., Groen, R., Dhimolea, E., Richardson, P.G., Anderson, K.C., & Mitsiades, C.S. (2013). Decoding the pathophysiology and the genetics of multiple myeloma to identify new therapeutic targets. *Seminars in Oncology, 40,* 537–548. doi:10.1053/j.seminoncol.2013.07.010

Lokhorst, H.M., Plesner, T., Gimsing, P., Nahi, H., Minnema, M., Lassen, U.N., ... Laubach, J. (2013). Phase I/II dose-escalation study of daratumumab in patients with relapsed or refractory multiple myeloma. Retrieved from http://meetinglibrary.asco.org/content/109895-132

Lonial, S., Vij, R., Harousseau, J.-L., Facon, T., Moreau, P., Mazumder, A., ... Jagannath, S. (2012). Elotuzumab in combination with lenalidomide and low-dose dexamethasone in relapsed or refractory multiple myeloma. *Journal of Clinical Oncology, 30,* 1953–1959. doi:10.1200/JCO.2011.37.2649

Millennium Pharmaceuticals Inc. (2014). Oncology development pipeline. Retrieved from http://www.millennium.com/ourScience/OurPipeline.aspx

Minami, J., Suzuki, R., Mazitschek, R., Gorgun, G., Ghosh, B., Cirstea, D., ... Anderson, K.C. (2014). Histone deacetylase 3 as a novel therapeutic target in multiple myeloma. *Leukemia, 28,* 680–689. doi:10.1038/leu.2013.231

Misso, G., Zappavigna, S., Castellano, M., De Rosa, G., Di Martino, M.T., Tagliaferri, P., ... Caraglia, M. (2013). Emerging pathways as individualized therapeutic target of multiple myeloma. *Expert Opinion on Biological Therapy, 13*(Suppl. 1), S95–S109. doi:10.1517/147125 98.2013.807338

Moreau, P. (2014). Oral therapy for multiple myeloma: Ixazomib arriving soon. *Blood, 124,* 986–987. doi:10.1182/blood-2014-06-581611

Moreau, P., & Touzeau, C. (2014). Elotuzumab for the treatment of multiple myeloma. *Future Oncology, 10,* 949–956. doi:10.2217/fon.14.56

National Cancer Institute. (2014). A phase 3 study comparing oral ixazomib plus lenalidomide and dexamethasone versus placebo plus lenalidomide and dexamethasone in adult patients with relapsed and/or refractory multiple myeloma. Retrieved from http://clinicaltrials.gov/show/NCT01564537

National Comprehensive Cancer Network. (2015). *NCCN Clinical Practice Guidelines in Oncology (NCCN Guidelines®): Multiple myeloma* [v.3.2015]. Retrieved from http://www.nccn.org/professionals/physician_gls/pdf/myeloma.pdf

Neri, P., Bahlis, N.J., & Lonial, S. (2012). Panobinostat for the treatment of multiple myeloma. *Expert Opinion on Investigational Drugs, 21,* 733–747. doi:10.1517/13543784.2012.668883

Offidani, M., Polloni, C., Cavallo, F., Liberati, A.M., Ballanti, S., Pulini, S., ... Palumbo, A. (2012). Phase II study of melphalan, thalidomide and prednisone combined with oral panobinostat in patients with relapsed/refractory multiple myeloma. *Leukemia and Lymphoma, 53,* 1722–1727. doi:10.3109/10428194.2012.664844

Podar, K., Chauhan, D., & Anderson, K.C. (2009). Bone marrow microenvironment and the identification of new targets for myeloma therapy. *Leukemia, 23,* 10–24. doi:10.1038/leu.2008.259

Reddy, N., Voorhees, P.M., Houk, B.E., Brega, N., Hinson, J.M., Jr., & Jillela, A. (2013). Phase I trial of the HSP90 inhibitor PF-04929113 (SNX5422) in adult patients with recurrent, refractory hematologic malignancies. *Clinical Lymphoma, Myeloma and Leukemia, 13,* 385–391. doi:10.1016/j.clml.2013.03.010

Richardson, P.G., Baz, R., Wang, M., Jakubowiak, A.J., Laubach, J.P., Harvey, R.D., ... Lonial, S. (2014). Phase 1 study of twice-weekly ixazomib, an oral proteasome inhibitor, in relapsed/refractory multiple myeloma patients. *Blood, 124,* 1038–1046. doi:10.1182/blood-2014-01-548826

Richardson, P.G., Chanan-Khan, A.A., Alsina, M., Albitar, M., Berman, D., Messina, M., ... Anderson, K.C. (2010). Tanespimycin monotherapy in relapsed multiple myeloma: Results of a phase 1 dose-escalation study. *British Journal of Haematology, 150,* 438–445. doi:10.1111/j.1365-2141.2010.08265.x

Richardson, P.G., Chanan-Khan, A.A., Lonial, S., Krishnan, A.Y., Carroll, M.P., Alsina, M., ... Anderson, K.C. (2011). Tanespimycin and bortezomib combination treatment in patients with relapsed or relapsed and refractory multiple myeloma: Results of a phase 1/2 study. *British Journal of Haematology, 153,* 729–740. doi:10.1111/j.1365-2141.2011.08664.x

Richardson, P.G., Hungria, V.T.M., Yoon, S., Beksac, M., Dimopoulos, M.A., Elghandour, A., ... Guenther, A. (2014). Panorama 1: A randomized, double-blind, phase 3 study of panobinostat or placebo plus bortezomib and dexamethasone in relapsed or relapsed and refractory multiple myeloma [Abstract No. 8510]. *Journal of Clinical Oncology, 32*(Suppl. 5). Retrieved from http://meetinglibrary.asco.org/content/125334-144

Richardson, P., Mitsiades, C., Colson, K., Reilly, E., McBride, L., Chiao, J., ... Siegel, D. (2008). Phase I trial of oral vorinostat (suberoylanilide hydroxamic acid, SAHA) in patients with advanced multiple myeloma. *Leukemia and Lymphoma, 49,* 502–507. doi:10.1080/10428190701817258

Richardson, P.G., Schlossman, R.L., Alsina, M., Weber, D.M., Coutre, S.E., Gasparetto, C., ... Lonial, S. (2013). PANORAMA 2: Panobinostat in combination with bortezomib and dexamethasone in patients with relapsed and bortezomib-refractory myeloma. *Blood, 122,* 2331–2337. doi:10.1182/blood-2013-01-481325

San-Miguel, J.F., Richardson, P.G., Günther, A., Sezer, O., Siegel, D., Bladé, J., ... Anderson, K.C. (2013). Phase Ib study of panobinostat and bortezomib in relapsed or relapsed and refractory multiple myeloma. *Journal of Clinical Oncology, 31,* 3696–3703. doi:10.1200/JCO.2012.46.7068

San-Miguel, J., Bladé, J., Shpilberg, O., Grosicki, S., Maloisel, F., Min, C.K., ... Orlowski, R.Z. (2014). Phase 2 randomized study of bortezomib-melphalan-prednisone with or without siltuximab (anti-IL-6) in multiple myeloma. *Blood, 123,* 4136–4142. doi:10.1182/blood-2013-12-546374

Siegel, D.S., Richardson, P., Dimopoulos, M., Moreau, P., Mitsiades, C., Weber, D., ... Anderson, K.C. (2014). Vorinostat in combination with lenalidomide and dexamethasone in patients with relapsed or refractory multiple myeloma. *Blood Cancer Journal, 4,* e182. doi:10.1038/bcj.2014.1

Spencer, A., Yoon, S.S., Harrison, S.J., Morris, S.R., Smith, D.A., Brigandi, R.A., ... Chen, C. (2014). The novel AKT inhibitor afuresertib shows favorable safety, pharmacokinetics, and clinical activity in multiple myeloma. *Blood, 124,* 2190–2195. doi:10.1182/blood-2014-03-559963

Traynor, K. (2013). Pomalidomide approved for multiple myeloma. *American Journal of Health-System Pharmacy, 70,* 474. doi:10.2146/news130020

U.S. Food and Drug Administration. (2015, February 23). FDA approves Farydak [panobinostat] for treatment of multiple myeloma [Press release]. Retrieved from http://www.fda.gov/NewsEvents/Newsroom/PressAnnouncements/ucm435296.htm

van der Veer, M.S., de Weers, M., van Kessel, B., Bakker, J.M., Wittebol, S., Parren, P.W., ... Mutis, T. (2011a). The therapeutic human CD38 antibody daratumumab improves the anti-myeloma effect of newly emerging multi-drug therapies. *Blood Cancer Journal, 1,* e41. doi:10.1038/bcj.2011.42

van der Veer, M.S., de Weers, M., van Kessel, B., Bakker, J.M., Wittebol, S., Parren, P.W., ... Mutis, T. (2011b). Towards effective immunotherapy of myeloma: Enhanced elimination of myeloma cells by combination of lenalidomide with the human CD38 monoclonal antibody daratumumab. *Haematologica, 96,* 284–290. doi:10.3324/haematol.2010.030759

van Rhee, F., Szmania, S.M., Dillon, M., van Abbema, A.M., Li, X., Stone, M.K., ... Afar, D.E. (2009). Combinatorial efficacy of anti-CS1 monoclonal antibody elotuzumab (HuLuc63) and bortezomib against multiple myeloma. *Molecular Cancer Therapeutics, 8,* 2616–2624. doi:10.1158/1535-7163.MCT-09-0483

Venner, C.P., Connors, J.M., Sutherland, H.J., Shepherd, J.D., Hamata, L., Mourad, Y.A., ... Song, K.W. (2011). Novel agents improve survival of transplant patients with multiple myeloma including those with high-risk disease defined by early relapse (< 12 months). *Leukemia and Lymphoma, 52,* 34–41. doi:10.3109/10428194.2010.531409

Vij, R., Horvath, N., Spencer, A., Taylor, K., Vadhan-Raj, S., Vescio, R., ... Jun, S. (2009). An open-label, phase 2 trial of denosumab in the treatment of relapsed or plateau-phase multiple myeloma. *American Journal of Hematology, 84,* 650–656. doi:10.1002/ajh.21509

Voorhees, P.M., Manges, R.F., Sonneveld, P., Jagannath, S., Somlo, G., Krishnan, A., ... Thomas, S.K. (2013). A phase 2 multicentre study of siltuximab, an anti-interleukin-6 monoclonal antibody, in patients with relapsed or refractory multiple myeloma. *British Journal of Haematology, 161,* 357–366. doi:10.1111/bjh.12266

Weber, D.M., Graef, T., Hussein, M., Sobecks, R.M., Schiller, G.J., Lupinacci, L., ... Jagannath, S. (2012). Phase I trial of vorinostat combined with bortezomib for the treatment of relapsing and/or refractory multiple myeloma. *Clinical Lymphoma, Myeloma and Leukemia, 12,* 319–324. doi:10.1016/j.clml.2012.07.007

Wolf, J.L., Siegel, D., Goldschmidt, H., Hazell, K., Bourquelot, P.M., Bengoudifa, B.R., ... Lonial, S. (2012). Phase II trial of the pan-deacetylase inhibitor panobinostat as a single agent in advanced relapsed/refractory multiple myeloma. *Leukemia and Lymphoma, 53,* 1820–1823. doi:10.3109/10428194.2012.661175

Zonder, J.A., Mohrbacher, A.F., Singhal, S., van Rhee, F., Bensinger, W.I., Ding, H., ... Singhal, A.K. (2012). A phase 1, multicenter, open-label, dose escalation study of elotuzumab in patients with advanced multiple myeloma. *Blood, 120,* 552–559. doi:10.1182/blood-2011-06-360552

Index

The letter f after a page number indicates that relevant content appears in a figure; the letter t, in a table.

A

absolute neutrophil count, 87
acquired (adaptive) immunity, 11–14, 12f, 15f
 cells involved in, 17–27, 22f
acute myeloid leukemia (AML), 198t
acute survival phase, 188. *See also* survivorship
adaptive immunity. *See* acquired (adaptive) immunity
adenoids, 14
adhesion molecules, 31–32, 44
adrenal insufficiency, 124, 196t
affinity of the interaction, 27
African Americans, MM in, 2, 53, 58–59, 63, 190–191
Agent Orange exposure, and MM risk, 60, 63
agricultural workers, MM risk in, 59–60
AIDS, 27, 62–63
alcohol use, 61, 193
alleles, 234
allogeneic SCT (alloSCT), 72–73, 94–97, 99f, 277t–278t
alopecia, 82
American Association for Cancer Research, 208f
American Cancer Society, 193, 208f, 254, 256f–257f, 281–282
American College of Sports Medicine, 282
American Psychosocial Oncology Society, 208f
American Society of Clinical Oncology, 208f, 256f, 299
anemia, 1, 56, 86, 169, 171, 201t, 222, 278t. *See also* fatigue
anorexia, 83t, 85
antibodies, 14, 19, 21–23
antibody-dependent cellular cytotoxicity (ADCC), 298
antigenic determinants, 18
antigen-presenting cells (APCs), 13, 19–21, 22f, 23, 48
antigens, 13, 18
anxiety, 83t
APEX clinical trial, 132, 158, 162
appendix, 15
APRIL (ligand), 38f, 48
arrhythmias, 168
atherosclerosis, 195t
atomic bomb survivors, MM risk in, 59
autocrines, 28
autoimmune disorders, in MM risk, 56, 62
autologous stem cell transplant (ASCT), 71–73, 114–115, 238
 collection process in, 80, 90–91, 115
 eligibility for, 115–116
 engraftment phase, 87–93
 induction phase of, 74–76, 75t, 77t–79t, 88–89, 92–93
 late effects of, 97–98, 99f, 104

in older adults, 97
optimal timing of, 74, 76t
patient education on, 274–279, 277t–278t
patient needs after, 98–103
pre-engraftment phase, 81f, 81–87, 83t–85t
radiation therapy and, 155
reduced-intensity, 116–117, 118t–120t
for relapsed MM, 156
single, 87–88
tandem, 88, 114
transplantation process, 73f, 73–93
avascular necrosis, 198t

B

bacterial infections, 86, 98
balloon kyphoplasty, 152, 263–264
Bandolier, 257f
basophils, 12, 17
B-cell activating factor (BAFF), 38f, 48
B-cell antigen receptors, 13
B-cell differentiation, 18
B-cell receptors (BCRs), 19
bendamustine, 158f
benzene, and MM risk, 60
beta-2 microglobulin (β2M), 92, 231, 233t, 238, 240f
Be the Match, 256f
biochemical relapse, 150. See also relapsed/refractory MM
biomarkers, 231–236, 233t, 239–241. See also genomics
bisphosphonates (BPs), 206f
patient education on, 262–263
for relapsed MM, 152–154. See also pamidronate; zoledronate
self-administration of, 220–221
side effects of, 153, 205
Black Swan Research Initiative (BSRI), 4
bleeding, 278t, 279–280. See also thrombosis
Blood and Marrow Transplant Information Network, 256f
B lymphocytes, 13–14, 15f, 17–20, 20f, 22f, 37
body mass index, and MM risk, 62
bone lesions/disease, 43–45, 44f, 151–154, 198t, 201t, 205, 219–220
patient education on, 261
bone marrow, 15

Bone Marrow Foundation, 256f
bone marrow microenvironment, 37–41, 38f, 40t, 41f–42f, 45, 231
bone marrow stromal cells (BMSCs), 37–39, 38f, 41–43
bone pain, 1, 6, 258, 261, 280–282
bone resorption, 43
Bort/Dex regimen, 88, 90, 124–125
bortezomib, 2, 71, 77t, 88–93, 97, 102–103, 117, 118t, 139–141, 149
with dexamethasone, 88, 90, 124–125, 159t
with dexamethasone and lenalidomide, 166–167
with dexamethasone and panobinostat, 166
with doxorubicin, 162–163
home administration of, 221
with lenalidomide, 238
with melphalan and prednisone, 129–133
with melphalan, prednisone, and thalidomide, 140
neuropathy with, 131
patient education on, 269–272, 273f
for relapsed MM, 157–162, 158f, 159t, 162–163
side effects of, 125, 130, 140, 161–163
BRCA1/BRCA2 mutations, and MM risk, 57
breast cancer, and MM risk, 57
BTD regimen, 90

C

calcium levels, 1. See also hypercalcemia
Cancer and Leukemia Group B (CALGB), 102
CancerCare, 208f, 254, 256f
Cancer Legal Resource Center, 256f
Cancer.Net, 256f
Cancer Survival Toolbox, 254
cardiomyopathy, 195t
Caregiver Action Network, 256f, 257
caregivers, 189, 207–208, 208f–209f, 257–258
carfilzomib, 2, 71, 77t, 92–93, 149–150, 158f, 159t–160t, 167–168
patient education on, 272–274, 275f
Caring Bridge, 256f
cataracts, 195t, 203t

Celgene Corporation, 126, 128, 164, 169, 267
cell-mediated immunity, 14, 15f
cellular immunity, 14, 15f
cereblon, 4
chemoattractants, 29
chemokines, 29–31, 31t
chromosomal abnormalities, 36
chromosomal analysis, 236–237
chromosomes, 36, 234
Chronic Disease Fund. *See* Good Days
cisplatin, 91, 156, 158f, 159t, 170–172
clarithromycin, 129
clinical relapse, 150. *See also* relapsed/refractory MM
clinical trials, 183, 238, 293–294, 294t, 295–299
 APEX, 132, 158, 162
 barriers to participation, 183
 on daratumumab, 298–299
 on elotuzumab, 295–297
 FIRST, 133–134, 141
 on ixazomib, 297–298
 on panobinostat, 294–295
 PANORAMA 2, 295
 patient education on, 283
 Total Therapy (TT), 91
 VISTA, 129, 131, 139–141
cluster of differentiation (CD), 18
cluster of differentiation-34+ (CD34+), 80
cluster of differentiation-40 (CD40), 48
Coalition of Cancer Cooperative Groups, 256f
Cochrane Review Organization, 257f
collectin receptors, 13
colony-stimulating factors (CSFs), 19, 29, 31t
communication styles, 189
comorbidities
 with MM, 55, 156, 185–186
 in survivorship, 194
complementary and alternative medicine (CAM), 255–256, 257f
complement-dependent cytotoxicity (CDC), 298
complete response (CR), 71–72, 89, 151
computed tomography (CT), 152
conditioning regimens, in ASCT, 81, 81f
congestive heart failure, 195t
constipation, 135, 161, 165, 201t

coronary artery disease, 195t
corticosteroids, 90, 103, 121–124
 side effects of, 122t–123t, 202t–203t, 266–267, 267f
CRAB criteria, 35, 150, 200
C-reactive protein (CRP), 222
creatinine level, 1. *See also* renal insufficiency
CTD regimen, 90, 134
CyBorD regimen, 90
cyclin D dysregulation, 36
CYCLONE regimen, 92–93
cyclophosphamide, 77t, 80, 90–93, 134, 156, 158f, 159t, 170–172
cytarabine, 91
cytochrome P450 enzymes, 161
cytogenetic abnormalities, 36
cytokines, 19, 27–31, 30t–31t, 45, 46f, 121
cytopenias, 198t

D

damage-associated molecular patterns (DAMPs), 13
daratumumab, 298–299
darbepoetin, 171
DCEP regimen, 91, 156, 158f, 159t, 170–171
decision making, 189–190, 226–227
 genomics and, 238–239, 240f
deep vein thrombosis, 3, 85t, 126, 136
dehydration, 277t
deletion, in chromosomes, 36
demographics, of MM, 1–2
dendritic cells, 16–17, 23
dental care, 154, 262–263
depression, 83t, 98–100
dexamethasone, 88–93, 103, 120t, 121–124, 122t–123t, 125
 with bortezomib, 88, 90, 124–125, 159t
 with bortezomib and lenalidomide, 166–167
 with bortezomib and panobinostat, 166
 with cyclophosphamide and thalidomide, 90, 134
 with cyclophosphamide, etoposide, and cisplatin, 91, 156, 158f, 159t, 170–171
 with lenalidomide, 90, 127–129, 159t, 163–166

with pomalidomide, 159t
for relapsed MM, 156, 158f, 159t, 163–166, 170–172
side effects of, 164
with vincristine and doxorubicin, 89, 136–138
diagnosis, of MM, 1, 188, 216–217
diarrhea, 6, 82–86, 83t, 130–131, 161, 165, 197t, 201t, 277t
diet, and MM risk, 61, 63
dietary supplements, 192
diffuse alveolar hemorrhage (DAH), 87
dimethyl sulfoxide (DMSO), 80, 82
DNA, 232–234
DNA methylation, 235
donor lymphocyte infusion (DLI), 96
double refractory MM, 149, 157f. *See also* relapsed/refractory MM
doxorubicin, 2, 89–91, 136–138, 156, 158f, 159t, 162–163, 171–172
side effects of, 162–163
DPACE regimen, 91
DT-PACE regimen, 156, 158f, 159t, 171–172
duration of remissions, with novel agents, 2
Durie, Brian, 3
dyes, and MM risk, 60–61
dyspnea, 168–169, 203t

E

early diagnosis, research on, 216–217
Eastern Cooperative Oncology Group (ECOG), performance status, 74
effector cells, 15f, 21, 22f
elotuzumab, 295–297
endocrines, 28
environmental factors, as MM risk, 59–61, 63
eosinophils, 12, 17
epigenetic changes, 235
epithelial cells, 13
epitopes, 14, 17–18
epoetin alfa, 171
erythropoiesis-stimulating agents (ESAs), 171
ESA APPRISE program, 171
esophagitis, 82–86
etiology, of MM, 53–63
etoposide, 91, 156, 158f, 159t, 170–172
European Group for Blood and Marrow Transplantation, response criteria, 74, 75t
European Organization for Research and Treatment of Cancer, 222
event-free survival (EFS), 2, 72
exercise
patient education on, 282–283
research on, 223, 225
during survivorship, 191–193
extended survival phase, 188. *See also* survivorship
extracellular matrix (ECM) proteins, 39

F

fall risk, 205–207
Family Caregiver Alliance, 256f, 257
family history, and MM, 56–58, 63. *See also* genetics
farmers, MM risk in, 59–60
fatigue, 6, 83t, 135, 169, 171, 201t
nursing research on, 222–226
patient education on, 258, 278t
febrile neutropenia, 86, 169
fertility, 197t, 255
fever, 84t
filgrastim. *See* granulocyte–colony-stimulating factor
FIRST clinical trial, 133–134, 141
five-year survival rates, 113, 149, 182, 182f, 215
fludarabine, 96
fluorescence in situ hybridization (FISH), 4, 36–37, 231, 236–237
free light chains (FLCs), 27, 232, 233t
Frieburg Comorbidity Index (FCI), 194
From Cancer Patient to Cancer Survivor: Lost in Transition (IOM), 181, 184. *See also* survivorship
Functional Assessment of Cancer Therapy–Fatigue (FACT-F), 222
fungal infections, 86

G

gastrointestinal side effects, 3, 6, 82–86, 83t, 130–131, 135, 161, 164–165, 197t
gene expression profiling (GEP), 4, 36, 92, 231, 233t, 237
genetics, 2, 35–48, 56–58, 63
genome-wide association study (GWAS), 2

genomics, 231–236, 234f. *See also* biomarkers
  nursing implications, 239–241
  risk stratification techniques, 236–237
glucocorticoids, 141. *See also* steroids, side effects of
Good Days, 208f
graft-versus-host disease (GVHD), 94, 99f, 278t
graft-versus-myeloma (GVM) effect, 94
granulocyte–colony-stimulating factor (G-CSF), 31t, 78t, 80, 96, 115
granulocyte macrophage–colony-stimulating factor (GM-CSF), 19, 31t

H

hair coloring/dyes, and MM risk, 60–61
hair loss, 82
hand-foot syndrome, 162–163
health promotion, during survivorship, 190–191
health-related quality of life (HRQOL), 181, 187. *See also* quality of life; survivorship
hearing loss, 195t
heavy-chain immunoglobulins, 24–27, 25t, 26f, 37
hematopoietic stem cells, 12, 19, 80
hematopoietic stem cell transplantation (HSCT), 3–4, 72–73, 73f. *See also* autologous stem cell transplant
  eligibility for, 115–116
  late effects of, 97–98, 99f, 104
  maintenance therapy after, 100–103, 138–141
  in older adults, 97
  patient education on, 274–279, 277t–278t
  patient needs after, 98–103
Hendrich II Fall Risk Model, 207
herpes zoster, 132–133
high-dose therapy (HDT), 71–73, 88–89, 95, 103, 238. *See also* melphalan; *specific agents*
histiocytes, 16
histone deacetylase (HDAC) inhibitors, 235
histones, 235
HIV infection, 63
HLA matching, 72–73

hope, concept of, 217–218
hospice, 283
Human Cell Differentiation Molecules, 18
Human Genome Project (HGP), 232
human leukocyte antigen (HLA), 20, 56, 72–73
humoral immunity, 13–14, 15f, 19
hybrid survivorship model, 186–187
hydroxyapatite, 153
hypercalcemia, 1, 201t
hyperdiploid group, of cytogenetic abnormalities, 36, 237
hyperglycemia, 124, 191–192
hypertension, 168, 196t
hyperviscosity, 201t
hypocalcemia, 153
hypotension, 202t
hypothyroidism, 196t

I

IL-6 receptor (IL6R), 235
imaging, with relapsed MM, 151–152
immune system, 11, 12f. *See also* acquired (adaptive) immunity; innate immunity
  organs of, 15
immunizations, 100, 101t, 132–133
immunoglobulin alpha/beta, 19
immunoglobulin domains, 24
immunoglobulin G (IgG), 25
immunoglobulins, 13–14, 19, 21–27, 26f, 37
  heavy-chain, 24–27, 25t, 26f, 37
  light-chain, 26f, 27
immunoglobulin superfamily (IgSF), 24
immunologic factors, in MM risk, 62–63
immunomodulatory drugs (IMiDs), 4, 89–90, 103, 126, 202t. *See also* lenalidomide; thalidomide
incidence, of MM, 1, 54, 55t, 215
incontinence, 197t
induction phase, of ASCT, 74–76, 75t, 77t–79t, 88–89, 92–93
infections, 202t
  diarrhea and, 131
  patient education on, 278t, 279
  with steroid use, 123
  in transplant recipients, 86, 98
  with VMP regimen, 132

infertility, 197*t*, 255
information needs priorities, 226–227
innate immunity, 11–14, 12*f*
  cells involved in, 16–17
insulin-like growth factor-1 (IGF-1), 39, 48
insulin receptor substrate type 1 (IRS1), 235
integrins, 31–32
interferon, 29, 30*t*, 91, 141
interferon regulatory factor 4, 4
Intergroupe Francophone du Myélome (IFM), 102, 114, 135
interleukin-1 (IL-1), 16, 19, 29, 43, 57
interleukin-6 (IL-6), 19, 29, 30*t*, 39, 41, 43, 45–46, 47*f*, 121, 222, 235
interleukin-12 (IL-12), 29, 30*t*
interleukins, 30*t*
International Association for Hospice and Palliative Care, 256*f*
International Myeloma Foundation (IMF), 3–4, 6, 200, 208*f*, 219, 254–255, 256*f*
International Myeloma Working Group (IMWG), 5, 150–151, 156, 200
International Myeloma Workshop Consensus Panel, 150
International Staging System (ISS), 4, 194, 231, 258
Internet use, for patient education, 253–257, 256*f*–257*f*
ionizing radiation, as MM risk, 59, 63
Italian Myeloma Group, 116
ixazomib, 297–298

J

The Joint Commission, Speak Up program, 251

K

Karnofsky Performance Status (KPS), 74
Kupffer cells, 16

L

large granular lymphocytes (LGLs), 21. *See also* natural killer cells
late effects
  patient education on, 293

of treatment, 97–98, 99*f*, 104, 194, 195*t*–199*t*
LD regimen, 90, 127–129, 159*t*, 163–166
learning needs assessment, 247–249, 248*f*–249*f*, 250*t*
lenalidomide, 2, 4, 71, 77*t*, 88–93, 97, 102–103, 115, 118*t*–119*t*, 139, 141, 149
  with bortezomib, 238
  with bortezomib and dexamethasone, 166–167
  with dexamethasone, 90, 127–129, 159*t*, 163–166
  with melphalan and prednisone, 133–134, 139
  patient education on, 268, 270*f*
  with prednisone, 139
  for relapsed MM, 158*f*, 159*t*, 163–166
  side effects of, 164–165
  teratogenic effects of, 128, 164
Leukemia and Lymphoma Society (LLS), 209*f*, 219, 255, 256*f*
lifestyle factors, and MM risk, 61–62, 193
light-chain immunoglobulins, 26*f*, 27
literacy skills, and patient education, 248
"lived experience" of MM, research on, 218–219
Livestrong Fertility, 255, 256*f*
Livestrong Foundation, 209*f*, 254, 256*f*, 282
loperamide, for diarrhea, 130–131
LP regimen, 97
lymph fluid, 15
lymph nodes, 14–15, 23
lymphocytes, 13, 17–21, 20*f*, 22*f*
lymphoid progenitor cells, 17–18

M

macrophage–colony-stimulating factor, 31*t*
macrophage inflammatory protein-1-alpha (MIP-1α), 43
macrophage inflammatory protein-1-beta (MIP-1β), 45
macrophages, 12, 14, 16, 23
magnetic resonance imaging (MRI), 152
maintenance therapy, 100–103, 138–141
major histocompatibility complex (MHC), 13, 20
malabsorption syndrome, 197*t*
malnutrition, 277*t*
mast cells, 12, 17

INDEX 311

Mayo Stratification of Myeloma and Risk-Adapted Therapy (mSMART) protocol, 37, 236–237, 239, 240*f*
MD Anderson Cancer Center, 257*f*
MedlinePlus, 256*f*, 265
MEL100-ASCT regimen, 97
melphalan, 77*t*, 81, 81*f*, 85, 88, 90–91, 95, 103, 115
  with bortezomib and prednisone, 129–133
  with bortezomib, prednisone, and thalidomide, 140
  with lenalidomide and prednisone, 133–134, 139
  with prednisone, 97, 113, 117–121, 120*t*
  reduced-intensity, 116–117
  side effects of, 120
  with thalidomide and prednisone, 117, 134–136, 137*f*
Memorial Sloan Kettering Cancer Center, 257*f*
memory cells, 19
MetaCancer Foundation, 256*f*
methotrexate, 96
methylation of cytosines, 235
microbial antigens, 18
minimal residual disease (MRD), 4–5, 151
mobilization, of stem cells, 80, 90–91
molecular classifications, of MM, 4
mollities ossium, 72
monoclonal gammopathy of undetermined significance (MGUS), 25, 35–36, 53–59, 61
monoclonal protein (M protein), 25
monoclonal (M) spike, 35
monocytes, 12, 28
mononuclear phagocytes, 17
monosomy, 36
motivational interviewing, 247, 248*f*
mouth rinses, 163
MP regimen, 97, 113, 117–121, 120*t*, 129
MPR-R regimen, 133–134
MPT regimen, 117, 134–136, 137*f*
mSMART (Mayo Stratification of Myeloma and Risk-Adapted Therapy) protocol, 37, 236–237, 239, 240*f*
mucositis, 82–86, 277*t*
Mullan, Fitzhugh, 188
multiparameter flow cytometry (MFC), 231
Multiple Myeloma Library, 256*f*

Multiple Myeloma Research Foundation (MMRF), 209*f*, 219, 255, 256*f*
multiple sclerosis, 27
Myeloma Research Consortium, 134
Myeloma Trialists' Collaborative Group, 113–114
myelosuppression
  after stem cell transplant, 86
  with bortezomib, 130
  with DCEP regimen, 170–171
  with lenalidomide, 129, 164
  NLB guidelines for, 3
myopathy, 203*t*
MyPRS (gene expression profiling), 233*t*, 237

N

National Alliance for Caregiving, 256*f*, 257
National Bone Marrow Transplant Link, 256*f*
National Cancer Institute (NCI), 256*f*
  on Internet resources, 254
  Office of Cancer Complementary and Alternative Medicine, 257*f*
  Office of Cancer Survivorship, 183, 209*f*
  on pain management, 281
  Surveillance, Epidemiology, and End Results (SEER) Program, 216
National Center for Complementary and Integrative Health, 257*f*
National Coalition for Cancer Survivorship, 183, 209*f*, 254, 256*f*
National Comprehensive Cancer Network (NCCN), 156, 200, 238, 256*f*, 258–259
National Marrow Donor Program, 209*f*, 256*f*
native immunity. *See* innate immunity
natural immunity. *See* innate immunity
natural killer (NK) cells, 12, 14, 18, 21, 22*f*
natural killer T (NKT) cells, 18, 20
Natural Medicines, 257*f*
nausea/vomiting, 82–86, 84*t*, 130, 161, 164–165, 277*t*
nephrotic syndrome, 197*t*
neuropathy/neurotoxicity, 131, 135–136, 172, 202*t*, 220–222, 227, 280. *See also* peripheral neuropathy
neutropenia, 86, 169

neutrophils, 12, 16
NOD-like receptors, 13
nonamyloid light-chain deposition disease (NALCDD), 27
nonhematopoietic cells, 12–13
nonhyperdiploid group, of cytogenetic abnormalities, 36, 237
nonmicrobial antigens, 18
nonmyeloablative alloSCT, 81*f*, 94–97
nonsteroidal anti-inflammatory drugs (NSAIDs), 280–281
Notch pathway, 41–42
novel agents, 2–3, 71–72, 88–92, 103, 117, 149, 215, 238. *See also* bortezomib; carfilzomib; doxorubicin; lenalidomide; panobinostat; pomalidomide; thalidomide
Novis, Susie, 3
nuclear factor–kappa-B (NF-κB), 57, 222
Nurse Leadership Board (NLB), 3–4, 6, 200
nursing guidelines, from NLB, 3–4
nursing research
  barriers to, 5
  on early diagnosis, 216–217
  on fatigue, 222–226
  future needs in, 227–228
  on MM, 5–6
  on pain management, 219–222
  on peripheral neuropathy, 221–222
  on psychosocial impact of MM, 217–219
  on symptom management, 219–226
nutrition, during survivorship, 191–193

O

obesity, and MM risk, 61–63, 192
occupational risk factors, as MM risk, 59–61, 63
Office of Cancer Complementary and Alternative Medicine (NCI), 257*f*
Office of Cancer Survivorship (NCI), 183, 209*f*
older adults
  survivorship in, 185–186
  transplantation in, 97, 116
OncoLink OncoLife Survivorship Care Plan, 256*f*
oral hygiene, 154, 163, 262–263

oral mucositis, 82–86, 277*t*
organs, of immune system, 15
osteoclastogenesis, 43
osteoclastogenesis inhibitory factor, 43
osteolytic bone resorption, 43
osteonecrosis, 198*t*
osteonecrosis of the jaw (ONJ), 153–154, 195*t*
  patient education on, 262–263
osteopenia, 151–152
osteoporosis, 198*t*
osteoprotegerin (OPG), 43
overall survival (OS), 2, 71, 89, 149, 151

P

PAD regimen, 90
pain, 84*t*, 85, 280–282
palliative care, 283
palmar-plantar erythrodysesthesia (PPE), 162–163
pamidronate, 78*t*, 153–154, 220–221, 262–263
pancreatic insufficiency, 197*t*
pancytopenia, after stem cell transplant, 86
panobinostat, 2, 158*f*, 159*t*, 166, 274, 294–295
PANORAMA 2 clinical trial, 295
paracrines, 28
partial response (PR), 151
Partnership for Prescription Assistance, 209*f*
pathogen-associated molecular patterns (PAMPs), 13
patient education, 245–247, 258–261, 260*f*
  assessment for, 247–249, 248*f*–249*f*, 250*t*
  evaluation of, 284–285
  goals/outcomes for, 250–252
  Internet use in, 253–257, 256*f*–257*f*
  methods/interventions for, 252–258
  on pain management, 280–282
  on pharmacologic treatments, 264–279, 265*f*
  topics for, 258–283
  on treatments, 262–279, 265*f*
percutaneous vertebroplasty, 152, 263–264
performance status, 74

peripheral neuropathy (PN), 6, 84*t*, 131, 135–136, 161–162, 167–168, 198*t*
 NLB guidelines for, 3
 nursing research on, 221–222
 patient education on, 280–282
permanent survivorship, 188. *See also* survivorship
pesticide exposure, and MM risk, 59–60, 63
Peyer patches, 14–15, 23
phagocytes, 14, 16–17
pharmacogenomics, 236
physical activity
 patient education on, 282–283
 research on, 223, 225
 during survivorship, 191–193
plain film radiography, 152
plasma cell labeling index (PCLI), 231
plasma cells, 1, 14, 20*f*, 21–23
 development/differentiation of, 23, 37
plasmacytomas, 151–152
plerixafor, 78*t*, 80, 91, 115
pluripotent stem cells, 29, 39
pneumococcal vaccination, 101*t*, 132–133
pneumonia, 132, 169
pneumonitis, 197*t*
POEMS syndrome, 27
pomalidomide, 2, 4, 71, 78*t*, 149–150, 158*f*, 159*t*, 168–170
 patient education on, 268–269, 271*f*
Pomalyst REMS, 169–170
positron-emission tomography (PET), 152
precursor cells, 29
prednisone, 97, 113, 117–121, 120*t*, 121–124, 122*t*–123*t*, 141
 with bortezomib and melphalan, 129–133
 with bortezomib, melphalan, and thalidomide, 140
 with lenalidomide, 139
 with melphalan and lenalidomide, 133–134, 139
 with melphalan and thalidomide, 117, 134–136, 137*f*
preexisting medical conditions, with MM, 55, 156, 185–186, 194
preexisting plasma cell disorders (PPCDs), 55
prevalence, of MM, 54

prevention, during survivorship, 190–191
primary care provider (PCP), 184–185
primary systemic amyloidosis, 27
primary translocation, of chromosomes, 36
progenitor cells, 29
progression-free survival (PFS), 117, 151
progressive disease (PD), 151
proinflammatory cytokines, 19
proteasome inhibitors (PIs), 89, 103, 202*t*. *See also specific agents*
psychosocial impact, of MM, 217–219, 278*f*
pulmonary complications, 86–87, 197*t*
pulmonary embolism, 85*t*
pulmonary fibrosis, 197*t*

Q

QLQ-C30 fatigue scale, 222
quality of life (QOL), 6
 with novel agents, 3
 nursing research on, 219–226

R

race, and MM incidence, 2, 53, 58–59, 63, 190–191
radiation, ionizing, as MM risk, 59, 63
radiation therapy
 for bone disease, 152, 264
 for relapsed MM, 154–155
RANKL signaling receptor, 43–45
RANK/RANKL signaling pathway, 43
rash, 202*t*
reading levels, for patient education, 248
receptor for advanced glycation end products (RAGE), 13
reduced-intensity alloSCT, 81*f*, 94–97
reduced-intensity ASCT, 116–117, 118*t*–119*t*
relapsed/refractory MM, 93–95, 149–150
 bisphosphonates for, 152–154
 clinical trials on, 294–295
 defined, 150
 imaging patients with, 151–152
 radiation therapy for, 154–155
 treatment choice for, 155–172, 157*f*–158*f*, 159*t*–160*t*
REMS (Risk Evaluation and Mitigation Strategy), 126, 128, 164, 169–171

renal dysfunction, 1, 86, 128–130, 153, 202t, 207
   patient education on, 261
renal insufficiency, 197t
resources, for MM survivors, 208f–209f
response rates (RR), with novel agents, 2
retinopathy, 195t
RevAssist program, 128, 164. See also Revlimid REMS
Rev/Dex regimen, 88
Revlimid REMS, 128, 164, 268
risk factors, for MM, 53–63, 190–191
RNA, 234
RP regimen, 139
RVD regimen, 103, 166–167

S

salvage transplant, 94
secondary malignancies, 194–200, 198t
secondary translocation, of chromosomes, 36
selectins, 31–32
self-management, during survivorship, 189–190
serum protein electrophoresis (SPEP), 232, 233t
shared decision making, 189–190
shingles, 132–133
Signal Genetics, 236
signaling cascades, 39
signaling pathways, 39, 40t
single autologous stem cell transplant, 87–88
single-nucleotide polymorphisms (SNPs), 57, 235
Sjögren disease, 27
sleep quality, 224–225
socioeconomic status, and MM risk, 61–62
solvents, and MM risk, 60
Speak Up program, 251
spleen, 14–15, 23
stable disease (SD), 151
Stages of Change model, 249, 250t
stem cell transplantation (SCT), 3–4, 72–73, 73f. See also autologous stem cell transplant
   eligibility for, 115–116
   late effects of, 97–98, 99f, 104
   maintenance therapy after, 100–103, 138–141

in older adults, 97
   patient education on, 274–279, 277t–278t
   patient needs after, 98–103
S.T.E.P.S. (System for Thalidomide Education and Prescribing Safety), 126, 128. See also Thalomid REMS
steroids, side effects of, 3, 122t–123t, 123, 202t–203t, 266–267, 267f
Stevens-Johnson syndrome, 127
stomatitis, 162–163
strength training, 225. See also exercise
strictures, 197t
stringent complete response (sCR), 151
stromal-derived factor-1-alpha (SDF-1α), 43
Stupid Cancer, 255, 256f
subcutaneous (SC) administration, 162
superfamilies, 24, 47–48
supportive care, during survivorship, 200–207, 201t–203t, 204f
Surveillance, Epidemiology, and End Results (SEER) Program, 216
survivorship, 181–183, 182f, 183–186, 184f
   cancer surveillance during, 194–200, 198t. See also survivorship care
   hybrid model for, 186–187
   phases of, 188–189
survivorship care, 181, 184f, 189–193, 190f, 194–200
   research needs in, 227–228
   resources for, 208f–209f
survivorship care plans (SCPs), 184–185, 204f
symptom clusters, 5–6
syngeneic SCT, 73
systemic lupus erythematosus, 27, 56

T

tacrolimus, 96
TAD regimen, 90
tandem autologous stem cell transplant, 88, 114
T-cell-dependent (TD) antibody responses, 23
T-cell-dependent pathways, 19
T-cell-independent (TI) antibody responses, 23
T-cell receptor (TCR), 13, 20

TD regimen, 90, 125–127
teratogenicity
  of lenalidomide, 128, 164
  of pomalidomide, 169–170
  of thalidomide, 125–126
testosterone deficiency, 197*t*
Thal/Dex regimen, 88
thalidomide, 2, 4, 71, 78*t*, 88–93, 100–102, 114, 116–117, 119*t*–120*t*, 140, 149
  with cyclophosphamide and dexamethasone, 90, 134
  with dexamethasone, 90, 125–127
  with melphalan and prednisone, 117, 134–136, 137*f*
  patient education on, 267–268, 269*f*
  for relapsed MM, 156, 158*f*, 159*t*, 171–172
  side effects of, 135, 140
  teratogenic effects of, 125–126
Thalomid REMS, 126, 267
therapy-related myelodysplastic syndrome (tMDS), 198*t*–199*t*
thrombocytopenia, 86, 169, 171, 203*t*
thromboembolism, 196*t*, 279–280
thrombosis, 3, 85*t*, 126–128, 136, 137*f*, 165–166, 203*t*
  patient education on, 278*t*, 279–280
thymus, 15, 20
time to progression (TTP), 91
T lymphocytes, 13–14, 15*f*, 17–21, 22*f*, 45, 48
TNF-alpha superfamily, 47–48
tobacco use, 193
Toll-like receptors, 13
tonsils, 14–15, 23
Total Therapy (TT) clinical trials, 91
transcription/translation, 234–235
translocation, of chromosomes, 36
treatment algorithm
  for MM, 76*f*
  for relapsed MM, 155–172, 157*f*–158*f*, 159*t*–160*t*
treatment decision making (TDM), 226–227
  genomics and, 238–239, 240*f*
treatment-emergent adverse events, 181
treatment-related mortality (TRM), 94
T regulatory cells (Tregs), 45
tumor necrosis factor (TNF), 16, 19, 29, 30*t*, 39, 47–48

U

urine protein electrophoresis (UPEP), 232, 233*t*
U.S. Preventive Services Task Force (USPSTF), 193

V

VAD regimen, 89, 136–138
vascular cell adhesion molecule-1 (VCAM-1), 44–45
vascular endothelial growth factor (VEGF), 39, 43, 47
VD regimen, 88, 90, 124–125
venous thromboembolism (VTE), 127–128, 136, 137*f*, 165–166, 279–280
vertebral compression fractures (VCFs), 152
vertebroplasty, 137*f*, 152, 201*t*, 263–264
very good partial response (VGPR), 72, 89, 151
Vietnam veterans, MM risk in, 60, 63
vincristine, 89, 136–138
viral infections, 86, 98
VISTA clinical trial, 129, 131, 139–141
visual changes, 195*t*, 203*t*
visual media, for patient education, 252–253
VMP regimen, 129–133
VMPT regimen, 140
VMPT-VT regimen, 140
vorinostat, 158*f*
VTD-PACE regimen, 91

W

Waldenström macroglobulinemia, 25
white blood cells, 16–17. *See also specific cells*
Wingless-type (Wnt) signaling pathway, 45

X

xerostomia, 195*t*
x-rays, 152

Z

zoledronate, 79*t*, 153–154, 205, 262–263

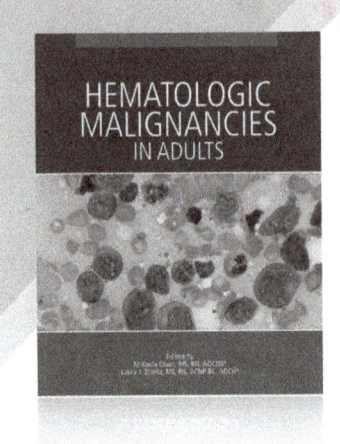

HEMATOLOGIC MALIGNANCIES IN ADULTS
Edited by M. Olsen and L.J. Zitella

More than 180 years since Thomas Hodgkin identified the first hematologic malignancy, nurses are still learning the best ways to treat patients with these complex cancers. *Hematologic Malignancies in Adults* enables you to

- Access up-to-date, comprehensive information on treatments, complications, and toxicity management for your everyday practice.
- Manage treatment-related side effects and toxicities with confidence.
- Keep pace with medical advances as you treat patients with hematologic malignancies.

Add it to your medical library today. 2013. 690 pages. Softcover.

ISBN: 9781935864264 • Item: INPU0627

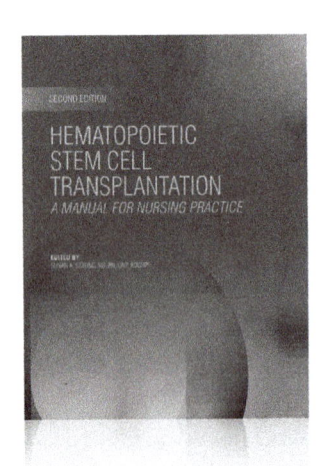

HEMATOPOIETIC STEM CELL TRANSPLANTATION: A MANUAL FOR NURSING PRACTICE (SECOND EDITION)
Edited by S.A. Ezzone

Patients undergoing hematopoietic stem cell transplantation need specialized care. This manual will help you

- Care for this unique population by providing a thorough explanation of the course of treatment and acute complications, graft-versus-host disease, and various complications from gastrointestinal to neurologic issues.
- Gain a better understanding of hematopoiesis and immunology, basic concepts of transplantation and stem cell collection, and stem cell processing and purging, all at your own pace.

Make sure you have the most up-to-date knowledge on this important subspecialty with the second edition. 2013. 340 pages. Softcover.

ISBN: 9781935864196 • Item: INPU0609

To order, visit www.ons.org/store, or contact customer service at help@ons.org or 866-257-4ONS.

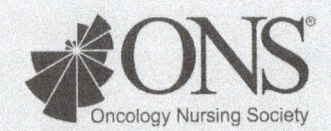

ONS Oncology Nursing Society